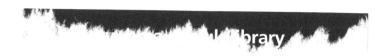

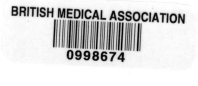

Pharmacogenomics in Clinical Therapeutics

Pharmacogenomics in Clinical Therapeutics

EDITED BY

Loralie J. Langman, PhD, DABCC, FACB, DABFT
Associate Professor of Laboratory Medicine
Mayo Clinic, Rochester, MN

Amitava Dasgupta, PhD, DABCC, FACB
Professor of Pathology and Laboratory Medicine
University of Texas Health Sciences Center at Houston
Houston, TX

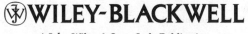

A John Wiley & Sons, Ltd., Publication

Library of Congress Cataloging-in-Publication Data

Pharmacogenomics in clinical therapeutics / edited by Loralie J. Langman and Amitava Dasgupta.
    p. ; cm.
  Includes bibliographical references and index.
  ISBN 978-0-470-65734-8 (cloth)
1. Pharmacogenetics. 2. Chemotherapy. I. Langman, Loralie J. II. Dasgupta, Amitava, 1958–
  [DNLM: 1. Pharmacogenetics–methods. 2. Drug Therapy–methods. 3. Pharmacological
Phenomena–genetics. QV 38]
  RM301.3.G45P4235 2012
  615.7–dc23

                                                                              2011021501

A catalogue record for this book is available from the British Library.

Wiley also publishes its books in a variety of electronic formats. Some content that appears in print may not be available in electronic books.

Set in 9/12pt Meridien by Thomson Digital, Noida, India
Printed and bound in Malaysia by Vivar Printing Sdn Bhd

1   2011

Contents

List of Contributors

Linnea M. Baudhuin, PhD
Department of Laboratory Medicine and Pathology
Mayo Clinic, Rochester, MN

Mark P. Borgman, PhD
Department of Pathology and Laboratory Medicine
University of Louisville, Louisville, KY

Amitava Dasgupta, PhD
Department of Pathology and Laboratory Medicine
University of Texas Health Sciences Center at Houston
Houston, TX

Christine M. Formea, PharmD
Department of Pharmacy
Mayo Clinic, Rochester, MN

Gideon Koren, MD
Division of Clinical Pharmacology and Toxicology
Hospital for Sick Children, Toronto, Canada

Matthew D. Krasowski, MD, PhD
Department of Pathology
University of Iowa Hospitals and Clinics, Iowa City

Loralie J. Langman, PhD
Department of Laboratory Medicine and Pathology
Mayo Clinic, Rochester, MN

Mark W. Linder, PhD
Department of Pathology and Laboratory Medicine
University of Louisville, Louisville, KY

Parvaz Madadi, PhD
Division of Clinical Pharmacology and Toxicology
Hospital for Sick Children, Toronto, Canada

Pierre Marquet, MD, PhD
Department of Medical Pharmacology
Université de Limoges, France

Wayne T. Nicholson, MD, PharmD
Department of Anesthesiology
Mayo Clinic, Rochester, MN

Nicolas Picard, PharmD, PhD
Department of Medical Pharmacology
Université de Limoges, France

Natella Y. Rakhmanina, MD, PhD
Department of Pediatrics
George Washington University
Children's National Medical Center
Washington, DC

Jorge L. Sepulveda, MD, PhD
Philadelphia VA Medical Center, Philadelphia, PA
Department of Pathology and Laboratory Medicine
University of Pennsylvania, Philadelphia, PA

Christine L.H. Snozek, PhD
Department of Laboratory Medicine and Pathology
Mayo Clinic, Rochester, MN

John N. van den Anker, MD, PhD
Departments of Pediatrics, Pharmacology and Physiology
George Washington University
Children's National Medical Center
Washington, DC

Preface

In recent years the media have focused on personalized medicine, thus increasing the general public's awareness regarding better therapy for various illnesses. After complete characterization of the human genome, there were expectations of translating these findings into better treatment of diseases as well as magic cures for genetically inherited diseases. In reality, there is always a significant time gap between discovery in basic science and its translation into application. The field of pharmacogenomics is no exception. In the 1970s, expansion of traditional therapeutic drug monitoring (TDM) services for drugs with narrow therapeutic indices certainly improved patient management by reducing incidences of drug toxicity by achieving personalized dosage of a particular drug for an individual. Pharmacogenomics is conceptually a step forward toward personalized medicine over TDM because it might be possible to predict the correct dosage. A good example is warfarin, where dosage based on a polymorphism of CYP2C9 and VCKOR1 has been stated in the package insert. Currently, in addition to warfarin, there is evidence that pharmacogenomics may be helpful in therapy with various antidepressants, immunosuppressants, cardioactive drugs, anesthetics, and analgesics. In addition, pharmacogenomics testing as well as TDM are both useful in managing patients infected with human immunodeficiency virus (HIV).

There are conflicting reports regarding the roles of pharmacogenomics in affecting therapy. This is particularly a problem with various psychoactive drugs because both genetic and environmental factors are known to affect the outcome of therapy. Other problems of pharmacogenomics testing are the costs of tests and reimbursement issues, especially from the federal government. Finding qualified technologists to perform these specialized tests is also challenging.

The goal of this book is to provide a comprehensive platform for readers to become familiar with the current state of pharmacogenomics in pharmacotherapy. Each chapter is written by experts in their field, covering all aspects of pharmacogenomics in clinical therapeutics which will be helpful for pharmacologists, toxicologists, clinical laboratory scientists, pathologists, and clinicians. Basic aspects of pharmacogenomics are discussed in Chapter 1 and also reviewed in each chapter as appropriate for the drugs discussed in these chapters for treating certain conditions. Therefore, readers do not need a background in pharmacogenomics to follow this book. However, readers with a background in pharmacogenomics will also be able to utilize this book as a quick handbook or reference, since at the end of each chapter, there is an extensive list of references for further advanced studies in this field.

We hope you enjoy reading this.

Loralie J. Langman, Rochester, Minnesota
Amitava Dasgupta, Houston, Texas

CHAPTER 1

Pharmacogenomics Principles: Introduction to Personalized Medicine

Parvaz Madadi, PhD and Gideon Koren, MD
Division of Clinical Pharmacology and Toxicology, Hospital for Sick Children, Toronto, Canada

Introduction

Interindividual variability in drug response is a clinical reality, and one that has been long recognized by physicians and healthcare professionals. The essence of personalized medicine is the act of tailoring a treatment regimen to an individual based on their unique characteristics. However, our increasing understanding and sophistication in elucidating the causes of variability provide a new opportunity for an integrative and holistic personalized medicine – one that can synchronize all these factors together to deliver the right treatment, at the right dose, for every patient.

Although medications are typically marketed based on standard doses that are associated with safe and efficacious profiles in controlled clinical trials, these trials are not always representative of the clinical setting. In reality, patients differ widely in their response to treatment; while many may benefit from drug therapy, a proportion of individuals may be nonresponders, while others may develop adverse drug reactions. To truly deliver personalized medicine, one must have a grasp on the factors that contribute to variable outcomes in patients (Table 1.1) and how these factors may interact together in an individual. In the following sections, we will consider these sources of variation in more detail.

Factors that contribute to variability in drug response

Adherence, the extent to which a person's behavior – taking medication, following a diet, and/or executing lifestyle changes – corresponds with agreed recommendations from a health care provider (World Health Organization, 2003) (1), is a major, sometimes unrecognized, source of variability in the clinical setting. The term *adherence* is preferred over *compliance*, which denotes a passiveness on the part of the patient to follow the doctor's orders rather than establish a therapeutic alliance with their physician (1, 2). However, in many circumstances, the two words may be used interchangeably. Most physicians are unable to recognize nonadherence in their patients (2). Poor medication adherence accounts for 33–69% of all medication-related hospital admissions, and costs approximately $100 billion a year in the United States alone (2).

Of the different disease modalities, adherence to medications in chronic conditions is particularly low. For example, survey results in North America, the United Kingdom, and Western European countries indicate that no more than 30% of patients maintain target blood pressure levels despite receiving pharmacotherapy. Using a pill container with a computerized microchip to record the date and time the container was accessed, researchers were able to

Pharmacogenomics in Clinical Therapeutics, First Edition. Edited by Loralie J. Langman and Amitava Dasgupta.
© 2012 John Wiley & Sons, Ltd. Published 2012 by John Wiley & Sons, Ltd.

Table 1.1 Factors Contributing to Variability in Drug Response

Adherence
Age of the patient
Disease state
Drug–drug interactions
Food–drug interactions
Formulation
Gender
Genetics
Pollutants (smoking, etc.)
Pregnancy
Route of administration

demonstrate that up to half of the "failures" in reaching these target blood pressure levels could be associated with inconsistent patterns of medication use, which was different from what was prescribed (3). Interestingly, these lapses were often unrecognized by patients. Similarly in India, more than half of type 2 diabetic patients in one study were nonadherent with their oral hypoglycemic treatment regiments. Considering that India has the highest number of people affected by diabetes in the world (expected to reach 79 million individuals by the year 2030), this is a substantial problem (4).

Clearly, adherence to pharmacotherapy is an international issue (4, 5). An essential step in this direction is to understand the factors that influence adherence in the first place. Some of these predictors are summarized in Table 1.2. These predictors could be social and economic factors, the health care team or system, characteristics of the disease and

Table 1.2 Predictors of Poor Adherence

Asymptomatic disease
Cognitive impairment
Complexity of treatment
Cost of medications
Inadequate follow-up or discharge
Patient lack of belief in the treatment
Psychiatric illness
Poor provider–patient relationship
Side effect of medication

disease-related therapies, and patient-related factors (1). Going back to our example of antihypertensive medications, one study in a cohort of over 80,000 Chinese patients prescribed antihypertensive identified the following factors that were associated with better adherence amongst patients: advanced age, female gender, payment of fees, adherence for attending appointments (i.e., attendance to specialist clinics and follow-up visits), and certain concomitant medications but not others (5). Overall, Chinese patients were more adherent to their antihypertensive medications (85% good compliance) than previously reported in studies of patients of Caucasian descent.

It has been postulated that increasing the effectiveness of adherence may have a far greater impact on population health than an improvement in a single area or specific treatment (6). Osterberg and Blaschke outlined four broad types of interventional methods to improve adherence: patient education (clear instructions that simplify the regimen, and information on the value of the treatment, side effects to be expected, and the effects of adherence toward achieving the health outcome), improved dosing schedules (minimizing total number of daily doses, and using medications with long half-lives or extended release formulations), increased accessibility to health care providers (longer clinic hours, shorter wait times, and removal of cost barriers), and improved communication between physicians and patients (2). Patient-tailored interventions that target adherence must be developed as part of the "personalized medicine" regimen.

Age is another important factor to consider in regard to variability in drug response. Throughout our life span, age-related physiological changes may affect the pharmacokinetics (absorption, distribution, metabolism, and elimination) of medications. Similarly, patients' response to medications (pharmacodynamics) may differ depending on age. The field of pediatric clinical pharmacology focuses on the developmental changes which influence pharmacokinetic profiles and drug response in infants and children. There are now many examples supporting the notion that children are not simply "small adults" when it comes to medication dosing requirements and response. For example, developmental changes in the gastrointestinal tract can influence the rate and extent of bioavailability (7). Gastric acidity does not reach that of adult capacity until around 3 years of age, resulting in relatively increased absorption of acid-labile drugs such as penicillin and ampicillin in neonates (8). On the other hand, neonates may require larger oral doses of drugs that are weak acids, such as phenobarbital, in order to achieve therapeutic plasma levels (7).

The ontogeny and expression profiles of transporters and drug-metabolizing enzymes, key determinants of drug distribution and metabolism respectively, are also important factors to consider in children (7). One well-studied example is the commonly prescribed opioid morphine. Age-related development in morphine glucuronidation and clearance has been shown to correspond to progressive functional maturation of the liver and kidney (9). The mean plasma morphine clearance rate is about 4–5 times higher in children as compared to neonates (10, 11), while the average rate of glucuronidation is about 6–10 times higher in the adult livers as compared to liver from second trimester fetuses (12). The expression of the primary enzyme involved in morphine glucuronidation, uridyl glucuronyl transferase 2B7 (UGT2B7) (13, 14), is expected to reach adult levels at 2 to 6 months of age (15–17). Similar developmentally regulated ontogenically profiles have been reported for transporters (such as p-glycoprotein), and other drug-metabolizing enzymes such as cytochrome P450 2D6 and 3A4.

Clearly, extrapolation from adult dose regimens to children (on mg/kg bases) is often not appropriate. Given the widening gap between the number of adult clinical trials and pediatric clinical trials (18), there are a number of new incentives and international advocacy groups that are devoting their attention to increasing the number of high-quality pediatric drug trials in children. The ultimate goal is to develop pediatric-specific data that will result in age-appropriate diagnostics and guidelines for children, while decreasing the current practice of off-label and/or unlicensed use of medications in the pediatric setting.

Underrepresentation in clinical trials also poses similar problems in the elderly population, who will account for over 20% of the U.S. population by the year 2050. Problems related to polypharmacy, affecting more than 40% of the geriatric population (19), contributes to a disproportionately high incidence of adverse drug reactions in this age group. The relative contribution of physiological changes associated with the normal aging process in these adverse outcomes is not clearly defined. Factors such as declining hepatic drug-metabolizing enzyme functionality and neuronal changes with aging (20) may account for some of the differences in medication response as compared to younger adults. The sensitivity to drug-related side effects also increases with older age, with poor tolerability and adherence issues interfering with the benefits of treatment (21). Geriatrics-oriented clinical pharmacology will be a pivotal component of the personalized medicine toolbox for future health care professionals.

A third important variable to consider is drug–drug interactions. These interactions can affect the absorption, distribution, biotransformation, or excretion of one drug by another, and/or have consequences on drug action and effectiveness depending on the therapeutic window of the substrate. Sometimes drug interactions are intentional and beneficial, such as inhibiting an efflux transporter at the blood–brain barrier by one drug to allow the therapeutic drug to reach its target. Most often however, the consequences of drug interaction are unintentional and unfavorable, and can be associated with serious clinical consequences, such as transplant rejection (22). About 50–75% of medications are substrates of the cytochrome P450 (CYP) 3A4 enzyme, 2C9, and/or 2D6 metabolizing enzymes. Therefore, knowledge of how and which drugs are subject to metabolism by the cytochrome P450 pathway is an important way to predict potential problems if certain drugs are coadministered (23, 24). Drug interactions which affect the activity of transporters, whose role is to modulate the uptake and efflux of medications into and out of cells, may also have important clinical consequences. Interestingly, there is a profound overlap (in terms of substrates and modulators) between CYP3A and the ubiquitously expressed P-efflux transporter (25). It is also important to keep in mind that CYP3A substrates are not limited to medications, but can include food products. The classic example of a food–drug interaction is that of felodipine with grapefruit juice, resulting in a clinically significant increase in plasma felodipine concentrations due to grapefruit juice's inhibitory effect on CYP3A4 (26). Smoking and exposure to pollutants, such as occupational exposure to pesticides, may also affect drug pharmacology due to the induction of drug-metabolizing enzymes.

In addition to adherence, age, and drug interactions, Table 1.1 lists other important sources of variation. The underlying disease or pathology is an important consideration as it may necessitate dosage adjustments depending on the scenario. Impaired renal function, for example, may result in toxicity with medications that rely primarily on renal clearance, such as digoxin (27). On the other hand, variances in drug formulations and manufacturing processes can affect the rate of drug entry *into* the system. Extended-release medications, for example, may rely on bead-based formulations that allow gastrointestinal fluid to dissolve and diffuse the drug out of the beads at a predetermined rate (28). The pharmacokinetic profile of such a medication will differ from its standard counterpart. The route of drug administration, whether enteral (oral or rectal) or parenteral (intravenous, intramuscular, inhalation, intradermal, subcutaneous, sublingual, or topical), can also affect the systemic concentration of the drug and its metabolites.

Gender differences refer not only to pharmacokinetic considerations such as differences in intramuscular absorption as a result of blood flow, but also to differences in health and lifestyle behaviors. The physiological changes associated with pregnancy, particularly, can substantially affect drug kinetics and response during the gestational and postpartum periods. Cardiovascular changes are particularly profound, including increases in maternal cardiac output by 30–50%, an increase in blood volume by 50%, increases in blood flow to the uterus and kidney, and increases in the resting heart rate (29). Increases in renal filtration and active drug transport affect the pharmacokinetics of renally cleared drugs such as amoxicillin (30) and digoxin. There are also alterations in the activity of maternal drug-metabolizing enzymes in the perinatal period.

Interindividual genetic variation

Patient genotype can account for a large proportion of drug response variability. Unfortunately, most physicians do not have knowledge of their patients' genotypes before prescribing medications. However, it is important to remember that genetic variation interacts with all the other sources of variability that influence drug response. Therefore, it best viewed as an integrative component of clinical pharmacology and therapeutics.

Genotype refers to an individual's full hereditary information. Genes can be viewed as the molecular blueprints that an individual is born with. *Phenotype* refers to the individual's actual, expressed properties. This could be molecules such as proteins, which are the products derived from the genetic blueprints. Phenotype can also refer to behaviors, actions, and diseases. Genetic studies try to deduce the associations between genotype and phenotype. While the majority of human genetic sequence is conserved between individuals, genetic variability does exist due to single-nucleotide polymorphisms (SNPs) and copy number variation (CNV).

A SNP is a base change in the genetic code that occurs at a population frequency above 1%. At the single nucleotide level, every two humans differ at 0.5–10 in 1000 bp (about 1 million SNP differences between individuals). Nucleotide base changes that occurs less commonly ($< 1\%$) are referred to as mutations. SNPs occur throughout the genome in both coding and noncoding regions. A SNP that occurs in the coding region may have functional consequences if the polymorphism changes amino acid composition (missense) or induces premature stop codons (nonsense), thereby affecting protein function. In contrast to these types of nonsynonymous polymorphisms, some SNPs in the coding region may not alter amino acid sequence and are thus silent (synonymous). Interestingly, it has been recently shown that even some synonymous SNPs can alter protein function and folding by altering the rate of ribonucleic acid (RNA) translation (31). In general, the majority of SNPs that occur in noncoding regions are silent, although they may affect gene expression (promoter SNPs) or RNA splicing (Figure 1.1).

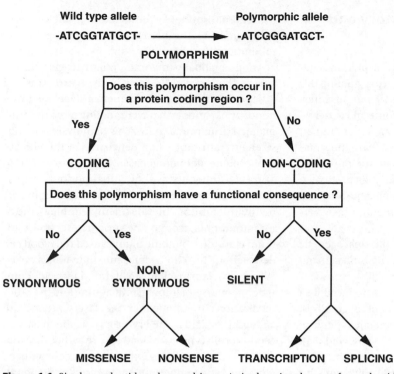

Figure 1.1 Single-nucleotide polymorphisms. A single point change of a nucleotide, here of the wild-type thymine (T) to a guanine (G), can occur throughout the genome in both coding and noncoding regions. More commonly, the polymorphism will not have a functional consequence (synonymous, or silent). However, functional consequences may arise if the polymorphism alters protein structure and function, or in noncoding regions, affects gene expression and splicing.

Copy number variation refers to DNA segments greater than 1,000 bases that are present at variable copy number (in comparison to the reference genome). CNVs are considered a substantial source of human genetic variation. Covering an estimated 12% of the human genome (32), the number of base pairs affected by CNVs is greater than the sum of all the SNPs across the genome combined (33). CNVs can consist of deletions and duplications which may arise from unequal crossover events during homologous recombination. There has been some success in our understanding of the clinical significance of certain CNVs with diseases, such as autism. Certainly in pharmacogenomics, CNVs have been identified in an important drug-metabolizing enzyme affecting the metabolism of many medications, as will be described below. However, complex disease–CNV associations are generally complicated by the fact that novel CNVs are found ubiquitously in each healthy control and patient that is genetically characterized. Therefore, the idea of the "reference genome" is constantly evolving. International repositories for human CNV data (such as the Database for Genomic Variants, hosted online by the Centre for Applied Genomics in Toronto, Canada) have been established to aid in this matter.

The field of pharmacogenetics and pharmacogenomics utilizes genetic information to predict both drug action (pharmacokinetics) and drug response (pharmacodynamics) for an increasing number of xenobiotics. While pharmacogenetic studies have traditionally focused on a single gene or several genes along a drug pathway, pharmacogenomic studies now more broadly utilize the entire or significant proportions of the genome. However in many contexts, the terms are used interchangeably.

Pharmacogenomics: history and current state

Despite the recent advancements in pharmacogenetics and genomics, the main principle guiding this field – that genetic variability can account for interindividual differences in drug response and toxicity– was established decades before the first human genome was sequenced (34). These early pharmacogenetic studies aimed to elucidate the molecular and functional mechanisms of variability between individuals. These early studied formed the basis and rational behind therapeutic drug monitoring of certain drugs.

One of the first and classical pharmacogenetic examples is the antituberculosis drug isoniazid and *N*-acetyltransferase 2 (NAT2) variability in individuals. In the 1950s, isoniazid was introduced as a breakthrough drug in the treatment of tuberculosis. Shortly after its introduction, a heritable difference in the rate of isoniazid metabolism was observed (35). This variability was due to a liver enzyme that remained in the supernatant after centrifugation – this enzyme was discovered to be an acetyltransferase (36, 37), later identified as NAT2 (N-acetyltransferase 2). Peripheral neuropathy was frequently observed in "slow acetylators" of isoniazid. Mechanistically, it was shown that isoniazid competed for an enzyme involved in the pyridoxine (vitamin B6) pathway, and that administration of pyridoxine could prevent and reverse isoniazid-induced peripheral neuropathy (38).

Currently, the most severe and delimiting adverse drug reaction associated with isoniazid is not peripheral neuropathy but hepatotoxicity. While the exact mechanism of how isoniazid induces hepatotoxicity is not known, there is some evidence that slow acetylation status may play a role in shifting the metabolism of isoniazid into an elimination pathway that favors the production of toxic metabolites. Genetic polymorphisms, as well as nongenetic factors such as age, concomitant medications, and underlying liver disease, have also been shown to potentiate the hepatotoxic effects of isoniazid treatment. Nonetheless, isoniazid remains an important and globally used medicine today. Knowledge of the factors which contribute to variability in isoniazid response, prior to the administration of the medication, will be useful in maximizing the benefits of this therapy while minimizing the risk of liver toxicity.

Another globally important pharmacogenetic discovery that started its roots in the 1950s was the observation that hemolytic anemia developed in a minority of patients that were administered the antimalarial drug primaquine. This hemolysis was subsequently attributed to a deficiency in the glucose 6-phosphate dehydrogenase (G6PD) enzyme (39, 40). Over time, it was shown that not only primaquine but also other medications such as dapsone, methylthioninium chloride (methylene blue), nitrofurantoin, phenazopyridine, rasburicase, and tolonium chloride (toluidine blue) caused red blood cell destruction in G6PD-deficient individuals (41). While the exact mechanism of drug-induced hemolytic anemia is not known, primaquine and the other medications mentioned in the last sentence are chemical oxidants. The erythrocyte is the most susceptible cell type to oxidative stress, because the G6PD–NADPH pathway is the only source of reduced glutathione, an important endogenous antioxidant. In G6PD-deficient individuals, this pathway is blocked and oxidative stress resulting in hemolysis occurs. Sporadic hemolytic crises are also caused by certain infections and the ingestion of the fava bean (favism) in individuals with the "Mediterranean" enzyme variant. Numerous biochemical and genetic studies to date have identified over 300 abnormal G6PD variants resulting from approximately 100 diverse mutations. G6PD deficiency is the most common enzymopathy in the world, affecting approximately 400 million people. Presumably, one of the reasons for its widespread frequency, particularly in endemic parts of the world, is its conferred resistance to malaria.

In the late 1950s, Kalow and colleagues, observing marked variability in drug action among individuals that had received the muscle relaxant succinylcholine, identified the basis for a third pharmacogenetic association. In most individuals, the effect of succinylcholine after injection would last for several minutes before rapid degradation of the drug by plasma cholinesterase. However in a minority of patients, this paralysis effect was observed for hours (referred to as *succinylcholine apnea*). Using the ultraviolet spectrophotometer, Kalow was able to demonstrate that in those patients who experienced succinylcholine apnea, there was a reduced cholinesterase binding affinity for its substrates, arising from a genetic alteration. Familial studies were also in line with this hypothesis of a genetic defect resulting in poor cholinesterase–succinylcholine binding interactions (42–47). This phenomenon was later linked to several functional variants in the butyrylcholinesterase gene (48, 49). The biochemical test Kalow developed to identify individuals susceptible to succinylcholine apnea is still used today (50).

The next wave of important pharmacogenetic studies came forth in the late 1970s and early 1980s. In Germany, Eichelbaum and colleagues were conducting pharmacokinetic studies on sparteine, an antiarrhythmic and uterine contractile (oxytocic) agent. In their study, two participants developed diplopia, blurred vision, dizziness, and headache following sparteine administration. Coincidentally, the plasma levels of sparteine in these two patients was several-fold higher than all the other subjects who had been administered the same dose of the drug. In addition, drug metabolites were not present in their urine and plasma, indicating minimal metabolism (51). Around the same time in Britain, Smith and colleagues were conducting pharmacokinetic studies on the new antihypertensive drug debrisoquine. In their study, it just so happened that the investigator, Smith, was also a study participant who took a standard oral dose of debrisoquine along with four other volunteers. Within 2 hours of drug administration, only Smith became dizzy, faint, and unable to stand, with blood pressure dropping to as low as 70/50 mmHg. While most symptoms improved, cardiovascular effects remained for several days after these events. Urine analysis revealed that Smith alone eliminated debrisoquine almost entirely as the parent compound with minimal metabolism, while the other subjects excreted the drug mainly in its metabolite form (52). These early studies illustrated the concept that the "dose of a drug was a poor predictor for patient response." Over the next several years, it was confirmed that sparteine and debrisoquine were metabolized by the same enzyme, aptly named sparteine/debrisoquine hydroxylase. Teams of researchers identified that this enzyme was a cytochrome P450, and that enzymatic deficiencies were inherited in an autosomal recessive fashion – the gene traced to chromosome 22 (53, 54). Today, this enzyme is more commonly referred to as cytochrome P450 2D6 (CYP2D6).

CYP2D6 is involved in the metabolism of a wide variety of medications (an estimated 25% of all drugs on the market) and has several recently suggested endogenous (55, 56) substrates (Table 1.3). However, CYP2D6 genetic variation has variable consequences for each of these listed substrates. Factors such as the reliance of the drug on the CYP2D6 pathway (i.e., the absence of other compensatory metabolic pathways), the therapeutic

Table 1.3 Substrates and Inhibitors of CYP2D6

CYP2D6 Substrates

For treatment of psychiatric and neurological disease
Amitriptyline, atomoxetine clomipramine, clozapine, desipramine, duloxetine, fluoxetine, fluvoxamine, haloperidol, imipramine, levomepromazine, mirtazapine, nortriptyline, olanzapine, paroxetine, risperidone, sertraline, tetrabenazine, venlafaxine

For treatment of cardiovascular disease and/or eye disease
Alprenolol, amiodarone, atenolol, bufuralol, bupranolol, debrisoquine, flecainide, indoramin, metoprolol, nimodipine, oxprenolol, propafenone, propranolol, quinidine, timolol

For treatment of pain
Codeine (metabolite is active), hydrocodone (metabolite is active), oxycodone (metabolite is active), tramadol (metabolite is active)

Others
Chlorpropamide, dextromethorphan, flunarizine, ondansetron, tamoxifen (metabolite is active), tropisetron, sparteine, 3,4-methylenedioxymethamphetamine ("Ecstasy"), amphetamine, methamphetamine

Endogenous substrates
5-methoxytryptamine (5-MT), 5-methoxy-N,N-dimethyltryptamine (5-MDMT), 6-methoxy-1,2,3,4-tetrahydro-β-carboline

CYP2D6 inhibitors
Fluoxetine, fluvoxamine, paroxetine, quinidine, sertraline

window of the drug, and the relationship between drug plasma concentration and drug effect are all predictors of the importance of CYP2D6 perturbations for each drug action.

While the discovery of the polymorphic nature of CYP2D6 was partly based on the administration of a probe drug and urine collection to determine drug and metabolite concentrations over time "phenotyping," there has been much effort to infer phenotype directly by genotyping, prior to administering the drug to the individual (Figure 1.2). A direct genotyping approach certainly has its advantages: the administration of the probe drug may be dangerous for some patients that cannot be identified beforehand, genotyping is less labor intensive on the part of the patient, and genotyping only needs to be performed once in a person's lifetime and is not subject to temporary sources of variation such as concomitant drug administration. On the other hand, CYP2D6 genotype to phenotype correlations is complicated by the highly polymorphic nature of CYP2D6, with over 70 alleles identified, and by gene duplication events resulting in as many as 13 CYP2D6 copy number variants. In addition, two individuals with the same genotype may not have the same phenotype due to basal differences in gene expression, dietary and ethnic influences, and the presence of yet undiscovered novel variants. However, clinical tools such as the CYP2D6 activity score have been developed and validated in some populations to optimize such correlations (57).

Although genotyping provides a long-term source of information pertaining to an individuals' metabolic capacity, genotype interpretations should always be made with the consideration of concomitant medications that the patient may be taking at the current time. Particularly, prescribers should be aware that drug interactions may interfere with the genotype to phenotype prediction, in a phenomenon referred to as phenocopying (a drug–drug

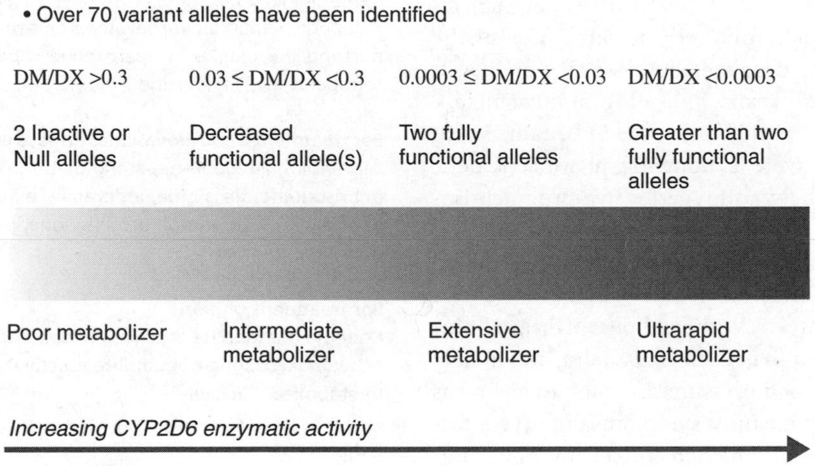

• Over 70 variant alleles have been identified

DM/DX >0.3	0.03 ≤ DM/DX <0.3	0.0003 ≤ DM/DX <0.03	DM/DX <0.0003
2 Inactive or Null alleles	Decreased functional allele(s)	Two fully functional alleles	Greater than two fully functional alleles
Poor metabolizer	Intermediate metabolizer	Extensive metabolizer	Ultrarapid metabolizer

Increasing CYP2D6 enzymatic activity →

Figure 1.2 A gradient of CYP2D6 enzymatic activity – characterizing activity levels by phenotyping or genotyping. Characterization of CYP2D6 enzymatic activity may be achieved by phenotyping an individual. Here, a CYP2D6 specific probe drug such as dextromethorphan is administered, and the relative ratio between the concentration of probe drug (dextromethorphan: DM) and its CYP2D6-specific metabolite (dextorphan: DX) is obtained. Those with higher DM:DX ratios have a higher proportion of unmetabolized parent drug to metabolite, thus exhibiting limited CYP2D6 metabolic capacity (poor metabolizers). Conversely, very small DM:DX ratios depict extensive CYP2D6 metabolic capacity in the individual (extensive to ultra-rapid metabolizers). Alternatively, one may indirectly infer enzymatic activity by genotyping the individual and assigning the individual to a metabolizer category (poor, intermediate, extensive, or ultra-rapid) based on the inferred functional consequence of their genotype. Although four phenotypic classes are commonly used, the cutoffs between the categories are not distinct, as there is a gradient of activity levels in the population. *Note*: DM: dextromethorphan, a CYP2D6 substrate. DX: dextrorphan, a CYP2D6-specific metabolite of dextromethorphan.

interaction can inhibit the CYP2D6 enzyme such that an individual with a genotype associated with extensive CYP2D6 metabolism will be phenotypically similar to an individual who has a poor metabolizer genotype).

The other important pharmacogenetic discovery that arose in the early 1980s was that of thiopurine S-methyltransferase (TPMT) polymorphisms. TPMT is a cytosolic enzyme involved in the metabolism of thiopurine drugs such as 6-mercaptopurine and azathioprine. Analyzing TPMT enzymatic activity from the red blood cells (RBC) of 298 randomly selected and unrelated Caucasian subjects, Weinshilboum and Sladek (58) reported three distinct activity profile cohorts (high-activity individuals [88.6%], intermediate-activity ones [11.1%], and those of undetectable activity [0.3%]). The authors also confirmed, via familial studies, that this variability in TMPT enzymatic activity was an inherited trait. Subsequently, it was shown that undetectable or low TPMT activity, occurring in about 1/300 individuals, was a major risk factor for the development of life-threatening azathioprine-induced myelosuppression in patients receiving "standard" doses of the drug (59). Similar adverse drug reactions were also reported in TMPT deficient patients receiving 6-mercaptopurine (60). Mechanistically, these adverse drug reactions develop as a result of an accumulation of cytotoxic thioguanine nucleotides, which are normally responsible for the therapeutic effect of thiopurines, but at high concentrations may cause severe toxicity. Thus, TMPT-deficient individuals require 10–15-fold lower doses than in those who possess high-functioning TMPT enzyme activity. Since the 1990s, the red blood cell (RBC) TPMT activity assay (61) and/or the RBC 6-thioguanine assay (which is inversely correlated to the RBC TMPT assay) (62) have been used in some institutions as a method to help determine optimal thiopurine doses in patients.

Following the cloning and characterization of the TMPT gene in the early 1990s, the molecular basis for the observed phenotypic variations has been better defined. Currently, there have been 30 SNPs identified in TPMT (63), most of which have been associated with decreased enzymatic activity. The frequency of these SNPs varies amongst different ethnic groups; TPMT*3A, for example, is the most common low activity variant in Caucasians (5% frequency), while the *3C is the major variant allele in African Americans and East Asian populations (64). In Caucasians, over 95% of cases of inherited TPMT deficiency can be detected by assaying for the TMPT*3A, *3C, and *2. Interestingly, trinucleotide repeat variants in the promoter of TPMT have recently been identified in a subset of individuals (1–2%), that exhibit extremely high enzyme activity (65). These individuals may actually require higher than standard thiopurine doses to achieve therapeutic effect.

Despite the well-established clinical significance of TPMT polymorphisms, the validated biomarkers for TPMT testing, and the safety information included on the FDA drug label, the uptake of TPMT genetic testing to determine optimal treatment for acute lymphocytic leukemia has been variable in the United States (66). Specifically in regard to TMPT, the rarity of the potentially fatal adverse drug reaction (1 in 300 to 400 patients) may mean that some physicians will never have a patient that experienced such toxicity in the absence of testing (66). Moreover, some oncologists argue that the pharmacodynamic response, measured as a decrease in leukocyte counts, has the same sensitivity and predictive value. Factors such as financial or logistical roadblocks to accommodate pharmacogenetic testing and patient and prescriber education in regard to treatment management options may contribute to this variable uptake and will be discussed in the subsequent section.

Pharmacogenomics and translational approaches

Although the terms *pharmacogenetics* and *pharmacogenomics* are used interchangeably, on a philosophical level, the word pharmacogenomics represents a more comprehensive way of thinking about the influence of genes on drug response. From the clinical pharmacology perspective, since the 1960s, when Dr. Werner Kalow wrote the first textbook in pharmacogenetics entitled *Pharmacogenetics: Heredity and the Response to Drugs,* to five decades later in the new millennium, our understanding of the multifactorial nature of drug response and variability has become more apparent. In the words of Kalow, "Pharmacogenetics arose with studies of single genes, which had major effects on the action of particular drugs. It turned into pharmacogenomics through realization that the controls of most drug responses are multifactorial" (67). From the genomics perspective, such realization was inextricably tied with the rapid advances in molecular biology based on user-friendly technological platforms that could scan large or complete proportions of the genome in a rapid and increasingly cost-effective manner.

Moving away from single gene studies, current approaches may involve genetic markers along an entire drug metabolism and response pathway. The polymorphisms in the major human drug-metabolizing enzymes and their pharmacokinetic effects have been well studied; the emphasis now is on the characterization of drug transporter and receptors polymorphisms and the synergistic effects of variation amongst the entire drug pathway. Another approach is genome-wide association studies (GWAS), which can assess over a million SNPs depending on the assay platform. This hypothesis-generating technique has contributed to over 800 unique SNP–trait associations for common diseases within the past decade (68). However, GWAS studies have traditionally been performed in those with European descent, and most commercially available SNP microarrays cannot capture variation in non-Caucasian ethnicities. Furthermore, rarer and novel variants are less likely to be identified. Thus, the more attractive, increasingly feasible, and comprehensive option, which is at the cutting edge of genomic science, is whole exome sequencing or whole genome sequencing.

By most predictions, as a consequence of the rapidly decreasing costs, whole genome sequencing will become routinely available within the next 5 to 10 years. Already, it has been demonstrated that clinically meaningful pharmacogenomic and disease risk information can be obtained in a clinic setting using the information derived from the sequencing of one patient's whole genome (69). Such comprehensive genomic techniques are able to identify novel variants and stimulate a revolution in our thinking of disease and drug response (70), though

Table 1.4 Use of Whole Genome Sequence in Clinical Practice

1. The broad scope of the results will require that patients receive complex and detailed information before they decide whether to be tested.
2. Interpretation of genome sequences should take into account the limits of the sequencing method used.
3. Easily accessible and well-curated information about the links between genomic sequences and diseases needs to be created, maintained, and frequently updated.
4. Physicians and patients will have to cope with enormous uncertainty in some results, particularly around variants of unknown importance, which might require analysis of genetic information from family members.
5. Effective ways to convey meaningful information to patients about the many implications of their whole genome sequences need to be developed and training for appropriate specialists to convey this information funded.
6. Whole genome sequences will need to be reviewed regularly to incorporate new information about disease risks, and changes in assessment will have to be conveyed to patients.

Source: From Ormond KE, Wheeler MT, Hudgins L, Klein TE, Butte AJ, Altman RB, *et al.* (2010). Challenges in the clinical application of whole-genome sequencing. *Lancet* 375 (9727):1749–51. Copyright Elsevier, Reprinted with permission.

not without its challenges (71) (Table 1.4). In contrast to the mechanistic approaches which assessed the causative effect of genetic polymorphisms in early "phenotype-to-genotype" pharmacogenetic studies, the functional effect of most variants that arise from a whole genome sequence is unknown. Thus, there is a significant diagnostic uncertainty about the meaning of the results. On one hand, the collection of large data sets from carefully phenotyped patients contributes to our knowledge of the clinical significance of these variants, which will ultimately advance our understanding of countless medical conditions in the future. In addition, the patient whose whole genome is sequenced today must be made aware that most sequence information obtained from their genome will be of unknown meaning, and under the pretense of a rapidly changing knowledge base.

This rapidly changing knowledge base will mean that genomic interpretations may change over time.

It also necessitates the need for publically available, user-friendly, and frequently updated databases for prescribers and patients, such as the Pharmacogenomics Knowledge Database (PharmGKB; see www.pharmgkb.org), supported by the National Institute of Health and the National Institute of General Medical Sciences. Such user-friendly translational interfaces are becoming an important component of an overall movement toward wide-scale educational and translational genomic strategies.

Educational and translational genomic strategies are needed in every aspect of science and medicine in this post-human genome sequencing era. Scientists and researchers will need to gain evaluative skills to be able to utilize the large quantities of data that are derived from genome sequencing. The emergent field of translational bioinformatics is uniquely positioned to make major advances in this area. Translational bioinformaticians integrate molecular and clinical data to enable novel translational hypotheses bidirectionally between the domains of biology and medicine (72). According to the American Medical Informatics Association, translational bioinformatics refers to "the development of storage, analytic, and interpretive methods to optimize the transformation of increasingly voluminous biomedical data, and genomic data in particular, into proactive, predictive, preventive, and participatory health." (73)

Major initiatives are currently underway to improve the competency of health care providers in the field of genomics. Traditionally, the field of medical genetics was devoted to the study of relatively rare single-gene or chromosomal disorders in primarily tertiary care settings by specialists. With advances in pharmacogenomics and the elucidation of multiple genomic contributions toward more common and complex conditions, genomic information is moving into the "medical mainstream" (74). However, the interpretation of genomic markers for these more common diseases is not as straightforward as rare, highly penetrant single gene–disease associations, given the interplay between genetic and environmental factors. Recognizing that health care professionals will increasingly use genetic and genomic information to meet the needs of their patients, essential genomic competencies, practice guidelines, and curricular resources in genetics and genomics are being developed across medical disciplines (75).

The literacy of the public in genomics also needs to be improved. The general public has limited knowledge of genetic risk factors as a cause of multifactorial disease and even less knowledge of how and why these factors affect health (76). These initiatives are particularly imperative in the current atmosphere of direct-to-consumer genetic testing companies, which bypass the medical system to deliver and market genetic information directly to the shopper. The public needs to develop an understanding of the limitations of genetic testing in order to critically appraise marketed genetic tests. They also need to be informed on the ethical, social, and legal issues surrounding genetic information and genetic testing.

References

1 World Health Organization Adherence to Long Term Therapies Project and the Global Adherence Interdisciplinary Network (2003) *Adherence to Long-Term Therapies: Evidence for Action*. World Health Organization, Geneva.

2 Osterberg, L., Blaschke, T. (2005) Adherence to medication. *New England Journal of Medicine*, **353**(**5**), 487–497.

3 Stephenson, J. (1999) Noncompliance may cause half of antihypertensive drug "failures." *Journal of the American Medical Association*, **282**(**4**), 313–314.

4 Sultana, G., Kapur, P., Aqil, M., Alam, M.S., Pillai, K.K. (2010) Drug utilization of oral hypoglycemic agents in a university teaching hospital in India. *Journal of Clinical and Pharmaceutical Therapies*, **35**(**3**), 267–277.

5 Wong, M.C., Jiang, J.Y., Griffiths, S.M. (2010) Factors associated with antihypertensive drug compliance in 83,884 Chinese patients: a cohort study. *Journal of Epidemiology and Community Health*, **64**(**10**), 895–901.

6 Haynes, R.B., McDonald, H., Garg, A.X., Montague, P. (2002) Interventions for helping patients to follow prescriptions for medications. *Cochrane Database Systems Review* (**2**) CD000011.

7 Kearns, G.L., Abdel-Rahman, S.M., Alander, S.W., Blowey, D.L., Leeder, J.S., Kauffman, R.E. (2003) Developmental pharmacology: drug disposition, action, and therapy in infants and children. *New England Journal of Medicine*, **349**(**12**), 1157–1167.

8 Koren, G. (1997) Therapeutic drug monitoring principles in the neonate. *Clinical Chemistry*, **43**(**1**), 222–227.

9 Assael, B.M. (1982). Pharmacokinetics and drug distribution during postnatal development. *Pharmacological Therapies*, **18**(**2**), 159–197.

10 Choonara, I.A., McKay, P., Hain, R., Rane, A. (1989) Morphine metabolism in children. *British Journal of Clinical Pharmacology*, **28**(**5**), 599–604.

11 Lynn, A.M., Slattery, J.T. (1987). Morphine pharmacokinetics in early infancy. *Anesthesiology*, **66**(**2**), 136–139.

12 Pacifici, G.M., Sawe, J., Kager, L., Rane, A. (1982) Morphine glucuronidation in human fetal and adult liver. *European Journal of Clinical Pharmacology*, **22**(**6**), 553–558.

13 Coffman, B.L., King, C.D., Rios, G.R., Tephly, T.R. (1998) The glucuronidation of opioids, other xenobiotics, and androgens by human UGT2B7Y(268) and UGT2B7H(268). *Drug Metabolism and Disposal*, **26**(**1**), 73–77.

14 Coffman, B.L., Rios, G.R., King, C.D., Tephly, T.R. (1997) Human UGT2B7 catalyzes morphine glucuronidation. *Drug Metabolism and Disposal*, **25**(**1**), 1–4.

15 Anderson, B.J., McKee, A.D., Holford, N.H. (1997) Size, myths and the clinical pharmacokinetics of analgesia in paediatric patients. *Clinical Pharmacokinetics*, **33**(**5**),313–327.

16 de Wildt, S.N., Kearns, G.L., Leeder, J.S., van den Anker, J.N. (1999) Glucuronidation in humans: pharmacogenetic and developmental aspects. *Clinical Pharmacokinetics*, **36**(**6**), 439–452.

17 McCarver, D.G., Hines, R.N. (2002) The ontogeny of human drug-metabolizing enzymes: phase II conjugation enzymes and regulatory mechanisms. *Journal of Pharmacological and Experimental Therapies*, **300**(**2**), 361–366.

18 Klassen, T.P., Hartling, L., Craig, J.C., Offringa, M. (2008) Children are not just small adults: the urgent need for high-quality trial evidence in children. *PLoS Medicine*, **5**(**8**), e172.

19 Barnett, S.R. (2009) Polypharmacy and perioperative medications in the elderly. *Anesthesiology Clinics*, **27**(**3**), 377–389.

20 Pollock, B., Forsyth, C., Bies, R. (2009) The critical role of clinical pharmacology in geriatric psychopharmacology. *Clinical and Pharmaceutical Therapies*, **85**(**1**), 89–93.

21 Meyers, B.S., Jeste, D.V. (2010) Geriatric psychopharmacology: evolution of a discipline. *Journal of Clinical Psychiatry*, **71**(**11**), 1416–1424.

22 Barone, G.W., Gurley, B.J., Ketel, B.L., Lightfoot, M.L., Abul-Ezz, S.R. (2000) Drug interaction between St. John's wort and cyclosporine. *Annals of Pharmacotherapy*, **34**(**9**), 1013–1016.

23 Wilkinson, G.R. (2005) Drug metabolism and variability among patients in drug response. *New England Journal of Medicine*, **352**(**21**), 2211–2221.

24 Flockhart, D.A. (2007) Drug interactions: cytochrome P450 drug interaction table [WWW document]. URL http://medicine.iupui.edu/clinpharm/ddis/table.asp [accessed on 17 June 2011]

25 Salphati, L., Benet, L.Z. (1998) Modulation of P-glycoprotein expression by cytochrome P450 3A inducers in male and female rat livers. *Biochemistry and Pharmacology*, **55**(**4**), 387–395.

26 Bailey, D.G., Malcolm, J., Arnold, O., Spence, J.D. (2004) Grapefruit juice–drug interactions. *1998. British Journal of Clinical Pharmacology*, **58**(**7**), S831–S840; discussion, S841-S843.

27 Mooradian, A.D. (1988) Digitalis: an update of clinical pharmacokinetics, therapeutic monitoring techniques and treatment recommendations. *Clinical Pharmacokinetics*, **15**(**3**), 165–179.

28 Amabile, C.M., Bowman, B.J. (2006) Overview of oral modified-release opioid products for the management of chronic pain. *Annals of Pharmacotherapy*, **40**(**7–8**), 1327–1335.

29 Haas, D.M., Hebert, M.F., Soldin, O.P., Flockhart, D.A., Madadi, P., Nocon, J.J., *et al.* (2009) Pharmacotherapy and pregnancy: highlights from the Second International Conference for Individualized Pharmacotherapy in Pregnancy. *Clinical and Translational Science*, **2**(**6**), 439–443.

30 Andrew, M.A., Easterling, T.R., Carr, D.B., Shen, D., Buchanan, M.L., Rutherford, T., *et al.* (2007) Amoxicillin pharmacokinetics in pregnant women: modeling and simulations of dosage strategies. *Clinical and Pharmaceutical Therapies*, **81**(**4**), 547–556.

31 Kimchi-Sarfaty C, Oh JM, Kim IW, Sauna ZE, Calcagno AM, Ambudkar SV, *et al.* (2007). A "silent" polymorphism in the MDR1 gene changes substrate specificity. *Science* **315**(**5811**):525–8.

32 Redon R, Ishikawa S, Fitch KR, Feuk L, Perry GH, Andrews TD, *et al.* (2006). Global variation in copy number in the human genome. *Nature* **444**(**7118**):444–54.

33 Eichler EE. (2008). Copy number variation and human disease. *Nature Education* **1**(**3**): http://www.nature.

com/scitable/topicpage/copy-number-variation-and-human-disease-741737.

34 Meyer UA. (2004). Pharmacogenetics – five decades of therapeutic lessons from genetic diversity. *Nat Rev Genet* **5**(9):669–76.

35 Evans DA. (1968). Genetic variations in the acetylation of isoniazid and other drugs. *Ann N Y Acad Sci* **151**(2):723–33.

36 Evans DA, White TA. (1964). Human Acetylation Polymorphism. *J Lab Clin Med* **63**:394–403.

37 Kalow W. (1971). Topics in pharmacogenetics. *Ann N Y Acad Sci;* **179**:654–9.

38 Krishnamurthy DV, Selkon JB, Ramachandran K, Devadatta S, Mitchison DA, Radhakrishna S, *et al.* (1967). Effect of pyridoxine on vitamin B6 concentrations and glutamic-oxaloacetic transaminase activity in whole blood of tuberculous patients receiving high-dosage isoniazid. *Bull World Health Organ* **36**(5):853–70.

39 Clayman CB, Arnold J, Hockwald RS, Yount EH, Jr., Edgcomb JH, Alving AS. (1952). Toxicity of primaquine in Caucasians. *J Am Med Assoc* **149**(17):1563–8.

40 Beutler E. (1994). G6PD deficiency. *Blood* **84**(11): 3613–36.

41 Youngster I, Arcavi L, Schechmaster R, Akayzen Y, Popliski H, Shimonov J, *et al.* (2010). Medications and glucose-6-phosphate dehydrogenase deficiency: an evidence-based review. *Drug Saf* **33**(9):713–26.

42 Kalow W. (1952). Hydrolysis of local anesthetics by human serum cholinesterase. *J Pharmacol Exp Ther* **104**(2):122–34.

43 Kalow W, Genest K. (1957). A method for the detection of atypical forms of human serum cholinesterase; determination of dibucaine numbers. *Can J Biochem Physiol* **35**(6):339–46.

44 Kalow W, Genest K, Staron N. (1956). Kinetic studies on the hydrolysis of benzoylcholine by human serum cholinesterase. *Can J Biochem Physiol* **34**(3):637–53.

45 Kalow W, Lindsay HA. (1955). A comparison of optical and manometric methods for the assay of human serum cholinesterase. *Can J Biochem Physiol* **33**(4):568–74.

46 Kalow W, Maykut MO. (1956). The interaction between cholinesterases and a series of local anesthetics. *J Pharmacol Exp Ther* **116**(4):418–32.

47 Kalow W, Staron N. (1957). On distribution and inheritance of atypical forms of human serum cholinesterase, as indicated by dibucaine numbers. *Can J Biochem Physiol* **35**(12):1305–20.

48 Kalow W. (1995). Life of a pharmacologist or the rich life of a poor metabolizer. *Pharmacol Toxicol* **76**(4):221–7.

49 Rubinstein HM, Dietz AA, Lubrano T. (1978). E1k, another quantitative variant at cholinesterase locus 1. *J Med Genet* **15**(1):27–9.

50 Daly AK. (2010). Pharmacogenetics and human genetic polymorphisms. *Biochem J* **429**(3):435–49.

51 Eichelbaum M, Spannbrucker N, Steincke B, Dengler HJ. (1979). Defective N-oxidation of sparteine in man: a new pharmacogenetic defect. *European Journal of Clinical Pharmacology*, **16**(3):183–7.

52 Smith RL. The Paton Prize Award. (2001). The discovery of the debrisoquine hydroxylation polymorphism: scientific and clinical impact and consequences. *Toxicology* **168**(1):11–9.

53 Gonzalez FJ, Matsunaga T, Nagata K, Meyer UA, Nebert DW, Pastewka J, *et al.* Debrisoquine 4-hydroxylase: characterization of a new P450 gene subfamily, regulation, chromosomal mapping, and molecular analysis of the DA rat polymorphism. *DNA* 1987; **6**(2):149–61.

54 Gonzalez FJ, Skoda RC, Kimura S, Umeno M, Zanger UM, Nebert DW, *et al.* (1988). Characterization of the common genetic defect in humans deficient in debrisoquine metabolism. *Nature* **331**(6155):442–6.

55 Yu AM, Idle JR, Gonzalez FJ. (2004). Polymorphic cytochrome P450 2D6: humanized mouse model and endogenous substrates. *Drug Metab Rev* **36**(2):243–77.

56 Yu AM, Idle JR, Herraiz T, Kupfer A, Gonzalez FJ. (2003). Screening for endogenous substrates reveals that CYP2D6 is a 5-methoxyindolethylamine O-demethylase. *Pharmacogenetics* **13**(6):307–19.

57 Gaedigk A, Simon SD, Pearce RE, Bradford LD, Kennedy MJ, Leeder JS. (2008). The CYP2D6 activity score: translating genotype information into a qualitative measure of phenotype. *Clinical and Pharmaceutical Therapies*, **83**(2), 234–242.

58 Weinshilboum RM, Sladek SL. (1980). Mercaptopurine pharmacogenetics: monogenic inheritance of erythrocyte thiopurine methyltransferase activity. *Am J Hum Genet* **32**(5):651–62.

59 Lennard L, Van Loon JA, Weinshilboum RM. (1989). Pharmacogenetics of acute azathioprine toxicity: relationship to thiopurine methyltransferase genetic polymorphism. *Clinical and Pharmaceutical Therapies*, **46**(2), 149–154.

60 Evans, W.E., Horner, M., Chu, Y.Q., Kalwinsky, D., Roberts, W.M. (1991) Altered mercaptopurine

metabolism, toxic effects, and dosage requirement in a thiopurine methyltransferase-deficient child with acute lymphocytic leukemia. *Journal of Pediatrics*, **119**(6), 985–989.

61 Weinshilboum, R.M., Sladek, S., Klumpp, S. (1979) Human erythrocyte thiol methyltransferase: radiochemical microassay and biochemical properties. *Clinica Chimica Acta: International Journal of Clinical Chemistry*, **97**(1), 59–71.

62 Lennard, L. (1987) Assay of 6-thioinosinic acid and 6-thioguanine nucleotides, active metabolites of 6-mercaptopurine, in human red blood cells. *Journal of Chromatography*, **423**,169–178.

63 Appell, M.L., Wennerstrand, P., Peterson, C., Hertervig, E., Martensson, L.G. (2010) Characterization of a novel sequence variant, TPMT*28, in the human thiopurine methyltransferase gene. *Pharmacogenetic Genomics*, **20**(11), 700–707.

64 Wang, L., Weinshilboum, R. (2006) Thiopurine S-methyltransferase pharmacogenetics: insights, challenges and future directions. *Oncogene*, **25**(11), 1629–1638.

65 Roberts, R.L., Gearry, R.B., Bland, M.V., Sies, C.W., George, P.M., Burt, M., *et al.* (2008) Trinucleotide repeat variants in the promoter of the thiopurine S-methyltransferase gene of patients exhibiting ultra-high enzyme activity. *Pharmacogenetic Genomics*, **18**(5), 434–438.

66 Freedman, A.N., Sansbury, L.B., Figg, W.D., Potosky, A. L., Weiss Smith, S.R., Khoury, M.J., *et al.* (2010) Cancer pharmacogenomics and pharmacoepidemiology: setting a research agenda to accelerate translation. *Journal of the National Cancer Institute*, **102**(22), 1698–1705.

67 Kalow, W. (2006) Pharmacogenetics and pharmacogenomics: origin, status, and the hope for personalized medicine. *Pharmacogenomics Journal*, **6**(3), 162–165.

68 Rotimi, C.N., Jorde, L.B. (2010) Ancestry and disease in the age of genomic medicine. *New England Journal of Medicine*, **363**(16), 1551–1558.

69 Ashley, E.A., Butte, A.J., Wheeler, M.T., Chen, R., Klein, T.E., Dewey, F.E., *et al.* (2010) Clinical assessment incorporating a personal genome. *Lancet*, **375**(9725), 1525–1535.

70 Butte, A.J. (2008). Medicine: the ultimate model organism. *Science*, **320**(5874), 325–327.

71 Ormond, K.E., Wheeler, M.T., Hudgins, L., Klein, T.E., Butte, A.J., Altman, R.B., *et al.* (2010) Challenges in the clinical application of whole-genome sequencing. *Lancet*, **375**(9727), 1749–1751.

72 Butte, A.J. (2009). Translational bioinformatics applications in genome medicine. *Genome Medicine*, **1**(6), 64.

73 American Medical Informatics Association (2011) AMIA strategic plan [WWW document]. URL https://www.amia.org/inside/initiatives [accessed on 17 June 2011].

74 Collins, F.S., Guttmacher, A.E. (2001) Genetics moves into the medical mainstream. *Journal of the American Medical Association*, **286**(18), 2322–2324.

75 National Human Genome Research Institute (2011) [Home page] [WWW document]. URL http://www.genome.gov/27527634 [accessed on 17 June 2011]

76 Smerecnik, C.M., Mesters, I., de Vries, N.K., de Vries, H. (2008) Educating the general public about multifactorial genetic disease: applying a theory-based framework to understand current public knowledge. *Genetics in Medicine*, **10**(4), 251–258.

CHAPTER 2

Traditional Therapeutic Drug Monitoring and Pharmacogenomics: Are They Complementary?

Christine L.H. Snozek, PhD[1], Loralie J. Langman, PhD[1], and Amitava Dasgupta, PhD[2]
[1]Department of Laboratory Medicine and Pathology, Mayo Clinic, Rochester, Minnesota
[2]Department of Pathology and Laboratory Medicine, University of Texas–Houston Medical School

Introduction

The practice of traditional therapeutic drug monitoring (TDM) started some 40 years ago. The International Association for Therapeutic Drug Monitoring and Clinical Toxicology adopted the following definition for therapeutic drug monitoring: "Therapeutic drug monitoring is defined as the measurement made in the laboratory of a parameter that, with appropriate interpretation, will directly influence prescribing procedures. Commonly, the measurement is in a biological matrix of a prescribed xenobiotic, but it may also be of an endogenous compound prescribed as a replacement therapy in an individual who is physiologically or pathologically deficient in that compound" (1). TDM most often takes the form of measuring serum or plasma concentrations of prescribed drugs, although there are a few laboratory tests such as the prothrombin time international normalized ratio (INR) that can also be used to monitor drug efficacy in a given patient.

Pharmacogenomics (PGX) is a branch of pharmacology that deals with the effects of genetic variations on a patient's response to a particular drug. The words *pharmacogenetics* and *pharmacogenomics* are often used interchangeably. In a stricter sense, pharmacogenetics is the study of inherent differences in drug metabolism and response due to genetic variations among different people, while pharmacogenomics refers to general study of all of the different genes that determine overall response of an individual to a particular drug. Therefore, pharmacogenomics is the whole genome application and includes genes which affect a drug's metabolism and disposition. The goal of PGX testing is to determine a patient's genetic background before initiation of drug therapy in order to optimize dosing, or to select a more appropriate drug, in order to get maximum benefit from the drug and minimum toxicity.

TDM and PGX testing are both clinical laboratory based methods for supporting pharmacotherapy. TDM is offered as routine tests in most hospital laboratories, whereas PGX testing is currently offered in relatively few major medical centers throughout the United States and the rest of the world. Both PGX and TDM are aspects of personalized medicine that are currently utilized in clinical practice. One must consider, however, that although traditional TDM is able to personalize dosage for a particular patient, this approach cannot determine prior to initiating therapy whether a person will respond to a particular drug, or how efficiently a patient might metabolize that drug. Currently TDM is sufficient for patient management during pharmacotherapy with many agents, but for certain drugs or drug classes PGX testing can provide more meaningful information for optimizing therapy.

Pharmacogenomics in Clinical Therapeutics, First Edition. Edited by Loralie J. Langman and Amitava Dasgupta.
© 2012 John Wiley & Sons, Ltd. Published 2012 by John Wiley & Sons, Ltd.

Pharmacology

A general understanding of the basics of pharmacology is required for a discussion of either TDM or PGX. Pharmacological response to a particular drug depends on many factors, including patient compliance, bioavailability, and drug clearance, as well as genetic and environmental factors that affect an individual's response to a drug. Conceptually, pharmacology can be divided into pharmacokinetics (PK; i.e., what the body does to the drug) and pharmacodynamics (PD; i.e., what the drug does to the body).

Pharmacokinetics

When a drug is administered, it undergoes several processes in the body which eventually determine concentration of that drug in serum or whole blood. These steps include liberation, absorption, distribution, metabolism, and elimination; together, these comprise the PK of a drug. *Liberation* of a drug refers to the quantity and timing of drug release from the dosing form (e.g., pill, liquid, or patch), and depends on the formulation. For example, with oral medications, immediate-release formulations release the active component very rapidly, whereas sustained- or controlled-release formulations release the drug over time.

Absorption of a drug depends on the route of administration. Intravenous injection places the full dose of the drug directly into circulation; all other routes require some form of absorption. Bioavailability is the ratio of absorbed drug relative to an intravenous dose, and reflects how readily the body takes up a particular compound. When a drug enters the blood it is distributed according to its affinity for various compartments (e.g., fatty tissue, lean tissue, or plasma). *Distribution* can greatly affect the ability of a therapeutic agent to reach its target site; for example, agents affecting the central nervous system must penetrate the blood–brain barrier. Binding to plasma proteins may limit movement into tissues, which may affect the amount of drug reaching the pharmacological target.

Finally, drugs are cleared through metabolism and/ or elimination. *Metabolism* generally increases the water solubility of a compound to facilitate *elimination*, and may occur in any tissue including the blood. The primary site of metabolism for most exogenous and endogenous compounds is the liver, which contains large amounts of Phase I (nonconjugating reactions) and Phase II (conjugating) enzymes (Table 2.1). The cytochrome P450 (CYP) family of Phase I enzymes are involved in the metabolism of most drugs; as discussed throughout this book, the genes encoding CYP enzymes are polymorphic and are therefore of great interest to PGX. The most common routes of elimination are through urine and feces, and elimination therefore may be affected by renal or gastrointestinal diseases. Management of conditions such as malabsorption or chronic kidney failure is a common rationale for performing TDM.

Pharmacodynamics

PD is the relationship between drug concentration and effect, and includes the description of variability in physiological responses despite equivalent drug delivery to effector sites (2). Many drugs interact

Table 2.1 Select Polymorphic Drug-Metabolizing Enzymes

Reaction	Phase	Name of Enzyme	Currently Useful in PGX or Clinical Testing?
Oxidation/reduction	Phase I	Cytochrome P450	Yes
		Alcohol dehydrogenase	No
		Monoamine oxidase	Possibly
Hydrolysis	Phase I	Butylcholinesterase	Yes
Glucuronidation	Phase II	Glucuronosyltransferase	Yes
Acetylation	Phase II	N-Acetyltransferase	Yes
Methylation	Phase II	Thiopurine methyltransferase	Yes
Amino acid conjugation	Phase II	Glutathione transferase	Possibly
Sulfation	Phase II	Sulfotransferase	No

with a receptor protein to initiate the steps leading to physiological response(s) to that particular compound. These receptors or drug targets can be intracellular, as in the case of steroid receptors, or transmembrane proteins. In theory, PD differences could be affected by genetic variation in not only the direct drug target but also downstream effectors, regulatory proteins, transcription factors, and a host of other molecules with the potential to modulate the cellular response to a particular drug.

One assumption in TDM is that the concentration of the drug at the receptor is reflected in the serum or blood concentrations. Drug transport plays a vital role in most PK processes. This has obvious implications in the penetration of drugs not only into the blood but also into compartments where the drug targets are (3). It has been suggested that during pharmacotherapy, 30–60% of patients may not respond to a particular drug (4). What component of that percentage is due to altered PK versus altered PD is not known.

Therapeutic drug monitoring

It has been suggested that serious adverse drug reactions cause up to 7% of all hospitalizations, and are a significant source of morbidity and (5). TDM can help avoid adverse drug reactions for certain drugs such as aminoglycosides (6). As mentioned, TDM is based on the hypothesis that the concentration of a drug in blood better reflects the amount of drug at the target site, clinical efficacy, and toxicity than do other parameters such as the administered dose. Some commonly monitored drugs are listed in Table 2.2.

Criteria for drugs to be candidates for TDM include the following:

A Narrow therapeutic range, that is, the amount of drug which produces the desired therapeutic effect is close to the concentration associated with toxicity.

B Absence of an easily measured clinical or biochemical parameter upon which to base dosing.

For example, blood pressure can be used to dose antihypertensives, which therefore do not require TDM.

C Variable PK leading to poor correlation between dose and clinical effect.

D Correlation of serum drug concentration with efficacy and/or toxicity.

E Significant risks associated with patient noncompliance.

Noncompliance is frequently a problem, particularly in long-term therapy for chronic conditions

Table 2.2 Drugs Commonly Monitored by TDM

Drug Class	Individual Drugs
Older Agents	
Anticonvulsants	Carbamazepine, Phenobarbital, Phenytoin, Valproic Acid
Antidepressants	Amitriptyline, Nortriptyline, Clomipramine, Doxepin, Imipramine, Desipramine
Antipsychotics	Lithium, Clozapine, Haloperidol
Antineoplastics	Methotrexate, Busulfan
Antibiotics	Vancomycin, Amikacin, Gentamicin, Tobramycin
Bronchodilators	Caffeine, Theophylline
Cardioactive Drugs	Digoxin, Digitoxin, Lidocaine, Procainamide, Quinidine
Immunosuppressants	Cyclosporine, Tacrolimus, Sirolimus
Newer Agents	
Anticonvulsants	Levetiracetam, Gabapentin, Lamotrigine, Zonisamide
Antidepressants	Fluoxetine, Sertraline, Venlafaxine
Antineoplastics*	5-Fluorouracil, Tamoxifen
Antifungals	Posaconazole, Voriconazole
Antiretrovirals	Amprenavir, Indinavir, Lopinavir, Nelfinavir, Saquinavir, Efavirenz, Nevirapine,
Immunosuppressant	Mycophenolic Acid, Everolimus**

*Although these drugs are not new, the practice of TDM has only recently been applied to them.
**Everolimus has been monitored for years in Europe, but was only FDA approved in 2010.

where compliance rates are often below 50% (7, 8). Measuring serum drug concentrations can assist physicians in ensuring patients take medications appropriately over time. In addition, TDM is useful to assess reasons for changes in an individual's response to a particular drug, or for dosage adjustments in children, the elderly, pregnant women, or critically ill patients where alterations in PK are a significant concern.

Requirements for valid TDM interpretation typically include the following: a patient who is at pharmacological steady state (i.e., drug input and output are in balance); blood samples drawn at trough, that is, immediately before the next scheduled dose; and knowledge of the individual's co-medications and clinical status. The analytical methodology is typically immunoassay for the limited selection of drugs with commercial assays available, or a chromatography-based platform such as high-performance liquid chromatography or liquid chromatography–mass spectrometry.

Pharmacogenomics

There is a great deal of interindividual variability at the DNA level which govern many aspects of pharmacology. Single-nucleotide polymorphisms (SNPs) account for over 90% of the genetic variation in the human genome, with the rest composed of insertions, deletions, variable number tandem repeats, and microsatellites (9). The science of PGX focuses on genetic variability in drug response due to germline alterations such as SNPs, gene deletions, or gene duplications, affecting molecules involved in PK and PD. To date, most PGX studies have focused on the impact of genetic variations in the expression and function of drug-metabolizing enzymes and transporter proteins.

Polymorphisms in metabolic enzymes

The cytochrome P450 (CYP) proteins comprise a superfamily of heme-containing proteins found in many organisms, with over 7,700 known members across all species studied. A relatively small number are associated with drug metabolism in humans,

most notably CYPs of the 1, 2, and 3 families (10). The major CYP isoforms responsible for metabolism of drugs include CYP1A2, CYP2B6, CYP2C9, CYP2C19, CYP2D6, CYP2E1, and CYP3A4/CYP3A5; many of the genes encoding these proteins are highly polymorphic (11, 12). Based on metabolism, individuals are classified as *extensive metabolizers* (EMs) who have "normal" function of the specific enzyme. Individuals lacking most or all of that enzyme's activity are called *poor metabolizers* (PMs); those with activity between EMs and PMs are *intermediate metabolizers* (IMs). Finally, individuals who have much higher function of certain enzymes are termed *ultrarapid metabolizers* (UMs). Differences in metabolism due to genetic polymorphism can lead to toxicity or therapeutic failure by altering the relationship between the administered dose and the steady-state concentration of the drug.

Polymorphisms in the CYP family greatly influence metabolism of many therapeutic drugs. *CYP2D6*, *CYP2C19*, and *CYP2C9* polymorphisms account for the most frequent variations in phase I metabolism of drugs; a large number of drugs are metabolized by these enzymes. Approximately 5–14% of Caucasians, 0–5% Africans, and 0–1% of Asians lack CYP2D6 activity, with many more individuals falling into the IM category (13). Although *CYP2D6* is the most highly polymorphic gene relevant to PGX, *CYP2C19* and *CYP2C9* also have catalytically inactive variants, with potential effects on common substrates such as omeprazole and propranolol (14), or warfarin and phenytoin, respectively.

Other metabolic enzymes with clinically significant polymorphisms include N-acetyltransferase (encoded by *NAT1* and *NAT2*), thiopurine-S-methyltransferase (*TPMT*), and the UGT family of glucuronide-conjugating enzymes. The slow acetylator phenotype of NAT1/2 results in isoniazid induced peripheral neuropathy and sulfonamide induced hypersensitivity reactions, while TPMT catalyzes inactivation of various anticancer and anti-inflammatory drugs (15). UGT family members metabolize a large number of drugs; the best characterized example of a pharmacologically relevant variant is the role of UGT1A1 in irinotecan metabolism. The TA promoter polymorphism in *UGT1A1* can result in reduced glucuronidation of the active metabolite of irinotecan, thus predisposing patients to potentially life-threatening toxicity.

Other clinically relevant polymorphisms

Although most literature is focused on the role of genetic variants in metabolic enzymes, genes related to drug transport and activity have also been studied for their importance to PGX. The best characterized drug transporter is the multidrug resistance protein MDR1 (also called P-glycoprotein). MDR1 is a glycosylated membrane-bound protein expressed mainly in the intestines, liver, kidneys, and brain. A large number of structurally unrelated drugs are substrates for MDR1, which regulates their intestinal absorption, hepatobiliary secretion, renal secretion, and brain transport (16, 17). A synonymous SNP in *MDR1* exon 26, C3435T, was found to affect duodenal expression of the protein despite the lack of an amino acid change. Subjects harboring the mutant T3435 allele had lower serum concentrations of digoxin after a single oral dose (18). Although over 25 SNPs have been found in *MDR1*, clinical investigations on the association of genotype with the expression and function of MDR1 have mainly focused on C3435T.

Compared to genes whose products are involved in PK much less is known about genetic polymorphism in PD such as drug targets and receptors. This is an important area for future study, as variations in drug targets can result in altered sensitivity of the individual to a therapeutic agent, with implications for both efficacy and toxicity. Some examples of PD-related molecules with potential relevance to PGX include the β1- and β2-adrenoreceptors (encoded by *ADBR1* and *ADRB2*) and the serotonin transporter (encoded by *5HTT*), which have variants associated with altered drug responses. One of the few PD genes to achieve significant clinical interest is *VKORC1*, which encodes vitamin K epoxide reductase, the molecular target of warfarin therapy (19); PGX for this gene will be discussed in a later section. Other examples where PGX has entered clinical practice (typically to a limited extent) are listed in Table 2.3.

Table 2.3 Examples of Some Drugs Where Pharmacogenomics Testing Has Clinical Significance

Drug	Polymorphic Gene(s)	Comments
Anticoagulant		
Warfarin	CYP2C19/VKORC1	Variants associated with both sensitivity and resistance have been described.
Antineoplastic drugs		
Irinotecan	UTG1A1	Accumulation of active metabolite SN-38 in patients with TA 7-repeat allele.
6-Mercaptopurine	TPMT	Neutropenia in poor metabolizers.
Tamoxifen	CYP2D6	Poor metabolizers have lower endoxifen, reduced response to therapy.
Antidepressants*		
Amitriptyline	CYP2D6	Poor metabolizers, possibly more adverse effects.*
Paroxetine	CYP2D6	Poor metabolizer, possibly more adverse effects. Ultra rapid metabolizers maybe nonresponsive.
Sertraline	CYP2C19	Poor metabolizers, possibly more adverse effects. Ultra-rapid metabolizers nonresponsive.
Cardioactive		
Clopidogrel	CYP2C19	Poor metabolizers have low levels of active metabolite in blood and show poor response.
Opiate analgesic		
Codeine	CYP2D6	Poor metabolizers unable to convert codeine to morphine, do not get pain relief.

*These are possible effects; please see Chapter 9 for in-depth discussion on this topic and references.

TDM versus PGX: phenotype, genotype, or both?

Commercial TDM assays are available for several commonly monitored therapeutic agents; these tests are typically compatible with autoanalyzers and require little or no specimen pretreatment. In addition, a wide variety of chromatographic techniques have been described for quantitating less commonly monitored compounds in biological matrices. These assays must be developed and validated in individual laboratories, and require greater technological expertise and resources than commercial methods. Test prices vary by analytical platform and laboratory, but are usually in the range of $50–200.

In marked contrast, PGX tests are less readily available and notably more expensive, often from several hundred to over a thousand dollars per sample. There are relatively few commercial assays; those that do exist often are not FDA cleared, require extensive preparation and technologist time, and cannot be readily automated. Furthermore, PGX assays frequently must be updated as new polymorphisms or clinical applications come to light. Interpretation of PGX results is rarely straightforward, and depending on the number of genes and polymorphisms involved, may require substantial training or complex algorithms to determine the clinical implications (20). Federal scrutiny and regulation of PGX assays have increased and likely will continue to do so, in part because of the difficulty in interpretation and the growing use of algorithms that may lack clinical validation studies.

Limitations of TDM and PGX

Although traditional TDM is successful in monitoring pharmacotherapy of certain drugs for a range of clinical needs, it does have several limitations. Genetic and nongenetic sources of variability often cannot be predicted prior to beginning therapy, thus traditional TDM is not able to tailor initial dose requirements or to predict risk of a serious adverse response. TDM also cannot provide the reason why a measured concentration is not in the desired range; for example, it is not possible to determine whether an unexpectedly low concentration reflects a patient with atypically rapid metabolism, or simply noncompliance. Finally, TDM is hampered by pre-analytical variables that are often out of the laboratory's control. Caregivers often do not realize the requirements for obtaining valid blood samples for TDM, thus many drug concentrations are reported for patients who are not yet at steady state, or who had taken a dose shortly before the supposedly "trough" sample was drawn.

In contrast to TDM, PGX measures aspects of an individual's inherent PK and PD, without being tied to a single drug. A priori knowledge of genetic variation, for example absence of a particular metabolic enzyme, may allow appropriate dose adjustment or alternate therapeutic selection to occur before the patient is exposed to a drug. Clinical adoption of this strategy in the case of warfarin therapy will be discussed below. PGX may also provide greater understanding of TDM results. In the above example of an unexpectedly low drug concentration, PGX tests might reveal variability in a drug transporter or metabolic enzyme that accounts for reduced drug exposure in a compliant patient.

PGX analyses have the advantage of being a one-time test: once an individual's genetic polymorphisms have been documented there is rarely a need to re-genotype unless new, clinically relevant variants are later described. Genetic tests are not affected by age, weight, hormonal status, disease state, or other confounding factors. TDM measurements, on the other hand, are designed to be serial assessments to give a real-time picture of the patient's current state, and ideally should be interpreted relative to previous results. When properly used, TDM can account for physiological or pathological conditions, co-medications, and so on by empirically demonstrating an individual's actual exposure to the drug of interest. PGX allows prediction of limited aspects of PK and PD, but cannot provide all the information that is relevant to pharmacotherapy – as a case in point, there is no genetic test for noncompliance.

Use of TDM as an indicator for PGX testing

Both PGX and TDM represent examples of personalized medicine: PGX delineates an individual's genotype, whereas TDM provides the phenotype that combines genetic and environmental variables. Phenotyping patients during pharmacotherapy is not a new concept; it can be done by measuring serum concentrations of the therapeutic agent, or in the case of compounds with significant risk for toxicity, through prospective use of a probe drug. An example of the latter practice is the use of dibucaine to assess function of the metabolic enzyme butylcholinesterase (also known as serum cholinesterase). Certain polymorphisms of the gene encoding butylcholinesterase reduce hydrolysis of the powerful muscle relaxants succinylcholine and mivacurium, resulting in prolonged muscular paralysis and potentially severe toxicity (21). Administration of the butylcholinesterase inhibitor dibucaine prior to use of these drugs can be helpful in assessing metabolic capacity with less risk of dangerous side effects, although the probe drug test is inadequate for identifying all cases of prolonged response to succinylcholine (22). Similar phenotyping studies have been performed for other metabolic enzymes, for example the use of omeprazole as a probe drug for CYP2C19. Initial testing using probe drugs for highly polymorphic enzymes can draw attention to a subset of individuals with aberrant metabolism, but given the substrate-specific effects of some variant alleles, results must be interpreted with caution.

TDM can also serve as a phenotypic indicator for potential genetic variability. Atypical serum drug concentrations require investigation into the cause; however, most unusual results stem from a nongenetic source. Once patient compliance, co-medications, laboratory error, or other pre-analytical and analytical factors have been ruled out, it becomes reasonable to consider PGX testing as a next step in the investigative process. Although there are some examples of drugs where the risk of early adverse effects (e.g., warfarin) or the lack of readily available biomarkers or serum drug assays to monitor therapy (e.g., tamoxifen) may warrant prospective genotyping of patients, most areas of pharmacotherapy are not yet ready for PGX as an initial step. A more cost-effective strategy for most drugs is to perform TDM once patients reach steady state, then following up with further investigation and possible PGX for the subset of patients who show atypical serum drug concentrations. The number of PGX assays available is currently rather small, given the wide array of genes that can potentially affect pharmacotherapy, thus prospective PGX is currently insufficient to prevent many of the PK and PD abnormalities that can be detected through TDM and clinical monitoring.

Can TDM and PGX be complementary?

Despite the promise of PGX, TDM is more widely used today in clinical practice. However, it is likely that future advances in personalized medicine will lead to the integration of PGX and TDM as complementary sources of information. One of the most important applications of PGX is the ability to prospectively assess an individual's probability of receiving benefit or experiencing toxicity from a particular drug. Currently, only a few drugs carry labels recommending genetic testing, all of which have significant risk of life-threatening adverse responses. For example, the effects of variant alleles are discussed in the package inserts for anti-neoplastic agents such as irinotecan (*UGT1A1* promoter polymorphism), azathioprine and mercaptopurine (*TPMT* genetic or protein activity analysis), and the antithrombotic warfarin (*CYP2C9* and *VKORC1*) (23). Aside from a handful of examples where PGX research has made the first steps toward inclusion in clinical practice, traditional TDM is far more widely applied to individualize dosing of a drug in patients. However, in several clinical fields the two approaches to personalized medicine have begun to fuse into a more holistic means of providing optimal patient care. The use of TDM and PGX as complementary strategies will be discussed below in the contexts of warfarin therapy, pain management, transplant immunosuppression, and other clinical settings.

Warfarin therapy

Warfarin is the most widely used oral anticoagulant for prevention of thrombotic events. It binds to the enzyme vitamin K 2, 3-epoxide reductase (encoded by *VKORC1*) to stop recycling of vitamin K, which is required for activation of several clotting factors.

Warfarin is highly prone to both PK and PD variability, thus therapy is monitored using the prothrombin time clotting assay, commonly reported as the international normalized ratio. This represents one of the relatively few situations where TDM is performed via measurement of a biological parameter other than drug concentration. Healthy, untreated individuals have an INR of 1; the target INR for warfarin anticoagulation is typically 2–3. However, the variability between individuals is so severe that a standard dose can lead to responses ranging from no clinical effect to double-digit INRs that place patients at high risk of potentially fatal hemorrhaging.

A large part of the interindividual variation in response to warfarin has been linked to polymorphisms in *CYP2C9* and *VKORC1*, which code for the drug's primary metabolic enzyme and molecular target respectively. Prospective genotyping has been suggested as a means of preventing much of the early morbidity and mortality associated with warfarin therapy. However, the INR is essential for long-term monitoring of the drug, due to the important role of environmental factors such as vitamin K intake and drug interactions (24). Genetic analysis cannot replace real-time assessment of physiological and environmental influences on response to warfarin. Chapter 3 will discuss the role of PGX in warfarin therapy.

Pain management

Chronic pain management is a growing concern in the United States and elsewhere; as a result, the use of opioids to treat noncancer pain is a topic of great discussion in the medical community. The fact that many opioid analgesics have a high risk of addiction and/or diversion potential makes their use both controversial and challenging. Many pain clinics have adopted the practice of monitoring their patients, typically with urine drug confirmations but sometimes with serum assays. Serum concentrations are not helpful in guiding dose adjustments because of the wide range of concentrations seen from opioid-naïve patients to those who have become tolerant. Urine analysis allows noninvasive collection of samples as well as a longer detection window for ensuring that the patient is both taking

the prescribed pain medication (rather than diverting it), and also is not taking anything that has not been prescribed (abuse of multiple drugs is common in addicts). Serum tests shorten the detection window, but have the advantage of ensuring that the sample donor cannot adulterate the specimen.

There has been substantial progress in understanding how genetic variations can influence the response to pain therapy, particularly with regard to metabolic enzymes and opioid receptors (25). In general, the majority of opioids used in pain management are metabolized by CYPs and/or UGT2B7. Codeine, for example, is metabolized by CYP2D6 to morphine, thus PM for this enzyme are unlikely to receive adequate analgesia from this drug. In the absence of TDM or PGX testing, the prescribing physician may well suspect a PM patient of drug diversion or exaggerating the level of perceived pain. TDM could confirm that the patient sample contains codeine, but does not guarantee that the individual is taking it as prescribed. However, addition of PGX analysis to demonstrate a PM genotype guides the physician toward better options for pain management in that patient. Genotyping following TDM assessment has been suggested to be beneficial in pain management (26). This topic is discussed in detail in Chapter 5.

Transplant immunosuppression

Organ transplant recipients receive immunosuppressive drugs in order to prevent graft rejection. Several of these, including cyclosporine, tacrolimus, sirolimus, mycophenolic acid, and the recently FDA-approved drug everolimus, are managed through routine TDM; recent reports indicate that PGX can complement this practice in certain patients. Immunosuppressants have narrow therapeutic windows and wide interindividual variations in blood concentrations after standard doses. Due to the long half-lives of most immunosuppressants, it may take 5–7 days for a patient to reach steady-state concentrations where TDM-guided dose adjustments can be made. However, the first 2–3 days after transplant are critical to patient outcome, thus the timeline of TDM bears the risk that transplant recipients may be exposed to either too little or too much immunosuppression.

Polymorphisms of *CYP3A5* and *MDR1* have been associated with individual responses to immunosuppressant therapy. CYP3A4 is the major metabolic enzyme for cyclosporine, tacrolimus, sirolimus, and everolimus; CYP3A5 shares many of the same substrates, but is not expressed in a large percentage of the population. Given the critical nature of the first few days after organ transplantation, it has been suggested that prospective PGX of *CYP3A5* and/or *MDR1* polymorphisms may improve initial dosing of immunosuppressants to allow more patients to achieve target concentrations as rapidly as possible (27). Concentration targets change with time from transplant, thus TDM would complement initial PGX-based dosing with long-term management of therapy. Chapter 6 has a more detailed discussion on this subject.

Antiretroviral drugs

The observed interindividual variation in antiretroviral PK results in a wide range of drug exposure in fixed-dose regimens. For this reason, TDM of certain antiretroviral drugs has been strongly recommended to optimize dosing for individual patients. Currently there is evidence that suggests TDM may improve therapy with nelfinavir, indinavir, ritonavir, amprenavir, saquinavir, lopinavir, efavirenz, delavirdine, zidovudine, and nevirapine (28). One study has concluded that TDM is useful in identifying toxic levels of nonnucleoside reverse transcriptase inhibitors (NNRTI) and subtherapeutic concentrations of protease inhibitors (29).

PGX tests can also be clinically useful for certain antiretroviral agents. The strong association of abacavir hypersensitivity reactions with the HLA-B*5701 allele permits prospective typing of patients to determine if an alternate therapy needs to be selected. Similarly, HLA-DRB*101 has been linked with hypersensitivity to nevirapine, while *UGT1A1* genotype appears to influence hyperbilirubinemia during atazanavir therapy (30) Additional PGX findings of interest include the association of *CYP2B6*6* with increased exposure to efavirenz resulting in higher risk of neuropsychological toxicity (31). PGX analysis is the cornerstone of avoiding hypersensitivity reactions to specific drugs, and may also prove useful in complementing TDM for other antiretro-

viral agents. These important topics are discussed in detail in Chapter 8.

Pharmacogenomics and therapeutic drug monitoring of psychoactive drugs

TDM of tricyclic antidepressants such as amitriptyline, clomipramine, and imipramine is a standard practice in patients receiving these medications. In addition, there are suggestions that TDM may be useful with newer antidepressants such as fluoxetine and venlafaxine. The objectives of TDM for old and new generation antidepressants differs, as older antidepressants have narrow therapeutic windows with concentration-dependent toxicity, while the newer antidepressants have wide therapeutic ranges and unclear relationships between plasma concentrations and physiological effects. Therefore, the purpose of TDM for newer antidepressants is largely monitoring patient compliance and investigating select groups such as the elderly, patients with liver and kidney impairment, or those at risk of drug interactions (32). At present, psychotropic medications for the treatment of mental illnesses, including antidepressants, mood stabilizers, and antipsychotics, are clinically suboptimal because they are effective in only a subset of patients or produce partial responses, and they are often associated with significant side effects that discourage adherence (33).

There are a number of PGX studies on antidepressants demonstrating the influence of CYP variants and polymorphic genes within the monoaminergic system on interindividual variability during psychoactive therapy. *CYP2D6* polymorphisms affect exposure to both older and newer antidepressants. Adverse drug reactions are more common in PM treated with amitriptyline or its active metabolite nortriptyline, due to the important role of that enzyme in nortriptyline metabolism. Paroxetine, a selective serotonin reuptake inhibitor (SSRI), is both a substrate and inhibitor of CYP2D6, thus PM are at risk for adverse effects from paroxetine and from other CYP2D6 substrates given simultaneously (34). PGX studies are revealing important variants for drug PD as well: variants in the serotonin transporter *5HTT* affect SSRI therapy, and there are suggestions that polymorphisms in genes regulating the hypothalamus-pituitary adrenal (HPA) axis can influence response to antidepressants (35). See Chapter 9 for an in-depth discussion on this topic.

Conclusions

Traditional TDM is useful for individualization of pharmacotherapy for certain drugs with narrow therapeutic ranges, but this approach has many limitations. PGX holds promise for prospectively predicting aberrant exposure or response to a drug, but cannot account for many of the environmental factors or patient compliance that is encompassed by TDM. Each approach can often make up for the shortcomings of the other, thus TDM and PGX are likely to grow together in a complementary fashion as individualized medicine becomes part of modern practice.

References

1 Watson, I., Potter, J., Yatscoff, R., *et al.* (1997) *Editorial. Therapeutic Drug Monitoring*, **19**, 125.

2 Roden, D.M. (2008) Principles of clinical pharmacology. In: A. Fauci, E. Braunwald, D. Kasper, S. Hauser, D. Longo, J. Jameson, J. Loscalzo (eds), *Harrison's Principles of Internal Medicine*, 17th ed. McGraw-Hill, New York.

3 Brinkmann, U., Eichelbaum, M. (2001) Polymorphisms in the ABC drug transporter gene MDR1. *Pharmacogenomics Journal*, **1**, 59–64.

4 Spear, B.B., Heath-Chiozzi, M., Huff, J. (2001) Clinical application of pharmacogenetics. *Trends in Molecular Medicine*, **7**, 201–204.

5 Lazarou, J., Pomeranz, B.H., Corey, P.N. (1998) Incidence of adverse drug reactions in hospitalized patients: a meta-analysis of prospective studies. *Journal of the American Medical Association*, **279**, 1200–1205.

6 Slaughter, R.L., Cappelletty, D.M. (1998) Economic impact of aminoglycoside toxicity and its prevention through therapeutic drug monitoring. *PharmacoEconomics*, **14**, 385–394.

7 Gillisen, A. (2007) Patient's adherence in asthma. *Journal of Physiology and Pharmacology*, **58** (Suppl. 5), 205–222.

8 Patsalos, P.N., Berry, D.J., Bourgeois, B.F., *et al.* (2008) Antiepileptic drugs: best practice guidelines for therapeutic drug monitoring: a position paper by the subcommission on therapeutic drug monitoring, ILAE Commission on Therapeutic Strategies. *Epilepsia*, **49**, 1239–1276.

9 Sachidanandam, R., Weissman, D., Schmidt, S.C., *et al.* (2001) A map of human genome sequence variation containing 1.42 million single nucleotide polymorphisms. *Nature*, **409**, 928–933.

10 Shimada, T., Yamazaki, H., Mimura, M., *et al.* (1994) Interindividual variations in human liver cytochrome P-450 enzymes involved in the oxidation of drugs, carcinogens and toxic chemicals: studies with liver microsomes of 30 Japanese and 30 Caucasians. *Journal of Pharmacology and Experimental Therapeutics*, **270**, 414–423.

11 Zanger, U.M., Fischer, J., Raimundo, S., *et al.* (2001) Comprehensive analysis of the genetic factors determining expression and function of hepatic CYP2D6. *Pharmacogenetics*, **11**, 573–585.

12 Smith, D.A., Abel, S.M., Hyland, R., *et al.* (1998) Human cytochrome P450s: selectivity and measurement in vivo. *Xenobiotica*, **28**, 1095–1128.

13 Zhou, S.F., Liu, J.P., Chowbay, B. (2009) Polymorphism of human cytochrome P450 enzymes and its clinical impact. *Drug Metabolism Reviews*, **41**, 89–295.

14 Jin, S.K., Kang, T.S., Eom, S.O., *et al.* (2009) CYP2C19 haplotypes in Koreans as a marker of enzyme activity evaluated with omeprazole. *Journal of Clinical Pharmacy and Therapeutics*, **34**, 437–446.

15 Ensom, M.H., Chang, T.K., Patel, P. (2001) Pharmacogenetics: the therapeutic drug monitoring of the future? *Clinical Pharmacokinetics*, **40**, 783–802.

16 Fardel, O., Payen, L., Courtois, A., *et al.* (2001) Regulation of biliary drug efflux pump expression by hormones and xenobiotics. *Toxicology*, **167**, 37–46.

17 Thiebaut, F., Tsuruo, T., Hamada, H., *et al.* (1987) Cellular localization of the multidrug-resistance gene product P-glycoprotein in normal human tissues. *Proceedings of the National Academy of Sciences of the United States of America*, **84**, 7735–7738.

18 Sakaeda, T., Nakamura, T., Horinouchi, M., *et al.* (2001) MDR1 genotype-related pharmacokinetics of digoxin after single oral administration in healthy Japanese subjects. *Pharmaceutical Research*, **18**, 1400–1404.

19 Daly, A.K. (2010) Pharmacogenetics and human genetic polymorphisms. *The Biochemical Journal*, **429**, 435–449.

20 Coleman, H., Ashcraft, K. (2008) Genelex Corporation. *Pharmacogenomics*, **9**, 469–475.

21 Gatke, M.R., Bundgaard, J.R., Viby-Mogensen, J. (2007) Two novel mutations in the BCHE gene in patients with prolonged duration of action of mivacurium or succinylcholine during anaesthesia. *Pharmacogenetics and Genomics*, **17**, 995–999.

22 Pantuck, E.J. (1993) Plasma cholinesterase: gene and variations. *Anesthesia and Analgesia*, **77**, 380–386.

23 Marsh, S., McLeod, H.L. (2006) Pharmacogenomics: from bedside to clinical practice. *Human Molecular Genetics*, **15**(**Spec. No. 1**), R89–R93.

24 Lurie, Y., Loebstein, R., Kurnik, D., *et al.* (2010) Warfarin and vitamin K intake in the era of pharmacogenetics. *British Journal of Clinical Pharmacology*, **70**, 164–170.

25 Stamer, U.M., Zhang, L., Stuber, F. (2003) Personalized therapy in pain management: where do we stand? *Pharmacogenomics*, **11**, 843–864.

26 Jannetto, P.J., Bratanow, N.C. (2009) Utilization of pharmacogenomics and therapeutic drug monitoring for opioid pain management. *Pharmacogenomics*, **10**, 1157–1167.

27 Ware, N., MacPhee, I.A. (2010) Current progress in pharmacogenetics and individualized immunosuppressive drug dosing in organ transplantation. *Current Opinion in Molecular Therapeutics*, **12**, 270–283.

28 Slish, J.C., Catanzaro, L.M., Ma, Q., *et al.* (2006) Update on the pharmacokinetic aspects of antiretroviral agents: implications in therapeutic drug monitoring. *Current Pharmaceutical Design*, **12**, 1129–1145.

29 Rendon, A., Nunez, M., Jimenez-Nacher, I., *et al.* (2005) Clinical benefit of interventions driven by therapeutic drug monitoring. *HIV Medicine*, **6**, 360–365.

30 Tozzi, V. (2010) Pharmacogenetics of antiretrovirals. *Antiviral Research*, **85**, 190–200.

31 Roca, B. (2008) Pharmacogenomics of antiretrovirals. *Recent Patents on Anti-Infective Drug Discovery*, **3**, 132–135.

32 Wille, S.M., Cooreman, S.G., Neels, H.M., *et al.* (2008) Relevant issues in the monitoring and the toxicology of antidepressants. *Critical Reviews in Clinical Laboratory Sciences*, **45**, 25–89.

33 Zandi, P.P., Judy, J.T. (2010) The promise and reality of pharmacogenetics in psychiatry. *Clinics in Laboratory Medicine*, **30**, 931–974.

34 Sheffield, L.J., Phillimore, H.E. (2009) Clinical use of pharmacogenomic tests in 2009. *The Clinical Biochemist*, **30**, 55–65.

35 Binder, E.B., Holsboer, F. (2006) Pharmacogenomics and antidepressant drugs. *Annals of Medicine*, **38**, 82–94.

CHAPTER 3

Pharmacogenomics Aspect of Warfarin Therapy

Matthew D. Krasowski, MD, PhD
Department of Pathology, University of Iowa Hospitals and Clinics

Introduction

Warfarin is the most widely used oral anticoagulant agent worldwide, with approximately 2 million prescriptions issued per year in the United States (1). Warfarin is currently the leading oral anticoagulant on the market in the United States, although dabigatran etexilate (oral thrombin inhibitor) and rivaroxaban (oral factor Xa inhibitor) recently gained Food and Drug Administration (FDA) approval (2, 3). The other alternatives for long-term anticoagulation are drugs that require parenteral administration such as unfractionated heparin, low-molecular weight heparins (e.g., enoxaparin), lepirudin, and argatroban (4–6). Although warfarin therapy has many potential negative effects, patients who require long-term anticoagulation often prefer oral therapy to therapies that require daily injections. Consequently, warfarin continues to be used extensively in patients who have had a thromboembolic event or who are at high risk for thromboembolism (e.g., atrial fibrillation, artificial heart valve replacement, or genetic risk factors for thromboembolism such as Factor V Leiden).

Warfarin is available as a racemic mixture of equimolar amounts of *R*- and *S*-warfarin. The *S*-isomer is four times more potent than the *R*-isomer as an anticoagulant. Warfarin is highly water soluble and rapidly absorbed after oral administration, with peak plasma concentrations achieved within 60 to 90 minutes. The maintenance doses of warfarin required to achieve stable yet safe anticoagulation vary considerably across the population with an average dose of 5 mg/day, but with some individuals requiring less than 1 mg/day or less and others requiring over 20 mg/day (1). The mechanism of action of warfarin is inhibition of the hepatic synthesis of vitamin K-dependent clotting factors (mainly factors II, VII, IX, and X).

Bleeding is the most common complication of warfarin, with an annual bleeding risk of 1–5% depending on patient comorbid conditions (7–11). There has been much research and effort to reduce the bleeding risk of warfarin, although such efforts have had limited success. Warfarin is cited as the second-leading drug-related cause for visits to the emergency room in the United States (12), and the most often cited reason for drug-related mortality (1). Gastrointestinal and intracranial hemorrhages represent the two most common life-threatening complications (13). The highest rate of adverse effects occurs during the first month of warfarin therapy (8, 14). Although warfarin is used most commonly in adults, pediatric patients receiving warfarin therapy may also experience severe adverse effects (15, 16).

Optimization of warfarin dosing is typically achieved by following the patient's prothrombin time (PT), which is standardized by the international normalized ratio (INR). The INR allows PT results to be comparable across different clinical laboratories that use a variety of PT assays. While the PT/INR test

Pharmacogenomics in Clinical Therapeutics, First Edition. Edited by Loralie J. Langman and Amitava Dasgupta.
© 2012 John Wiley & Sons, Ltd. Published 2012 by John Wiley & Sons, Ltd.

is easy to perform and widely available, including on some point-of-care devices (17), it is worth keeping in mind that the PT/INR assay reflects a complex physiologic endpoint that is affected by both vitamin K-dependent (II, VI, and X) and K-independent (I, V) clotting factors. An INR value of 1.0 is the average value for healthy individuals not receiving anticoagulant therapy. The target INR value for patients on warfarin is often 2.5, a target that has been demonstrated effective and relatively safe in clinical trials, although certain patients may warrant target INR values greater than 2.5 (18, 19). The risk of hemorrhage increases proportionally to higher PT/INR, with INR values greater than 4.0 associated with markedly elevated risk of hemorrhagic complications. Consequently, there is always a delicate risk–benefit tradeoff between adequate anticoagulation and risk of hemorrhagic complications.

Depending on the patient, determination of the warfarin dose that provides a stable, target INR may take days to weeks or even months. Flexible protocols, computer aids, and nomograms have helped to improve control, but there is often room for improvement (20–24). Warfarin serum and plasma levels are rarely determined for clinical purposes and are typically available only at large reference or academic medical center clinical laboratories. In terms of therapeutic monitoring, warfarin is somewhat unique compared to other medications in being followed by a laboratory test that measures physiologic function as opposed to concentration of drug in the serum or plasma.

Factors affecting warfarin dosing

Various factors should be taken into account for proper dosing of warfarin. These factors are discussed in this section.

Polymorphism in cytochrome P-450

Cytochrome P450 (CYP) 2C9 is an enzyme that is involved in the oxidative metabolism of a number of clinically important drugs (e.g., warfarin, phenytoin, glipizide, and losartan) as well as endogenous molecules such as arachidonic acid and serotonin (5-hydroxytryptamine). CYP2C9 accounts for

approximately 18% of the total CYP protein content in the human liver (25, 26). Over the years, a number of polymorphisms have been discovered in the gene for CYP2C9 (27–31). Two of the more common polymorphisms result in missense mutations in the coding region of the CYP2C9 gene. CYP2C9*2 isoform is due to replacement of arginine at amino acid residue 144 by cysteine. This mutation reduces the catalytic activity of the enzyme to about 12% of the wild-type enzyme. CYP2C9*3 results in a substitution of leucine for isoleucine at amino acid position 359, which results in a reduction of catalytic activity to about 5% of wild type. Both CYP2C9*2 and *3 genetic variants are common in Caucasian populations, with allele frequencies varying from 3.3% to 18% (32, 33). Both CYP2C9*2 and *3 exhibit markedly impaired hydroxylation of warfarin compared to the wild-type CYP2C9 enzyme and are associated with decreased warfarin dose requirements, longer time to achieve stable warfarin dosing, a higher risk of bleeding during initiation phase of warfarin therapy, and an overall higher bleeding risk (27, 34–42).

Genetic variation in the gene for CYP2C9 accounts for approximately 12% of the variation in warfarin maintenance dose requirements (27, 30, 36). One limitation of genotyping for CYP2C9*2 and *3 is that these alleles are uncommon in many non-Caucasian populations (43–46). One study estimated that rare variants of CYP2C9 (i.e., alleles other than *2 and *3) collectively account for approximately 5% of the total variability in warfarin dose requirements (47).

Polymorphisms in VKORC1

While it was known for many years that the mechanism of warfarin involved vitamin K, the molecular target of warfarin proved elusive until 2004, when two independent groups discovered a previously unknown protein that was then named vitamin K epoxide reductase complex subunit 1 (VKORC1) (48, 49). The discovery of VKORC1 utilized cases of warfarin resistance in either rodents or humans. The designation of VKORC1 as subunit 1 followed from the small size of the protein and the hypothesis that this protein formed part of a larger complex of proteins involved in vitamin K recycling. It now appears that VKORC1 acts by itself, leading to the shortened, informal designation as VKOR.

VKORC1 recycles reduced vitamin K which is essential for posttranslational γ-carboxylation of vitamin K-dependent clotting factors II (prothrombin), VII, IX, and X. Two reports have described patients with extreme warfarin resistance (even to very high doses) who were then found to have rare mutations leading to amino acid changes in VKORC1 (49, 50). Warfarin resistance in rats was also described over 50 years ago, when warfarin itself was commonly used as a rodenticide (51–55). Two different research groups independently discovered VKORC1 using positional cloning approaches that capitalized on warfarin resistance in human kindreds or rats (48, 49). Several common polymorphisms in the gene for VKORC1 have been described. Overall, genetic variation of the VKORC1 gene accounts for approximately 30% of the interindividual variation in warfarin maintenance dosing (48, 49, 56–59).

Three single nucleotide VKORC1 polymorphisms (especially the $-1638G > A$ allele) have been associated with higher dose requirements for warfarin to achieve target INR. Approximately 55% of the variability in warfarin dose can be explained by equations incorporating VKORC1 and CYP2C9 genotypes, age, body weight, concomitant drugs, and medical indication for warfarin anticoagulation (59). Similar results have been obtained in studies in Chinese (60) and Japanese (61) subjects, although genotyping for VKORC1 and CYP2C9 alleles uncommon in Caucasian populations (e.g., CYP2C9*6 or *11) was required.

Other genetic polymorphisms affecting warfarin

In addition to CYP2C9 and VKORC1, researchers have attempted to identify other proteins that have genetic variation affecting warfarin effect (34, 59, 62–64). Two studies have implicated variation in the gene for CYP4F2 as accounting for approximately 1–2% of the interindividual variation in stable warfarin dose requirement (41, 65, 66). CYP4F2 is widely distributed in human liver and other tissues, and catalyzes ϖ-hydroxylation of lipoxygenase-derived eicosanoids as well as oxidation of vitamin K_1 (67). A genetic variant of CYP4F2 which results in replacement of valine-433 by methionine results in decreased oxidation of vitamin K_1 and increased requirements for warfarin, presumably secondary to higher hepatic concentrations of vitamin K_1 (68).

Multiple studies have found that a microsatellite variant in the gene for γ-glutamyl carboxylase (GGCX) is associated with increased sensitivity to warfarin (59, 69–71). GGCX is an enzyme that plays a critical role in the vitamin K cycle by catalyzing the γ-carboxylation of vitamin K-dependent proteins in the coagulation cascade. Patients who have the GGCX microsatellite variant exhibit a modest ($\sim$6%) reduction in warfarin dose requirements. Overall, however, genetic variation in GGCX accounts for less than 1% of variation in warfarin dose requirements (70).

A number of studies have searched for variation in additional genes that might underlie variation in dose response. One study found weak but significant association of factor VII and X polymorphisms with higher warfarin dose requirements, although these polymorphisms likely account for only a very small amount of the variability of warfarin dosing (34). A single-nucleotide variation in the gene for microsomal epoxide reductase 1 (EPHX1) shows statistically significant or near significant associations with lower warfarin dose; however, this variant also accounts for only a very small fraction of warfarin dose variation (72, 73).

Diet and warfarin therapy

The term *vitamin K* actually refers to a family of compounds of which vitamin K_1 (phylloquinone) and vitamin K_2 (menaquinone) are of most relevance to human health and disease (74). Vitamin K_1 is found in diet (especially green leafy vegetables and certain vegetable oils) and supplements, and typically comprises the majority of vitamin K stores in humans (75). Vitamin K_2 is synthesized by gut bacteria and generally has a minor role in fulfilling human daily requirements. Vitamin K has the lowest total body stores of the four main fat-soluble vitamins (A, D, E, and K), with depletion of vitamin K stores occurring within several weeks of restricted dietary intake. Interindividual variation in vitamin K intake and hepatic concentrations has often been invoked as a factor in warfarin sensitivity or resistance (76). However, vitamin K plasma or serum concentrations in humans are rarely measured and, even if assayed, only provide a limited estimation of vitamin K levels in the liver. Surrogate laboratory markers of vitamin K status have been explored in research studies but have not been found routine clinical use.

Numerous case reports have described reduced therapeutic response to warfarin following high vitamin K intake (76). In larger clinical trials, the estimated contribution of vitamin K intake to warfarin response has been quite varied, a finding which in part may relate to the common clinical practice of instructing patients to limit vitamin K intake while on warfarin. Two studies have shown interindividual differences in vitamin K intake to be a significant contributor to variation in response to warfarin during initiation phase of dosing (77, 78).

Concomitant medications and warfarin

A prodigious number of medications have the potential to alter the dosing requirements for warfarin. The main mechanisms by which these drug–drug interactions occur are by induction or inhibition of hepatic CYP2C9, or by competition for the plasma protein binding sites of warfarin. A number of drugs are known to increase (induce) the expression of CYP2C9; these compounds often induce expression of other liver drug-metabolizing enzymes as well (79–81). Well-characterized inducers include the antimycobacterial drug rifampin, carbamazepine, phenobarbital, phenytoin, and the herbal antidepressant St. John's wort. Patients taking inducer medication concomitantly with warfarin may require higher doses of warfarin to achieve the desired clinical effect.

There are numerous described inhibitors of CYP2C9 (25). Commonly used medications that can inhibit CYP2C9 include azole antifungal medications (e.g., fluconazole and voriconazole), amiodarone, sulfamethoxazole (found in the common combination antibiotic trimethoprim-sulfamethoxazole), statins (e.g., fluvastatin and lovastatin), and some antidepressants (e.g., fluvoxamine and sertraline). Patients taking medications that inhibit CYP2C9 risk overdose of warfarin due to reduced metabolism and clearance of warfarin. Multiple studies have shown that amiodarone and the statins have the highest impact on warfarin dose requirements in terms of

drug–drug interactions (34, 82). The website warfarindosing.org, which predicts warfarin dosing based on clinical and demographic factors, includes concomitant therapy with amiodarone, statins, azole antifungals, and sulfamethoxazole and trimethoprim as factors used in estimating warfarin dosing (83).

Warfarin is highly bound to plasma proteins (typically albumin) with a free fraction of approximately 3%. Lovastatin and indomethacin are two medications that compete with warfarin for plasma protein-binding sites, potentially increasing the active free fraction of warfarin. Other medications known to compete with warfarin for protein-binding sites include chloral hydrate, chloramphenicol, and phenylbutazone, medications rarely or no longer used in the United States.

Other factors influencing warfarin response

A number of other clinical and demographic factors are associated with warfarin dose requirements. For example, in a study published in 2008, age, gender, race (white compared to African American), body surface area, and creatinine clearance were significant factors in a multiple regression analysis of warfarin dose requirements (82). Specifically, warfarin dose requirements are 13% lower per decade of life, 15% lower in Caucasians versus African Americans, 12% lower in females versus males, 15% greater per standard deviation increase in body surface area, and 10% greater per standard deviation increase in creatinine increase. A formula that incorporated these five factors, use of amiodarone, use of simvastatin, the target INR, and CYP2C9 genotyping explained approximately 39% of variation in warfarin steady-state dosing (82).

Thyroid hormone status is also known to influence warfarin dosing. The mechanism of this interaction is complex and not entirely understood. Hyperthyroidism is known to be a hypermetabolic state with increased liver catabolism via higher expression of CYP and other enzymes. Under this theory, warfarin sensitivity increases in patients with hyperthyroidism due to increased metabolism and clearance of vitamin K-dependent clotting factors (84). Conversely, warfarin sensitivity decreases in hypothyroid states.

Cigarette smoking can also affect warfarin disposition. Multiple case reports or case series have described increases in PT/INR in cigarette smokers who discontinue smoking while on chronic warfarin therapy (85–88). Cigarette smoking is included in the algorithm for estimating warfarin dosage in the online calculator warfarindosing.org (83). A recent case report described a patient who experienced supratherapeutic PT/INR when he began smoking marijuana while on warfarin therapy (89).

Lastly, liver failure can lead to markedly increased sensitivity to warfarin (90). One main mechanism underlying this is reduced synthesis of vitamin K-dependent clotting factors, which in itself leads to increased tendency for bleeding. Additionally, in severe liver failure, CYP enzyme (including 2C9)

expression is compromised, leading to decreased clearance of warfarin (91).

A summary of the various factors that affect warfarin dosing is illustrated in Figure 3.1.

Application of genetic variation to predict warfarin dosing

Dose models incorporating pharmacogenomics

Given the multitude of factors that can affect warfarin dosing, models that utilize pharmacogenomic information to predict warfarin dosing generally include other factors such as age, gender, race, concomitant medications, and some measure of

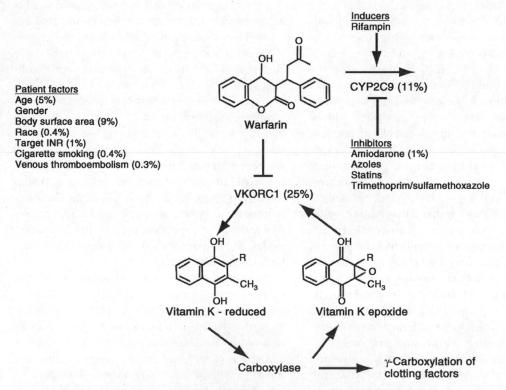

Figure 3.1 A summary of the major known factors that affect warfarin dosing. Warfarin dosing requirements are affected by patient factors (e.g., age, gender, and cigarette smoking), concomitant medications, and genetic variation. The percentages included in parentheses next to some factors are the R^2 contribution of these factors to a multiple regression model of warfarin maintenance dosing prediction (82).

body size (40, 64, 82, 92–97). Three algorithms derived from data from large studies of over 1,000 patients seem most likely to achieve widest use (64, 82, 94). Several studies have attempted to compare the available algorithms based on retrospective data (37, 95, 96, 98); however, no one algorithm has emerged as the clear, consensus choice, with ongoing research into how to best incorporate pharmacogenetic-guided dosing into the PT/INR-based warfarin dose adjustment regimens that health care providers have used for decades (99, 100).

One of the most commonly used algorithms is available at the free website warfarindosing.org (83), a collaborative effort by the International Warfarin Pharmacogenetics Consortium and the Warfarin Dose Refinement Collaboration (82, 94). This site incorporates anonymous data from thousands of patients. The nonpharmacogenomic variables included in the algorithm are age, sex, ethnicity (non-Hispanic, Hispanic, unknown), race (African American, Native American, Asian/Indian subcontinent, native Pacific Islander, and Caucasian or Middle Eastern), weight, height, cigarette smoking, presence of liver disease, baseline INR, target INR, and concomitant medications (amiodarone, statins, azoles, trimethoprim/sulfamethoxazole). The pharmacogenomic variables include VKORC1 ($-1639/3673$), CYP4F2 (V433M), GGCX (microsatellite), and CYP2C9 (*2, *3, *5, and *6). The website assigns a code to each patient and requests that the user provide information on the daily warfarin dose, INR, occurrence of new thrombotic or ischemic event, and occurrence of bleeding after 30 days of therapy. Warfarindosing.org also uses a clinical prediction algorithm known as HEMORR$_2$HAGES to estimate bleeding risk (101). For the HEMORR$_2$HAGES prediction tool, risk factors that increase risk of bleeding while on warfarin include renal disease, liver disease, ethanol use, recent metastatic cancer, age > 75 years, thrombocytopenia, antiplatelet therapy (e.g., aspirin), prior hospitalization for bleeding, uncontrolled hypertension, anemia (hemoglobin $< 10\,g/dL$), CYP2C9 variants (*2 and *3), neurologic or other conditions that increase risk of falls, and prior ischemic stroke.

The algorithm found in warfarindosing.org was applied to a validation cohort of 1,009 subjects (94). A model that included both clinical and pharmaco-genetics factors identified a larger proportion of patients that needed less than 21 mg or greater than 49 mg of warfarin per week. For the 54% of patients whose weekly warfarin dose requirements was between 21 and 49 mg, the two models did not differ from each other, and in fact were not superior to a fixed-dose warfarin dosing approach. The results of this study suggest that pharmacogenetic-guided dosing of warfarin has most benefit in those patients who have warfarin dose requirements that deviate from the average (102).

Practical considerations in testing for warfarin variants

The diagnostic industry and clinical laboratories have made considerable progress in warfarin pharmacogenetic testing (37, 103–105). As of November 2010, four FDA-cleared assay systems are available in the United States for genotyping of the most common allelic variants that influence warfarin response. These include the Verigene® Warfarin Metabolism Nucleic Acid Test (Nanosphere, Inc., Northbrook, IL), eSensor® Warfarin Sensitivity Test (Osmetech Molecular Diagnostics, Pasadena, CA), INFINITI® 2C9 & VKORC1 Multiplex Assay for Warfarin (AutoGenomics, Inc., Carlsbad, CA), and eQ-PCR™ LC Warfarin Genotyping Kit (TrimGen Corporation, Sparks, MD). These four FDA-cleared systems all target CYP2C9*2 and *3 alleles and either of two common VKORC1 variants (1173C $>$ T or 1639G $>$ A). In addition to these FDA-cleared assays, there are also a growing number of research-use only diagnostic assays that may receive FDA 510(k) clearance in the future. The College of American Pathologists offers a proficiency testing program for pharmacogenetics testing with 56 clinical laboratories participating in September 2009. Most of the clinical laboratories that currently perform warfarin pharmacogenetics testing in the United States are commercial reference laboratories or clinical laboratories associated with larger hospitals and medical centers.

Limitations of pharmacogenomics-based dosing models

There are several main limitations to pharmacogenomics-based dosing models for warfarin (106–108). Perhaps the most difficult hurdle is that testing for genetic variants of CYP2C9 and VKORC1 or any other genes does not remove the necessity of following the PT/INR. Warfarin dosing algorithms that utilize pharmacogenomic information at best more accurately predict initiation and maintenance dosing of warfarin but still cannot account for approximately ~45% of the interindividual variation in warfarin response. The complexity of warfarin response means that those prescribing or managing warfarin therapy need to be cautious in not over-hyping what genotyping can do (109). The general public in particular may also find it challenging to distinguish between the promised goal of "personalized medicine" (110–112), whereby genomics can facilitate individualized therapies, and the messier challenge of dealing with a drug like warfarin that has many nongenetic factors (some as yet uncharacterized) that complicate therapy.

The second main challenge to adopting warfarin pharmacogenomics is the practical and economic issue of performing the genetic testing. Many hospitals and clinics do not have the clinical laboratory resources to perform the genetic testing and therefore would need to refer the testing to outside laboratories, with relatively higher costs of the genotyping assays relative to most common laboratory tests. Even hospitals or medical center clinical laboratories that commonly perform genetic testing would be unlikely to perform warfarin genotyping with a fast turnaround time. Due to a variety of factors including patents covering genotyping methods or reagents, genetic tests have relatively high per unit costs favoring batch analysis (to conserve reagent used for testing of positive and negative controls) as opposed to more frequent testing sche-dules. Consequently, unless the patient genotype status for CYP2C9 and VKORC1 is known from previous studies, genetic results would generally not be available with fast turnaround time for initial dosing of warfarin, a limitation especially important in patients who have already experienced thromboembolism and thus need to be started quickly on warfarin therapy.

In the debate surrounding the relabeling of the package insert for warfarin, the FDA and manufacturers of warfarin formulations had to contend with how strongly to recommend genotyping in the dosing and safety guidelines of the package inserts. In the January 2010 revision of the package insert for Coumadin®, a genotype-based dosing table for different CYP2C9 and VKORC1 allelic variants was included based on data from multiple studies (Table 3.1); however, the labeling does not state that genotyping must be performed as part of standard of care (113). In part, this reflects caution given uncertainty of whether genotyping actually contributes to better outcomes and/or reduced overall cost in clinical practice. There are also the economic and medicolegal implications of "mandating" expensive genetic testing for a medication used by millions of patients. Nevertheless, the package insert revision represents an important development in providing a guide to health care professionals for translating genotype results into estimated warfarin doses, consistent with ongoing FDA efforts to provide guidance in bringing pharmacogenetic information to clinical practice (114).

No large-scale, randomized controlled clinical trial with adequate power has yet demonstrated that pharmacogenetic-guided algorithms significantly

Table 3.1 FDA Guide to Initial Dosing of Warfarin Based on VKORC1 and CYP2C9 Genotypes*

VKORC1-1639	CYP2C9					
	*1/*1	*1/*2	*1/*3	*2/*2	*2/*3	*3/*3
GG	5–7 mg	5–7 mg	3–4 mg	3–4 mg	3–4 mg	0.5–2 mg
AG	5–7 mg	3–4 mg	3–4 mg	3–4 mg	0.5–2 mg	0.5–2 mg
AA	3–4 mg	3–4 mg	0.5–2 mg	0.5–2 mg	0.5–2 mg	0.5–2 mg

*From the package insert for Coumadin® (Bristol-Myers-Squibb) (113). The package insert has more detailed dosing information (http://packageinserts.bms.com/pi/pi_coumadin.pdf).

reduce major adverse effects of warfarin such as hemorrhage or thrombosis (107, 114–118). One randomized trial showed that patients receiving pharmacogenetic-guided dosing required fewer INR determination and less frequent and smaller dose adjustments, although the percent INR values out of therapeutic range did not differ compared to the control group (92). A second randomized trial showed that pharmacogenetic-guided dosing reached a stable warfarin more quickly than the control group (119). A third randomized trial utilized CYP2C9 genotyping and showed that incorporation of CYP2C9 allelic variants in predicting warfarin dosing allowed patients to reach a stable warfarin dose more quickly and to spend more time within the therapeutic PT/INR range (35). Lastly, a large, prospective observational trial utilizing pharmacogenetic-guided dosing demonstrated an approximate 30% reduction in hospitalizations of warfarin-treated patients during the first six months of therapy compared to historical controls (120). However, the dramatic results obtained in this study have been questioned in light of the trial design, especially the selection of historical controls and differences in the control versus observed populations (108). The trials to date have not yet shown clear evidence that pharmacogenetics-guide warfarin dosing saves costs relative to other warfarin-dosing strategies (121–129).

Conclusions

Over the last decade, considerable progress has been made in defining the genetic variation that influences warfarin dosing. Genetic variation in the main warfarin-metabolizing enzyme (CYP2C9) and the molecular target of warfarin (VKORC1) accounts for roughly one-third of the interindividual variation in warfarin dosing. Algorithms that use pharmacogenetic and other factors can now account for approximately 55% of the variation in warfarin dosing. Several clinical trials have demonstrated that pharmacogenetic information can be combined with other variables to better predict warfarin maintenance dose and reduce adverse effects, although larger trials are needed to determine whether phar-

macogenetic-guided strategies actually improve patient outcomes and reduce health care costs. Overall, pharmacogenomic approaches offer the promise of reducing adverse events in patients on warfarin therapy.

References

1 Wysowski, D.K., Nourjah, P., Swartz, L. (2007) Bleeding complications with warfarin use: a prevalent adverse effect resulting in regulatory action. *Archives of Internal Medicine*, **167**, 1414–1419.

2 Garcia, D. (2009) Novel anticoagulants and the future of anticoagulation. *Thrombosis Research*, **123**(**Suppl. 4**), S50–S55.

3 Gross, P.L., Weitz, J.I. (2009) New antithrombotic drugs. *Clinical and Pharmacological Therapies*, **86**, 139–146.

4 Bauer, K.A. (2008) New anticoagulants. *Current Opinions on Hematology*, **15**, 509–515.

5 Connolly, S.J., Ezekowitz, M.D., Yusuf, S., Eikelboom, J., *et al.* (2009) Dabigatran versus warfarin in patients with atrial fibrillation. *New England Journal of Medicine*, **361**, 1139–1151.

6 Weitz, J.I., Bates, S.M. (2005) New anticoagulants. *Journal of Thrombosis and Haemostasis*, **3**, 1843–1853.

7 Fihn, S.D., McDonell, M., Martin, D., Henikoff, J., *et al.* (1993) Risk factors for complications of chronic anticoagulation: a multicenter study: Warfarin Optimized Outpatient Follow-up Study Group. *Annals of Internal Medicine*, **118**, 511–520.

8 Landefeld, C.S., Beyth, R.J. (1993) Anticoagulant-related bleeding: clinical epidemiology, prediction, and prevention. *American Journal of Medicine*, **95**, 315–328.

9 Levine, M.N., Hirsh, J., Landefeld, S., Raskob, G. (1992) Hemorrhagic complications of anticoagulant treatment. *Chest*, **102**, 352S–363S.

10 Palareti, G., Leali, N., Coccheri, S., Poggi, M., *et al.* (1996) Bleeding complications of oral anticoagulant treatment: an inception-cohort, prospective collaborative study (ISCOAT): Italian Study on Complications of Oral Anticoagulant Therapy. *Lancet*, **348**, 423–428.

11 van der Meer, F.J., Rosendaal, F.R., Vandenbroucke, J. P., Briet, E. (1993) Bleeding complications in oral anticoagulant therapy: an analysis of risk factors. *Archives of Internal Medicine*, **153**, 1557–1562.

12 Budnitz, D.S., Pollock, D.A., Weidenbach, K.N., Mendelsohn, A.B., *et al.* (2006) National surveillance of

emergency department visits for outpatient adverse drug events. *Journal of the American Medical Association*, **296**, 1858–1866.

13 Moore, T.J., Cohen, M.R., Furberg, C.D. (2007) Serious adverse drug events reported to the Food and Drug Administration, 1998–2005. *Archives of Internal Medicine*, **167**, 1752–1759.

14 Douketis, J.D., Foster, G.A., Crowther, M.A., Prins, M.H., *et al.* (2000) Clinical risk factors and timing of recurrent venous thromboembolism during the initial 3 months of anticoagulant therapy. *Archives of Internal Medicine*, **160**, 3431–3436.

15 Cohen, A.L., Budnitz, D.S., Weidenbach, K.N., Jernigan, D.B., *et al.* (2008) National surveillance of emergency department visits for outpatient adverse drug events in children and adolescents. *Journal of Pediatrics*, **152**, 416–421.

16 Thornburg, C.D., Jones, E., Bomgaars, L., Gage, B.F. (2010) Pediatric warfarin practice and pharmacogenetic testing. *Thrombosis Research*, **126**, e144–e146.

17 Franke, C.A., Dickerson, L.M., Carek, P.J. (2008) Improving anticoagulation therapy using point-of-care testing and a standardized protocol. *Annals of Family Medicine*, 6(**Suppl. 1**), S28–S32.

18 Pengo, V., Cucchini, U., Denas, G., Davidson, B.L., *et al.* (2010) Lower versus standard intensity oral anticoagulant therapy (OAT) in elderly warfarin-experienced patients with non-valvular atrial fibrillation. *Thrombosis and Haemostasis*, **103**, 442–449.

19 Singer, D.E., Albers, G.W., Dalen, J.E., Fang, M.C., *et al.* (2008) Antithrombotic therapy in atrial fibrillation: *American College of Chest Physicians Evidence-Based Clinical Practice Guidelines* (8th Edition) *Chest*, **133**, 546S–592S.

20 Bon Homme, M., Reynolds, K.K., Valdes, R., Jr., Linder, M.W. (2008) Dynamic pharmacogenetic models in anticoagulation therapy. *Clinics in Laboratory Medicine*, **28**, 539–552.

21 Crowther, M.A. (2003) Oral anticoagulant initiation: rationale for the use of warfarin dosing nomograms. *Seminars in Vascular Medicine*, **3**, 255–260.

22 Lazo-Langner, ARRCR.R. Kovacs, M.J. (2010) Predicting warfarin dose. *Current Opinions in Pulmonary Medicine*, **16**, 426–431.

23 Lazo-Langner, A., Monkman, K., Kovacs, M.J. (2009) Predicting warfarin maintenance dose in patients with venous thromboembolism based on the response to a standardized warfarin initiation nomogram. *Journal of Thrombosis and Haemostasis*, **7**, 1276–1283.

24 Le Gal, G., Carrier, M., Tierney, S., Majeed, H., *et al.* (2010) Prediction of the warfarin maintenance dose after completion of the 10 mg initiation nomogram: do we really need genotyping? *Journal of Thrombosis and Haemostasis*, **8**, 90–94.

25 Rettie, A.E., Jones, J.P. (2005) Clinical and toxicological relevance of CYP2C9: drug–drug interactions and pharmacogenetics. *Annual Review of Pharmacology and Toxicology*, **45**, 477–494.

26 Van Booven, D., Marsh, S., McLeod, H., Carrillo, M.W., *et al.* (2010) Cytochrome P450 2C9-CYP2C9. *Pharmacogenetic Genomics*, **20**, 277–281.

27 Aithal, G.P., Day, C.P., Kesteven, P.J., Daly, A.K. (1999) Association of polymorphisms in the cytochrome P450 CYP2C9 with warfarin dose requirement and risk of bleeding complications. *Lancet*, **353**, 717–719.

28 Crespi, C.L., Miller, V.P. (1997) The R144C change in the CYP2C9*2 allele alters interaction of the cytochrome P450 with NADPH:cytochrome P450 oxidoreductase. *Pharmacogenetics*, **7**, 203–210.

29 Haining, R.L., Hunter, A.P., Veronese, M.E., Trager, W.F., *et al.* (1996) Allelic variants of human cytochrome P450 2C9: baculovirus-mediated expression, purification, structural characterization, substrate stereoselectivity, and prochiral selectivity of the wild-type and I359L mutant forms. *Archives of Biochemistry and Biophysics*, **333**, 447–458.

30 Rettie, A.E., Wienkers, L.C., Gonzalez, F.J., Trager, W.F., *et al.* (1994) Impaired (S)-warfarin metabolism catalysed by the R144C allelic variant of CYP2C9. *Pharmacogenetics*, **4**, 39–42.

31 Steward, D.J., Haining, R.L., Henne, K.R., Davis, G., *et al.* (1997) Genetic association between sensitivity to warfarin and expression of CYP2C9*3. *Pharmacogenetics*, **7**, 361–367.

32 Kirchheiner, J., Brockmoller, J. (2005) Clinical consequences of cytochrome P450 2C9 polymorphisms. *Clinical Pharmacology & Therapeutics*, **77**, 1–16.

33 Ross, K.A., Bigham, A.W., Edwards, M., Gozdzik, A., *et al.* (2010) Worldwide allele frequency distribution of four polymorphisms associated with warfarin dose requirements. *Journal of Human Genetics*, **55**, 582–589.

34 Aquilante, C.L., Langaee, T.Y., Lopez, L.M., Yarandi, H.N., *et al.* (2006) Influence of coagulation factor, vitamin K epoxide reductase complex subunit 1, and cytochrome P450 2C9 gene polymorphisms on warfarin dose requirements. *Clinical Pharmacology & Therapeutics*, **79**, 291–302.

35 Caraco, Y., Blotnick, S., Muszkat, M. (2008) CYP2C9 genotype-guided warfarin prescribing enhances the efficacy and safety of anticoagulation: a prospective randomized controlled study. *Clinical Pharmacology & Therapeutics*, **83**, 460–470.

36 Higashi, M.K., Veenstra, D.L., Kondo, L.M., Wittkowsky, A.K., *et al.* (2002) Association between CYP2C9 genetic variants and anticoagulation-related outcomes during warfarin therapy. *Journal of the American Medical Association*, **287**, 1690–1698.

37 Langley, M.R., Booker, J.K., Evans, J.P., McLeod, H.L., *et al.* (2009) Validation of clinical testing for warfarin sensitivity: comparison of CYP2C9-VKORC1 genotyping assays and warfarin-dosing algorithms. *Journal of Molecular Diagnostics*, **11**, 216–225.

38 Puehringer, H., Loreth, R.M., Klose, G., Schreyer, B., *et al.* (2010) VKORC1–1639G>A and CYP2C9*3 are the major genetic predictors of phenprocoumon dose requirement. *European Journal of Clinical Pharmacology*, **66**, 591–598.

39 Sanderson, S., Emery, J., Higgins, J. (2005) CYP2C9 gene variants, drug dose, and bleeding risk in warfarin-treated patients: a HuGEnet systematic review and meta-analysis. *Genetics in Medicine*, **7**, 97–104.

40 Sconce, E.A., Khan, T.I., Wynne, H.A., Avery, P., *et al.* (2005) The impact of CYP2C9 and VKORC1 genetic polymorphism and patient characteristics upon warfarin dose requirements: proposal for a new dosing regimen. *Blood*, **106**, 2329–2333.

41 Takeuchi, F., McGinnis, R., Bourgeois, S., Barnes, C., *et al.* (2009) A genome-wide association study confirms VKORC1, CYP2C9, and CYP4F2 as principal genetic determinants of warfarin dose. *PLoS Genetics*, **5**, e1000433.

42 Wells, P.S., Majeed, H., Kassem, S., Langlois, N., *et al.* (2010) A regression model to predict warfarin dose from clinical variables and polymorphisms in CYP2C9, CYP4F2, and VKORC1: derivation in a sample with predominantly a history of venous thromboembolism. *Thrombosis Research*, **125**, e259–e264.

43 Cavallari, L.H., Langaee, T.Y., Momary, K.M., Shapiro, N.L., *et al.* (2010) Genetic and clinical predictors of warfarin dose requirements in African Americans. *Clinical Pharmacology & Therapeutics*, **87**, 459–464.

44 Lee, C.R., Goldstein, J.A., Pieper, J.A. (2002) Cytochrome P450 2C9 polymorphisms: a comprehensive review of the in-vitro and human data. *Pharmacogenetics*, **12**, 251–263.

45 Schelleman, H., Limdi, N.A., Kimmel, S.E. (2008) Ethnic differences in warfarin maintenance dose requirement and its relationship with genetics. *Pharmacogenomics*, **9**, 1331–1346.

46 Scott, S.A., Khasawneh, R., Peter, I., Kornreich, R., *et al.* (2010) Combined CYP2C9, VKORC1 and CYP4F2 frequencies among racial and ethnic groups. *Pharmacogenomics*, **11**, 781–791.

47 Sagreiya, H., Berube, C., Wen, A., Ramakrishnan, R., *et al.* (2010) Extending and evaluating a warfarin dosing algorithm that includes CYP4F2 and pooled rare variants of CYP2C9. *Pharmacogenetic Genomics*, **20**, 407–413.

48 Li, T., Chang, C.Y., Jin, D.Y., Lin, P.J., *et al.* (2004) Identification of the gene for vitamin K epoxide reductase. *Nature*, **427**, 541–544.

49 Rost, S., Fregin, A., Ivaskevicius, V., Conzelmann, E., *et al.* (2004) Mutations in VKORC1 cause warfarin resistance and multiple coagulation factor deficiency type 2. *Nature*, **427**, 537–541.

50 Orsi, F.A., Annichino Bizzacchi, J.M., de Paula, E.V., Ozelo, M.C., *et al.* (2010) VKORC1 V66M mutation in African Brazilian patients resistant to oral anticoagulant therapy. *Thrombosis Research*, **126**, e206–e210.

51 Cuthbert, J.H. (1963) Further evidence of resistance to warfarin in the rat. *Nature*, **198**, 807–808.

52 Kohn, M.H., Pelz, H.J. (2000) A gene-anchored map position of the rat warfarin-resistance locus, Rw, and its orthologs in mice and humans. *Blood*, **96**, 1996–1998.

53 Kohn, M.H., Pelz, H.J., Wayne, R.K. (2000) Natural selection mapping of the warfarin-resistance gene. *Proceedings of the National Academy of Sciences of the United States of America*, **97**, 7911–7915.

54 Lund, M. (1964) Resistance to warfarin in the common rat. *Nature*, **203**, 778.

55 O'Reilly, R.A., Pool, J.G., Aggeler, P.M. (1968) Hereditary resistance to coumarin anticoagulant drugs in man and rat. *Annals of the New York Academy of Sciences*, **151**, 913–931.

56 D'Andrea, G., D'Ambrosio, R.L., Di Perna, P., Chetta, M., *et al.* (2005) A polymorphism in the *VKORC1* gene is associated with an interindividual variability in the dose–anticoagulant effect of warfarin. *Blood*, **105**, 645–649.

57 Flockhart, D.A., O'Kane, D., Williams, M.S., Watson, M.S., *et al.* (2008) Pharmacogenetic testing of CYP2C9 and VKORC1 alleles for warfarin. *Genetics in Medicine*, **10**, 139–150.

58 Rieder, M.J., Reiner, A.P., Gage, B.F., Nickerson, D.A., *et al.* (2005) Effect of VKORC1 haplotypes on transcriptional regulation and warfarin dose. *New England Journal of Medicine*, **352**, 2285–2293.

59 Wadelius, M., Chen, L.Y., Downes, K., Ghori, J., *et al.* (2005) Common VKORC1 and GGCX polymorphisms associated with warfarin dose. *Pharmacogenomics Journal*, **5**, 262–270.

60 Veenstra, D.L., You, J.H., Rieder, M.J., Farin, F.M., *et al.* (2005) Association of Vitamin K epoxide reductase complex 1 (VKORC1) variants with warfarin dose in a Hong Kong Chinese patient population. *Pharmacogenetic Genomics*, **15**, 687–691.

61 Takahashi, H., Wilkinson, G.R., Nutescu, E.A., Morita, T., *et al.* (2006) Different contributions of polymorphisms in VKORC1 and CYP2C9 to intra- and interpopulation differences in maintenance dose of warfarin in Japanese, Caucasians and African-Americans. *Pharmacogenetic Genomics*, **16**, 101–110.

62 Cooper, G.M., Johnson, J.A., Langaee, T.Y., Feng, H., *et al.* (2008) A genome-wide scan for common genetic variants with a large influence on warfarin maintenance dose. *Blood*, **112**, 1022–1027.

63 Wadelius, M., Chen, L.Y., Eriksson, N., Bumpstead, S., *et al.* (2007) Association of warfarin dose with genes involved in its action and metabolism. *Human Genetics*, **121**, 23–34.

64 Wadelius, M., Chen, L.Y., Lindh, J.D., Eriksson, N., *et al.* (2009) The largest prospective warfarin-treated cohort supports genetic forecasting. *Blood*, **113**, 784–792.

65 Caldwell, M.D., Awad, T., Johnson, J.A., Gage, B.F., *et al.* (2008) CYP4F2 genetic variant alters required warfarin dose. *Blood*, **111**, 4106–4112.

66 Pautas, E., Moreau, C., Gouin-Thibault, I., Golmard, J.L., *et al.* (2010) Genetic factors (VKORC1, CYP2C9, EPHX1, and CYP4F2) are predictor variables for warfarin response in very elderly, frail inpatients. *Clinical Pharmacology & Therapeutics*, **87**, 57–64.

67 Zordoky, B.N., El-Kadi, A.O. (2010) Effect of cytochrome P450 polymorphism on arachidonic acid metabolism and their impact on cardiovascular diseases. *Pharmacological Therapies*, **125**, 446–463.

68 McDonald, M.G., Rieder, M.J., Nakano, M., Hsia, C.K., *et al.* (2009) CYP4F2 is a vitamin K1 oxidase: An explanation for altered warfarin dose in carriers of the V433M variant. *Molecular Pharmacology*, **75**, 1337–1346.

69 Kimura, R., Miyashita, K., Kokubo, Y., Akaiwa, Y., *et al.* (2007) Genotypes of vitamin K epoxide reductase, gamma-glutamyl carboxylase, and cytochrome P450 2C9 as determinants of daily warfarin dose in Japanese patients. *Thrombosis Research*, **120**, 181–186.

70 King, C.R., Deych, E., Milligan, P., Eby, C., *et al.* (2010) Gamma-glutamyl carboxylase and its influence on warfarin dose. *Thrombosis and Haemostasis*, **104**, 750–754.

71 Rieder, M.J., Reiner, A.P., Rettie, A.E. (2007) Gamma-glutamyl carboxylase (GGCX) tagSNPs have limited utility for predicting warfarin maintenance dose. *Journal of Thrombosis and Haemostasis*, **5**, 2227–2234.

72 Schelleman, H., Brensinger, C.M., Chen, J., Finkelman, B.S., *et al.* (2010) New genetic variant that might improve warfarin dose prediction in African Americans. *British Journal of Clinical Pharmacology*, **70**, 393–399.

73 Wang, T.L., Li, H.L., Tjong, W.Y., Chen, Q.S., *et al.* (2008) Genetic factors contribute to patient-specific warfarin dose for Han Chinese. *Clinica Chimica Acta: International Journal of Clinical Chemistry*, **396**, 76–79.

74 Booth, S.L., Al Rajabi, A. (2008) Determinants of vitamin K status in humans. *Vitamins and Hormones*, **78**, 1–22.

75 Thane, C.W., Paul, A.A., Bates, C.J., Bolton-Smith, C., *et al.* (2002) Intake and sources of phylloquinone (vitamin K1): variation with socio-demographic and lifestyle factors in a national sample of British elderly people. *British Journal of Nutrition*, **87**, 605–613.

76 Lurie, Y., Loebstein, R., Kurnik, D., Almog, S., *et al.* (2010) Warfarin and vitamin K intake in the era of pharmacogenetics. *British Journal of Clinical Pharmacology*, **70**, 164–170.

77 de Assis, M.C., Rabelo, E.R., Avila, C.W., Polanczyk, C.A., *et al.* (2009) Improved oral anticoagulation after a dietary vitamin k-guided strategy: a randomized controlled trial. *Circulation*, **120**, 1115–1122.

78 Kurnik, D., Lubetsky, A., Loebstein, R., Almog, S., *et al.* (2003) Multivitamin supplements may affect warfarin anticoagulation in susceptible patients. *Annals of Pharmacotherapy*, **37**, 1603–1606.

79 Dickins, M. (2004) Induction of cytochromes P450. *Current Topics in Medicinal Chemistry*, **4**, 1745–1766.

80 Schuetz, E.G. (2001) Induction of cytochromes P450. *Current Drug Metabolism*, **2**, 139–147.

81 Xu, C., Li, C.Y., Kong, A.T. (2005) Induction of phase I, II and III drug metabolism/transport by xenobiotics. *Archives of Pharmacal Research*, **28**, 249–268.

82 Gage, B.F., Eby, C., Johnson, J.A., Deych, E., *et al.* (2008) Use of pharmacogenetic and clinical factors to predict the therapeutic dose of warfarin. *Clinical Pharmacology & Therapeuticsapies*, **84**, 326–331.

83 *Warfarin dosing online calculator* [WWW document]. URL http://www.warfarindosing.org [accessed on 28 June 2011]

84 Kellett, H.A., Sawers, J.S., Boulton, F.E., Cholerton, S., *et al.* (1986) Problems of anticoagulation with warfarin in hyperthyroidism. *Quarterly Journal of Medicine*, **58**, 43–51.

85 Bachmann, K., Shapiro, R., Fulton, R., Carroll, F.T., *et al.* (1979) Smoking and warfarin disposition. *Clinical Pharmacology & Therapeutics*, **25**, 309–315.

86 Colucci, V.J., Knapp, J.F. (2001) Increase in international normalized ratio associated with smoking cessation. *Annals of Pharmacotherapy*, **35**, 385–386.

87 Evans, M., Lewis, G.M. (2005) Increase in international normalized ratio after smoking cessation in a patient receiving warfarin. *Pharmacotherapy*, **25**, 1656–1659.

88 Mitchell, A.A. (1972) Smoking and warfarin dosage. *New England Journal of Medicine*, **287**, 1153–1154.

89 Yamreudeewong, W., Wong, H.K., Brausch, L.M., Pulley, K.R. (2009) Probable interaction between warfarin and marijuana smoking. *Annals of Pharmacotherapy*, **43**, 1347–1353.

90 Demirkan, K., Stephens, M.A., Newman, K.P., Self, T. H. (2000) Response to warfarin and other oral anticoagulants: effects of disease states. *Southern Medical Journal*, **93**, 448–454, quiz 455.

91 Villeneuve, J.P., Pichette, V. (2004) Cytochrome P450 and liver diseases. *Current Drug Metabolism*, **5**, 273–282.

92 Anderson, J.L., Horne, B.D., Stevens, S.M., Grove, A. S., *et al.* (2007) Randomized trial of genotype-guided versus standard warfarin dosing in patients initiating oral anticoagulation. *Circulation*, **116**, 2563–2570.

93 Ferder, N.S., Eby, C.S., Deych, E., Harris, J.K., *et al.* (2010) Ability of VKORC1 and CYP2C9 to predict therapeutic warfarin dose during the initial weeks of therapy. *Journal of Thrombosis and Haemostasis*, **8**, 95–100.

94 Klein, T.E., Altman, R.B., Eriksson, N., Gage, B.F. *et al.* (2009) Estimation of the warfarin dose with clinical and pharmacogenetic data. *New England Journal of Medicine*, **360**, 753–764.

95 Schelleman, H., Chen, J., Chen, Z., Christie, J., *et al.* (2008) Dosing algorithms to predict warfarin maintenance dose in Caucasians and African Americans. *Clinical Pharmacology & Therapeutics*, **84**, 332–339.

96 Wu, A.H., Wang, P., Smith, A., Haller, C., *et al.* (2008) Dosing algorithm for warfarin using CYP2C9 and VKORC1 genotyping from a multi-ethnic population: comparison with other equations. *Pharmacogenomics*, **9**, 169–178.

97 Zhu, Y., Shennan, M., Reynolds, K.K., Johnson, N.A., *et al.* (2007) Estimation of warfarin maintenance dose based on VKORC1 (-1639 G>A) and CYP2C9 genotypes. *Clinical Chemistry*, **53**, 1199–1205.

98 Roper, N., Storer, B., Bona, R., Fang, M. (2010) Validation and comparison of pharmacogenetics-based warfarin dosing algorithms for application of pharmacogenetic testing. *Journal of Molecular Diagnostics*, **12**, 283–291.

99 Crowther, M.A., Ginsberg, J.B., Kearon, C., Harrison, L., *et al.* (1999) A randomized trial comparing 5-mg and 10-mg warfarin loading doses. *Archives of Internal Medicine*, **159**, 46–48.

100 Kovacs, M.J., Rodger, M., Anderson, D.R., Morrow, B., *et al.* (2003) Comparison of 10-mg and 5-mg warfarin initiation nomograms together with low-molecular-weight heparin for outpatient treatment of acute venous thromboembolism. A randomized, double-blind, controlled trial. *Annals of Internal Medicine*, **138**, 714–719.

101 Gage, B.F., Yan, Y., Milligan, P.E., Waterman, A.D., *et al.* (2006) Clinical classification schemes for predicting hemorrhage: results from the National Registry of Atrial Fibrillation (NRAF). *American Heart Journal*, **151**, 713–719.

102 Woodcock, J., Lesko, L.J. (2009) Pharmacogenetics: tailoring treatment for the outliers. *New England Journal of Medicine*, **360**, 811–813.

103 Babic, N., Haverfield, E.V., Burrus, J.A., Lozada, A., *et al.* (2009) Comparison of performance of three commercial platforms for warfarin sensitivity genotyping. *Clinica Chimica Acta: International Journal of Clinical Chemistry*, **406**, 143–147.

104 King, C.R., Porche-Sorbet, R.M., Gage, B.F., Ridker, P. M., *et al.* (2008) Performance of commercial platforms for rapid genotyping of polymorphisms affecting warfarin dose. *Am J Clin Pathol*, **129**, 876–883.

105 Maurice, C.B., Barua, P.K., Simses, D., Smith, P., *et al.* (2010) Comparison of assay systems for warfarin-related CYP2C9 and VKORC1 genotyping. *Clinica Chimica Acta: International Journal of Clinical Chemistry*, **411**, 947–954.

106 Bussey, H.I., Wittkowsky, A.K., Hylek, E.M., Walker, M.B. (2008) Genetic testing for warfarin dosing? Not yet ready for prime time. *Pharmacotherapy*, **28**, 141–143.

107 Garcia, D.A. (2008) Warfarin and pharmacogenomic testing: the case for restraint. *Clinical Pharmacology & Therapeutics*, **84**, 303–305.

108 Ginsburg, G.S., Voora, D. (2010) The long and winding road to warfarin pharmacogenetic testing. *Journal of the American College of Cardiology*, **55**, 2813–2815.

109 Limdi, N.A., Veenstra, D.L. (2010) Expectations, validity, and reality in pharmacogenetics. *Journal of Clinical Epidemiology*, **63**, 960–969.

110 Ashley, E.A., Butte, A.J., Wheeler, M.T., Chen, R., *et al.* (2010) Clinical assessment incorporating a personal genome. *Lancet*, **375**, 1525–1535.

111 Evans, W.E., Relling, M.V. (2004) Moving towards individualized medicine with pharmacogenomics. *Nature*, **429**, 464–468.

112 Feero, W.G., Guttmacher, A.E., Collins, F.S. (2008) The genome gets personal: almost. *Journal of the American Medical Association*, **299**, 1351–1352.

113 Coumadin® (warfarin sodium) Tablets [Package insert]. (2010) Coumadin® for Injection. Bristol-Myers Squibb, Princeton, NJ. URL http://packageinserts.bms.com/pi/pi_coumadin.pdf [accessed on 28 June 2011]

114 Lesko, L.J. (2008) The critical path of warfarin dosing: finding an optimal dosing strategy using pharmacogenetics. *Clinical Pharmacology & Therapeutics*, **84**, 301–303.

115 Rosove, M.H., Grody, W.W. (2009) Should we be applying warfarin pharmacogenetics to clinical practice? No, not now. *Annals of Internal Medicine*, **151**, 270–273, W295.

116 Shurin, S.B., Nabel, E.G. (2008) Pharmacogenomics: ready for prime time? *New England Journal of Medicine*, **358**, 1061–1063.

117 Wadelius, M. (2009) Point: use of pharmacogenetics in guiding treatment with warfarin. *Clin Chem*, **55**, 709–711.

118 Wu, A.H. (2009) Pharmacogenomic testing for warfarin dosing: we are ready now. *Expert Reviews in Cardiovascular Therapy*, **7**, 1483–1485.

119 Huang, S.W., Chen, H.S., Wang, X.Q., Huang, L., *et al.* (2009) Validation of VKORC1 and CYP2C9 genotypes on interindividual warfarin maintenance dose: a pro-spective study in Chinese patients. *Pharmacogenetic Genomics*, **19**, 226–234.

120 Epstein, R.S., Moyer, T.P., Aubert, R.E., DJ, O.K., *et al.* (2010) Warfarin genotyping reduces hospitalization rates results from the MM-WES (Medco-Mayo Warfarin Effectiveness study). *Journal of the American College of Cardiology*, **55**, 2804–2812.

121 Conti, R., Veenstra, D.L., Armstrong, K., Lesko, L.J., *et al.* (2010) Personalized medicine and genomics: challenges and opportunities in assessing effectiveness, cost-effectiveness, and future research priorities. *Medical Decision Making*, **30**, 328–340.

122 Dervieux, T., Meshkin, B., Neri, B. (2005) Pharmacogenetic testing: proofs of principle and pharmacoeconomic implications. *Mutation Research*, **573**, 180–194.

123 Eckman, M.H., Rosand, J., Greenberg, S.M., Gage, B.F. (2009) Cost-effectiveness of using pharmacogenetic information in warfarin dosing for patients with non-valvular atrial fibrillation. *Annals of Internal Medicine*, **150**, 73–83.

124 Epstein, R.S., Teagarden, J.R. (2010) Comparative effectiveness research and personalized medicine: catalyzing or colliding? *Pharmacoeconomics*, **28**, 905–913.

125 Meckley, L.M., Gudgeon, J.M., Anderson, J.L., Williams, M.S., *et al.* (2010) A policy model to evaluate the benefits, risks and costs of warfarin pharmacogenomic testing. *Pharmacoeconomics*, **28**, 61–74.

126 Meckley, L.M., Neumann, P.J. (2010) Personalized medicine: factors influencing reimbursement. *Health Policy*, **94**, 91–100.

127 Phillips, K.A., Van Bebber, S.L. (2004) A systematic review of cost-effectiveness analyses of pharmacogenomic interventions. *Pharmacogenomics*, **5**, 1139–1149.

128 Phillips, K.A., Van Bebber, S.L. (2005) Measuring the value of pharmacogenomics. *Nature Reviews Drug Discovery*, **4**, 500–509.

129 Veenstra, D.L. (2007) The cost-effectiveness of warfarin pharmacogenomics. *Journal of Thrombosis and Haemostasis*, **5**, 1974–1975.

CHAPTER 4

Pharmacogenetics and Cancer Chemotherapy

Christine L.H. Snozek
Department of Laboratory Medicine and Pathology, Mayo Clinic, Rochester, Minnesota

Introduction

Chemotherapy is unique from traditional pharmacological therapy in a number of ways. First, the drugs involved are often highly toxic and only moderately selective, frequently causing adverse effects even at "therapeutic" doses. Second, many protocols are designed to administer chemotherapeutics at levels near the threshold of intolerability, in order to achieve maximum response from the malignancy. Finally, because of the life-threatening nature of most cancers, both providers and patients are willing to accept side effects and toxicities so severe as to be inconceivable in any other field of medicine, without any guarantee of lasting clinical response.

It is increasingly being recognized that there is substantial room for patient-specific improvement of these factors (1). Population-derived administration protocols do not address a given individual's unique pharmacokinetics, pharmacodynamics, and disease characteristics; thus, mechanisms to personalize chemotherapy for each patient could potentially enhance clinical response and minimize toxicity. Pharmacogenetics, that is, the understanding of genetic variation as it pertains to pharmacokinetics and pharmacodynamics, is a powerful tool for individualization of therapy (2). Once again, though, the treatment of cancer has unique challenges: specifically, the fact that genetic mutation is an inherent component of malignancies, thus application of pharmacogenetics requires knowledge of both germline and somatic variations.

The field of pathology has taken up this challenge, going beyond the traditional categorization of cancer by histological type to elucidate molecular markers of pathogenesis and prognosis. At the same time, the rapid growth of molecular diagnostics has permitted evaluation of genetic factors affecting response to therapy. Together, detailed characterization of an individual cancer alongside a profile of germline and somatic genetics may hold the key for providing the proper therapy at the right dose for each patient.

Although historically chemotherapeutics were nonspecific poisons with some degree of selectivity (e.g., for rapidly proliferating cells), modern advances in drug design and molecular understanding have allowed the development of agents aimed at specific oncogenic targets. Hormonal therapies such as tamoxifen are early examples of drugs aimed at specific pathways capable of driving cancer progression (3). However, the first truly targeted chemotherapy was imatinib (Gleevec), designed specifically to inhibit the chimeric protein product of the *BCR-ABL* translocation associated with chronic myelogenous leukemia (4). Following the remarkable therapeutic success of imatinib, many other targeted drugs have been brought to clinical trials and standard practice (1, 4).

Targeted chemotherapies have the advantage that much of their molecular mechanism tends to be

Pharmacogenomics in Clinical Therapeutics, First Edition. Edited by Loralie J. Langman and Amitava Dasgupta.
© 2012 John Wiley & Sons, Ltd. Published 2012 by John Wiley & Sons, Ltd.

known by the time the drug is in clinical trials (4), which should in theory simplify the process of evaluating potential pharmacogenetic influences. Older or nontargeted agents may require more thorough study of their mechanisms of action before the effect of genetic variation in pharmacodynamics or pharmacokinetics can be assessed. For most chemotherapeutics, the best-characterized pharmacogenetic players are polymorphic metabolic enzymes such as the cytochrome P450 (CYP) family; however, pharmacodynamic variants are increasingly being studied in the context of chemotherapy.

This chapter will focus on the current state of knowledge and clinical utility of pharmacogenetic variants in predicting response to treatment, toxicity, and outcome in cancer therapy. The emphasis will be on solid tumors, although certain therapeutics used in hematological malignancies will also be discussed.

Germline genetic variation

Germline genetic variations affect therapy with several anticancer agents, including thiopurines, irinotecan, and tamoxifen.

Thiopurines

Thiopurines such as azathioprine and 6-mercaptopurine (6-MP) are antimetabolites used to treat hematological malignancies such as acute lymphoblastic anemia, as well as inflammatory and immune disorders (5). These drugs are at the heart of one of the oldest and best-characterized pharmacogenetic phenomena, namely, the role of thiopurine S-methyltransferase (TPMT) in patient response to thiopurine therapy (6). The clinical observation that a subset of patients responded differently to standard doses lead to the identification of genetic polymorphisms in *TPMT* associated with reduced metabolism of thiopurines and increased risk of toxicity.

Thiopurines require extensive modification in vivo to become activated. Azathioprine is a prodrug for 6-MP, which is further metabolized by a series of enzymes to active thioguanine nucleotides. These are incorporated into DNA and induce cell cycle arrest and cytotoxicity. A variety of inactive metabolites are also produced, some of which are implicated in adverse responses to thiopurine therapy (7). A newer thiopurine drug, 6-thioguanine, bypasses many of the initial stages of biotransformation including metabolism by TPMT (5), and will not be discussed here.

One of the primary factors determining the success of thiopurine therapy is TPMT activity. TPMT methylates several intermediate products in the thiopurine activation cascade, reducing the amount available for conversion to active thioguanine nucleotides. Roughly 90% of individuals have "normal" TPMT activity, though average enzymatic activity varies between ethnicities (5). Over 20 variant alleles have been described, resulting in approximately 10% of the population having reduced (intermediate) activity, and a small (<1%) but highly clinically relevant fraction exhibiting minimal TPMT activity (6). Such individuals do not efficiently metabolize and eliminate thiopurine drugs and are thus at high risk for toxicity, including life-threatening myelosuppression.

Three *TPMT* variants account for the vast majority of reduced-activity alleles across most ethnic groups: *TPMT*2* (G238C, Ala80Pro), *TPMT*3A* (G460A, Ala154Thr; and A719G, Tyr240Cys), and *TPMT*3C* (A719G, Tyr240Cys) (5). These mutations appear to drastically increase the rate of TPMT proteolysis, leading to a vast reduction in protein quantity and half-life. A variety of other mutant alleles have been characterized as resulting in decreased TPMT activity, but these are much less prevalent than the three described above, and are often not included in studies.

There are both genotyping and phenotyping assays available to determine TPMT status (7, 8). Genetic tests generally focus on *TPMT*2*, *3A*, and *3C*, whereas phenotyping characterizes TPMT function without assessing whether an atypical result is due to heritable mutations (i.e., is likely a permanent condition) or nongenetic causes such as inhibition by other drugs (and therefore may change over time). Average TPMT activity varies between ethnic groups (5); although the reason for this remains unclear, the implication is that prediction of TPMT functional status from genetic information is difficult without further knowledge of each individual's ethnic origin. These factors complicate use of TPMT characterization assays in clinical practice.

Clinical uptake of *TPMT* genotyping prior to thiopurine therapy is limited somewhat by the availability of phenotyping assays that may provide better correlation with the risk of thiopurine toxicity (6). Genotyping has the advantage of being unaffected by recent blood transfusion, which can falsely increase or lower phenotyping results based on the relative TPMT activities of the donor and recipient. The disadvantages of genotyping include is that, although three alleles account for the majority of reduced-function mutations, ethnic variation and other factors affecting TPMT activity can lead to imperfect correlation of *TPMT* alleles to in vivo enzyme function.

Regardless of whether genotyping or phenotyping is performed, clinical utilization has the potential to benefit patients, and several studies have shown a cost benefit to prospectively screening for TPMT function prior to initiating thiopurine therapy (6, 9). Reports from the United States and Europe agree on this, despite the wide range of costs reported for TPMT testing and medications in the various countries included in the analyses. Genotyping was the preferred assay in these studies, despite acknowledgment of the lower cost and greater availability of phenotyping methods (9).

TPMT is only one of several areas of pharmacogenetic interest relevant to therapy with 6-MP and azathioprine. The first step in the activation of 6-MP (Figure 4.1) is catalyzed by hypoxanthine guanine phosphoribosyl transferase (HGPRT), while TPMT and xanthine oxidase (XO) compete with for 6-MP as a substrate (5). TPMT converts 6-MP to the hepatotoxin 6-methylmercaptopurine (7), while XO catabolizes 6-MP to the inactive metabolite thiouric acid. HGPRT action on 6-MP creates 6-thioinosine monophosphate (6-thio-IMP), an intermediate product which can be further transformed by a series of enzymes to form thioguanine nucleotides. Alternately, 6-thio-IMP can be phosphorylated to the triphosphate 6-thio-ITP, a pathway which is counteracted by inosine triphosphate pyrophosphatase (ITPase), which converts 6-thio-ITP back to 6-thio-IMP (5).

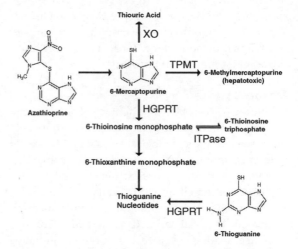

Figure 4.1 Metabolic and activation pathways of thioguanine drugs. HGPRT: hypoxanthine guanine phosphoribosyltransferase; ITPase: inosine triphosphatase; TPMT: thiopurine S-methyltransferase; and XO: xanthine oxidase.

In theory, polymorphisms in any of the enzymes involved in thiopurine metabolism could affect patient outcome. Genetic variants of ITPase have been investigated for association with thiopurine toxicity, with conflicting results. At least two mutations in *ITPA* result in enzyme deficiency – C94A (Pro32Thr) and IVS2 + A21C – which range in prevalence from 1% to 19% in different ethnic groups. ITPase deficiency leads to accumulation of 6-thio-ITP, which is thought to contribute to immunosuppression and myelotoxicity (10). The C94A mutant substantially reduces phosphorylase function, with hetero- and homozygous carriers of this allele demonstrating <25% and 0% residual activity, respectively (5). In contrast, even homozygous expression of the intronic mutant results in approximately 60% ITPase activity. The C94A allele is therefore the more promising variant for study with respect to thiopurine therapy, but the few reports currently in the literature are inconsistent as to whether there is (11) or is not (12) an association with toxicity.

Although *ITPA* and possibly other genes may allow for better individualization of thiopurine therapy, *TPMT* characterization currently represents one of the best-established clinical applications for pharmacogenetics. Cost-benefit analyses and clinical studies support the use of prospective genotyping or phenotyping prior to administering azathioprine or 6-MP, and provide evidence for adopting *TPMT* testing as a best practice in oncology.

Irinotecan

Irinotecan (CPT-11) is a topoisomerase I poison used to treat metastatic colorectal cancer and a number of other solid and hematological tumors (13). Several different combination therapy protocols incorporate irinotecan, including FOLFIRI (leucovorin [folinic acid], 5-fluorouracil, and irinotecan) and two-agent regimens with various chemotherapeutics such as cetuximab or oxaliplatin. Its major dose-limiting toxicities include severe diarrhea and potentially life-threatening neutropenia. A host of clinical factors contribute to the risk for toxicity, such as age, weight, sex, and hepatic function (14).

Once administered, irinotecan is converted by carboxylesterase to the highly active metabolite SN-38 (Figure 4.2) (14). This metabolite is eliminated largely through glucuronide conjugation (SN-38-G), mediated by uridine diphosphate glucuronyl transferase (UGT) enzymes (14, 15). The primary enzyme responsible for forming SN-38-G is UGT1A1, although more recent studies are elucidating roles for UGT1A7 and UGT1A9 as well (16). Irinotecan can also be metabolized by CYP3A4/5 to 7-ethyl-10-[4-*N*-(5-aminopentanoic acid)-1-piperidino]-carbonyloxycamptothecin (APC) and 7-ethyl-10-[4-amino-1-piperidino]-carbonyloxycamptothecin (NPC), which

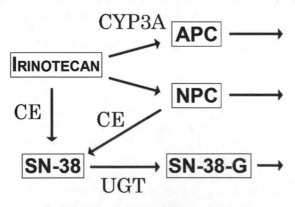

Figure 4.2 Metabolism of irinotecan. CE: carboxylesterase; CYP3A: cytochrome P450 3A; and UGT: uridine diphosphate glucuronyltransferase.

are only weakly active compared to SN-38 (17). Carboxylesterase activity can convert NPC to SN-38 (14).

Increased exposure to SN-38 is associated with increased likelihood of severe (grade 3–4) toxicity, thus a reduction in UGT activity can potentially lead to adverse responses to irinotecan therapy. This phenomenon has been demonstrated with variant alleles of *UGT1A1*: the best-characterized example to date is *UGT1A1*28*, a promoter polymorphism wherein a variable number of tandem repeats (VNTR) domain contains 7 TA repeats rather than the typical 6, resulting in reduced UGT1A1 expression (15). Homozygotes for this allele (*28/*28*, also referred to as 7/7) are at greater risk for toxicity when administered irinotecan, leading to a recommendation to reduce irinotecan doses for *28/*28* individuals (13). Two other variants involving 5 (*UGT1A1*36*) or 8 (*UGT1A1*37*) tandem repeats at the same promoter VNTR site are found at low prevalence, primarily in individuals of African descent (15). Limited studies suggest that the 5-repeat allele produces roughly normal UGT1A1 activity, whereas the 8-repeat allele confers reduced enzyme function (18).

The majority of clinical studies to date have focused on *UGT1A1*28*, yet the effect of this variant on irinotecan therapy remains somewhat unclear. Several trials of high-dose ($>200\,\text{mg/m}^2$) irinotecan regimens demonstrated reduced SN-38 glucuronidation and clearance in *28* carriers; some reported increased incidence or severity of neutropenia, while others showed association with diarrhea but no effect on hematological toxicity (15). It is possible that differences in co-prescribed medications or the ethnic backgrounds of the populations studied play a role in this inconsistency (19). In contrast, a trial comparing single-agent and combination therapies in unpretreated metastatic colorectal cancer examined molecular markers for over 400 patients administered irinotecan, but showed no significance for the *UGT1A1*28* allele in risk for toxicity (20). Only roughly 40% received a high dose of irinotecan ($350\,\text{mg/m}^2$) but there was no apparent utility for *UGT1A1*28* genotyping in the high-dose subset.

Despite this negative finding, many studies examining high-dose irinotecan show increased risk of toxicity in *UGT1A1*28* homozygotes. However, the case is not so simple with low- or medium-dose regimens. Results from trials of these protocols range from corroborating the findings of high-dose studies, to showing no association at all between *UGT1A1*28* and irinotecan toxicity (15). Several of these reports were relatively small (<50 patients) and likely underpowered; a recent, larger trial studied patients treated with the IFL (irinotecan dose 100–125 mg/m^2, n = 109) or IROX (irinotecan dose 200 mg/m^2, n = 103) protocols. This study demonstrated significantly higher incidence of grade 4 + neutropenia in **28/*28* homozygotes treated with IROX, but no significant association was seen with the lower-dose IFL regimen (21). To date, it remains unclear whether it is necessary to reduce irinotecan dosing for *UGT1A1*28* patients enrolled in low- or medium-dose irinotecan protocols.

An intriguing complement to the finding that carriers of *UGT1A1*28* alleles might experience greater toxicity, is the suggestion that patients with wild-type UGT1A1 expression may actually be underdosed because current protocols were established without excluding homozygotes for low-activity variants. A study of "genotype-driven" dosing concluded that **1/*1* and **1/*28* patients could successfully tolerate escalation of irinotecan in the FOLFIRI regimen, up to 420 and 370 mg/m^2, respectively (22). Although all patients received irinotecan doses above the standard (180 mg/m^2) for FOLFIRI, tumor response was significantly greater in those treated with the highest doses (310–420 mg/m^2), and in heterozygous carriers of the *UGT1A1*28* allele. This study suggests that current therapeutic protocols may be improved by reexamining recommended doses for all *UGT1A1* genotypes, not just low-activity homozygotes.

Despite being the best-studied variant, the *UGT1A1*28* allele is not the whole story when it comes to irinotecan pharmacogenetics. Promoter polymorphisms are relatively common in individuals of Caucasian or African descent, but are less prevalent in other ethnicities. Another low-activity allele, *UGT1A1*6*, encodes a nonsynonymous mutation in exon 1 (G211A, Gly71Arg) and is found in roughly 20% of Asian populations (15). The presence of a *UGT1A1*6* allele reduces glucuronidation capacity to roughly the same degree as *UGT1A1*28*,

and dosing adjustments are similar to those recommended for *UGT1A1*28*. There are also a variety of lower prevalence mutations thought to affect UGT1A1 activity, including *UGT1A1*27* (C686A, Pro229Gln), *UGT1A1*60* (T-3279G), and *UGT1A1*93* (G-3156A), although there are currently few studies examining their significance on irinotecan therapy (23). The *UGT1A1*93* promoter polymorphism is intriguing: despite high linkage disequilibrium with other UGT1A1 variants, a *UGT1A1*93* genotype has been suggested as a better predictor of irinotecan toxicity (23) or tumor response (16) than the *UGT1A1*28* allele.

Further studies have implicated other UGT family members as pharmacogenetic players in irinotecan therapy, most notably *UGT1A7* and *UGT1A9* (14). Recent, comparatively larger studies have compared the predictive capabilities of individual polymorphisms in *UGT1A1*, *1A7*, and *1A9*, as well as haplotypes of those genes (16, 24). These reports found that *UGT1A7*3* (Asp129Lys, Arg131Lys, Trp208Arg) was predictive of hematological or gastrointestinal toxicity after the first round of FOLFIRI or irinotecan + fluorouracil therapy, respectively. Haplotype analysis in both showed an association between all variant alleles except *UGT1A9* with toxicity (24) or response rate (16); the latter report also saw a link between hematological toxicity and the haplotype with all wild-type alleles except *UGT1A9*. The implications of the *UGT1A9*22* (del T-118) variant were contradictory in these studies, with **22/*22* status as a risk factor for severe hematological toxicity in one report (16), while in contrast the **1/*1* genotype was linked to nonhematological toxicity in the other (24). These findings reinforce the need for further studies with sufficient patient numbers to explore the implications of *UGT1A* genes and haplotypes in the many chemotherapeutic protocols incorporating irinotecan.

There are a number of other candidate genes that have been examined for their influence on irinotecan therapy. ATP-binding cassette (ABC) transporters such as ABCB1, ABCC1, ABCC2, and ABCG2, as well as the organic anion transporter OATP1B3 (encoded by *SLCO1B1*) have the potential to affect uptake or elimination of irinotecan and its metabolites. The combination of *ABCC1 IVS11* (C-48T),

SLCO1B1*1b, and *UGT1A1*93* was found to account for nearly a third of the variability in neutrophil nadir in a study that also linked *ABCB1*, *ABCC1*, *ABCC2*, and *SLCO1B1* polymorphisms to alterations in pharmacokinetics after irinotecan administration (23). This study mainly included whites and African Americans, but such associations have also been found in Asian patients (17).

Other candidates currently of interest in irinotecan pharmacogenetics include the drug target topoisomerase I and metabolic enzymes such as carboxylesterase and CYP3A4/5. Few solid findings have emerged thus far, although the *CYP3A5*3C* allele (encoding a splice variant that severely decreases expression) was significantly associated with rate of response to irinotecan plus 5-fluorouracil (21). Given the highly inducible nature of CYP3A4 activity, phenotyping might be a viable alternative to genotyping for *CYP3A4/5* variants. A recent prospective study examined whether irinotecan dosing could be optimized using a CYP3A4 phenotype-based equation to predict clearance of the drug (25). Although the range of doses administered in the equation-dosed group was considerably wider than with body surface area based dosing, the authors noted less interindividual variability after phenotyping, with a reduction in severe adverse effects.

Individualized irinotecan therapy is an evolving process, beginning with *UGT1A1*28* and expanding to include additional variants in *UGT1A* and other genes. Both toxicity and efficacy of the drug have been associated with genetic polymorphisms, which hold the promise to further improve use of irinotecan in chemotherapy. However, several outstanding questions must be more thoroughly addressed for this to occur, including the impact of the irinotecan dose, co-prescribed medications, and patient ethnicity.

Tamoxifen

A mainstay of breast cancer therapy for over 25 years, tamoxifen is a selective estrogen receptor modulator (SERM) used in treatment and prophylaxis against hormone receptor-positive (estrogen receptor, ER$^+$, or progesterone receptor, PR$^+$) tumors (26). Administration of tamoxifen disrupts ER-dependent signaling, which is a major oncogenic driver in receptor-positive tumors. Use of this drug

has shown substantial benefit in improving patient outcome, and long-term therapy with tamoxifen is thought to be a major contributing force to the reduction of breast cancer-related deaths (27). However, not all patients respond to tamoxifen, thus there is a clinical demand to ascertain which patients would be better served by alternate treatments such as aromatase inhibitors.

Tamoxifen undergoes extensive metabolism to other active compounds (Figure 4.3). Several CYP isoforms, most notably CYP3A4/5, can catalyze formation of the major metabolite N-desmethyltamoxifen (NDT) (28, 29). Hydroxylation of tamoxifen or NDT by CYP2D6 creates the highly active metabolites 4-hydroxytamoxifen (4OHT) and endoxifen, respectively. Both of these are notably more potent (~100×) than tamoxifen; however, endoxifen is typically present at higher concentrations than 4OHT and downregulates ER signaling via additional mechanisms, thus it is believed to be the primary determinant of therapeutic success (29). Metabolism by CYP2D6 is a key step in the formation of endoxifen, thus variants of this enzyme are of great pharmacogenetic interest.

CYP2D6 is a highly polymorphic gene, with over 75 alleles described to date. The resulting enzyme activities of variants range from virtually zero to many times greater than average (27). Homozygosity or compound heterozygosity for alleles that confer minimal residual activity gives rise to the *poor metabolizer* (PM) phenotype. Individuals with roughly "normal" CYP2D6 activity are termed *extensive metabolizers* (EMs), while those with greater than average enzyme function are *ultra-rapid metabolizers* (UMs). One final category, termed *intermediate*

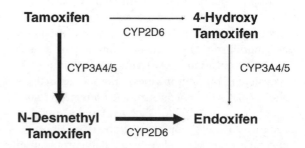

Figure 4.3 Metabolism of tamoxifen.

metabolizers (IMs), is an amorphous collection of individuals either heterozygous for low-activity alleles or homozygous (and sometimes heterozygous) for reduced-activity alleles. The clinical importance of the IM phenotype remains to be determined, but categorization of this group confounds comparison of different studies, which may consider IM with PM, EM, or independently (28).

The prevalence of CYP2D6 PM and IM alleles varies greatly between ethnicities. Null (including *3, *4, and *5) and low-activity (e.g., *9, *10, *41) alleles are common in individuals of European descent, with approximately 10% considered PMs and 10–15% IMs (27). UMs (typically duplication of *1 or *2) comprise 10–15% of this population, leaving only 60–70% classified as EMs. In contrast, most Asian ethnicities show higher prevalence of IM alleles, particularly *CYP2D6*10*, whereas Northern Africans have a higher proportion of UM individuals (27). The differences between populations and the constant expansion of knowledge regarding *CYP2D6* variants must be kept in mind when comparing studies, particularly because a number of early reports genotyped for only one or two variants (typically *4 or *10), and categorized all other alleles as "wild type" (28).

CYP2D6 genotype and its relationship to tamoxifen therapy have been examined in a variety of contexts, including monotherapy, combination therapies, and familial and sporadic cancers. Many studies have demonstrated a significant correlation between reduced CYP2D6 activity and poor outcome with tamoxifen therapy, while some have shown contradictory results. Unfortunately, very few studies have sufficient numbers for statistical power, and even fewer include multiple PM and IM alleles. A recent meta-review compiled data from 10 studies, and found no significant association between *CYP2D6* and disease-free survival or overall survival (28). However, out of the 10 studies included, seven examined a single variant allele, and only two reports were rated as having good quality design and data. One of the two good-quality studies included some prospectively collected data, and found significant correlations between *CYP2D6* genotype and time to recurrence, event-free survival, and disease-free survival; notably, this study

was limited to ER⁺/PR⁺ patients (30). The other good-quality report included in the meta-review examined metastatic familial breast cancer (*BRCA1* and *BRCA2*) (31). No significant association was seen with BRCA1 tumors, only 57.5% of which were ER⁺, but there was a significant association between *CYP2D6* and overall survival in BRCA2 tumors, 91% of which were ER⁺ (31). Tamoxifen is known to have minimal impact on ER⁻ cancer (27), thus including data from ER⁻ tumors likely reduced the statistical power of the study, and may have masked any true association between genotype and outcome. This highlights the difficulty of comparing studies with very different inclusion criteria, and reinforces the need for more prospective trials limited to relevant patient populations.

Important progress in the study of *CYP2D6* and tamoxifen has been made recently. As mentioned above, Schroth *et al.* published some of the first prospectively collected data: this multicenter trial was designed with sufficient patient numbers and specific inclusion criteria to provide statistical power while removing confounding influences such as hormone receptor status and combination chemotherapy (30). The authors reported significantly shorter time to recurrence for both PMs and IMs, with an apparent gene–dose effect (i.e., worse hazard ratio for PMs than for IMs). Both reduced-function groups showed poorer event-free and disease-free survival. Additional studies have begun to examine the importance of various factors that confound interpretation of many reports, such as combination chemotherapy and adherence to the tamoxifen regimen (32, 33). This latter is especially important given the alarming finding that functional *CYP2D6* alleles are associated with discontinuation of tamoxifen therapy, indicating that the very patients who would benefit from the drug are more likely to stop taking it (34).

The effect of *CYP2D6* genotype must be considered in light of other variables, most notably the concomitant use of medications that inhibit CYP2D6 activity. Several common antidepressants (e.g., paroxetine and fluoxetine) are potent inhibitors of the enzyme; there are a variety of other strong inhibitors, and many more weak-to-moderate inhibitors (29). Antidepressants are of particular interest because they are frequently prescribed in breast cancer patients, both for clinical depression and to alleviate the hot flashes that often accompany tamoxifen therapy. Although studies are still limited, there is evidence that CYP2D6 inhibition by co-medications can affect mortality and recurrence in tamoxifen-treated breast cancer (35, 36). Current recommendations suggest that, when available, alternate medications that do not inhibit CYP2D6 should be prescribed during tamoxifen use (26, 29). If this is not possible, replacing tamoxifen with aromatase inhibitors is an option for postmenopausal women; premenopausal women require ovarian suppression to use aromatase inhibitors, but studies regarding efficacy and outcomes for this strategy are lacking (29). Endoxifen as a stand-alone drug is in the pharmaceutical pipeline, which may provide a remedy for both genetic and functional problems with tamoxifen conversion to its active metabolite (37).

Somatic mutations

Somatic mutation affects therapy with anticancer drugs such as imatinib and drugs that target epidermal growth factor receptor (EGFR).

Imatinib

Imatinib, the first true designer drug, was originally developed to specifically inhibit the chimeric Bcr-Abl kinase responsible for chronic myeloid leukemia (CML) (38). By targeting the mutant protein, inhibition of native Abl activity was minimized; however, subsequent data revealed that imatinib also inhibits the c-Kit and platelet-derived growth factor receptor-α (PDGFR-A) kinases (39). This discovery is fortuitous for patients with a different type of cancer, namely, gastrointestinal stromal tumors (GIST), the vast majority of which are driven by signaling through c-Kit and/or PDGFR-A. In both cancers, somatic mutations can affect susceptibility to imatinib therapy.

The progression of CML can be characterized in three phases (38). Chronic phase (CP) patients exhibit few or no symptoms, whereas accelerated phase (AP) involves worsening of biomarkers such as increased percentage of myeloblasts or acquisition of new cytogenetic abnormalities. This eventually converts to blast phase (BP), which is marked by further expansion of the malignant cell population, and short patient survival. The introduction of imatinib vastly changed the prognosis of CML from a typical life expectancy of 3–5 years after diagnosis to, in some cases, a manageable chronic condition (38, 40). However, resistance to imatinib is a common phenomenon, especially in long-term therapy, and presents a clinical challenge.

Resistance to imatinib can be primary (i.e., no response to initial treatment) or secondary (i.e., occurring after an initial response), and most frequently arises due to Bcr-Abl mutations that diminish its susceptibility to inhibition (38). Many imatinib-resistant mutants are susceptible to the newer Bcr-Abl inhibitors dasatinib and nilotinib, while either high-dose imatinib or a second-line agent are therapeutic options for imatinib resistance due to other mechanisms (40). In general, mutations in the adenosine triphosphate-binding P-loop (e.g., G250E, Y253F/H, and E255K/V) appear to have the most detrimental effect on patient response to imatinib, with substantially poorer outcomes compared to mutations outside of the P-loop (38). However, most P-loop mutants are vulnerable to other Bcr-Abl inhibitors, whereas the non-P-loop mutation T315I confers resistance to all currently approved agents and remains a therapeutic challenge in CML (38, 40).

The development of imatinib for use in CML was an unintentional but welcome breakthrough for treatment of GIST. Although it is the most common gastrointestinal sarcoma, GIST is a rare cancer and previously lacked viable therapeutic options (41). The vast majority of these tumors express the tyrosine kinase receptors c-Kit and/or PDGFR-A, which are frequently mutated to cause gain of function in the neoplastic cells. *KIT* mutations typically affect the protein's juxtamembrane/extracellular regulatory regions or the tyrosine kinase domain, whereas *PDGFRA* mutations are most often located in the activation loop of the receptor kinase domain (39). Both c-Kit and PDGFR-A can drive oncogenic signaling through a variety of pathways, resulting in dysregulation of proliferation, apoptosis, and chemotaxis (42).

Some of the most common primary (pathogenic) mutations in *KIT* and *PDGFRA* appear to increase the receptors' susceptibility to imatinib inhibition (39, 42). Exon 11 *KIT* mutations, found in over half of all GISTs, are associated with better response to standard-dose imatinib therapy than either exon 9 mutant or *KIT* wild type tumors. Higher doses (600–800 mg/day) may improve outcomes for patients with exon 9 mutations. In contrast, a Asp842Val mutation in PDGFR-A eliminates the ability of imatinib to inhibit this receptor (42).

Mutations acquired after imatinib therapy is initiated can cause secondary resistance. In *KIT*, most secondary mutations are located in the tyrosine kinase regions; many have not been described in GIST prior to exposure to imatinib, although there is some overlap with primary pathogenic mutations (39, 42). Development of resistance through secondary alterations in *PDGFRA* is much less common, with the exception of the Asp842Val mutant described above (42). Other mechanisms leading to imatinib resistance include upregulation of target receptor expression through gene amplification, or increased reliance on alternate oncogenic pathways (39). Increased doses of imatinib may overcome these latter mechanisms, whereas secondary mutations typically require use of an alternate therapy such as sunitinib, a broad-spectrum inhibitor of c-Kit, PDGFR, and a variety of other tyrosine kinases (39, 42).

The development of imatinib was a giant step forward in targeting chemotherapy to specific oncogenic pathways, and it revolutionized the management of two previously difficult-to-treat cancers. CML can now often be stabilized into a chronic disease, while patients with GIST have finally been provided with a viable therapeutic option. The success of imatinib was the proof of principle that drug development could be specifically tailored for a target molecule, and it has led the way for a wave of new, targeted chemotherapeutic agents.

EGFR-targeted therapies

The epidermal growth factor receptor (EGFR) family of proteins are membrane-bound tyrosine kinase receptors, with powerful effects on signaling cascades involved in cellular growth, proliferation, and

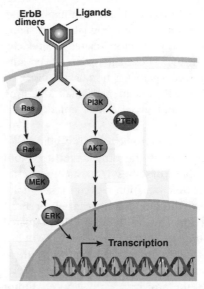

Figure 4.4 Simplified cartoon of epidermal growth factor receptor (EGFR)–mediated signaling networks.

differentiation (43). The first (EGFR or ErbB1) and second (HER2/neu or ErbB2) members of this family have been heavily implicated in a number of cancers (44). HER2/neu is the antigen target of trastuzumab (Herceptin), a humanized antibody used for treatment of breast cancers overexpressing the strongly oncogenic protein, and one of the earliest and most successful examples of drugs designed to inhibit a specific molecule (3).

EGFR is thought to be a driving force in a variety of different tumor types. It activates several very potent signaling networks (Figure 4.4) including the mitogen-activated protein kinase (MAPK) and phosphoinositol 3-kinase (PI3K) pathways, typically resulting in suppression of apoptosis and enhancement of growth and proliferation (43, 44). Signaling is initiated within the cell by EGFR homo- or heterodimerization with another ErbB protein, which initiates the phosphorylation cascade through these pathways. A number of cancer therapeutics have therefore been designed to diminish EGFR-mediated signaling, including kinase inhibitors (e.g., gefitinib and erlotinib) and antibodies targeting the extracellular domain of the protein (e.g., cetuximab and panitumumab) (44). The inhibitors bind to the cytoplasmic region to prevent phosphorylation of

EGFR targets, whereas anti-EGFR antibodies may act via disrupting intracellular signaling, engaging the antibody-dependent cell-mediated cytotoxicity system, or both (4). These agents have been successfully employed against a number of diseases, including colorectal cancer, non-small cell lung cancer (NSCLC), and glioblastoma, among others (43–46).

The most obvious pharmacogenetic candidate for anti-EGFR therapies is the drug target itself, but predicting likelihood of success is not simply a matter of examining *EGFR* variation. Several other molecules both upstream and downstream of the ErbB receptors can modify the efficacy EGFR-targeted agents, including *KRAS*, *BRAF*, and *PTEN* (47). Intriguingly, though somatic alterations in these genes are common to many cancers, their effects on anti-EGFR therapy can vary between tumor types; thus, results from clinical trials in one area of oncology must be cautiously interpreted when applied to another.

Both amplification and mutation of the *EGFR* gene are common in tumors, as is overexpression driven by mechanisms other than increased gene copy number. Although not all studies have shown definitive associations, *EGFR* gene copy number in tumor cells appears to correlate positively with response to the antibodies cetuximab and panitumumab in metastatic colorectal cancer (43). Amplification of *EGFR* is found in approximately 12% of colorectal carcinomas, whereas mutation of the gene is rare in this disease (47). In contrast, there was no correlation between *EGFR* copy number and response to erlotinib or gefitinib in glioblastoma, despite the much higher prevalence (~40%) of amplification in these tumors (44).

Although all EGFR-targeted therapies can exert their pharmacological activity on the wild-type protein, somatic mutations present in tumors affect the response to certain agents. A deletion in the extracellular ligand-binding domain results in a constitutively active protein termed EGFRvIII that is resistant to endogenous regulation; gefitinib is ineffective against this mutant, whereas erlotinib maintains its activity in vitro (44). EGFRvIII is common in glioblastoma, which likely contributes to the poor success of gefitinib against this cancer. In contrast,

gefitinib is very effective against certain EGFR kinase domain mutations that enhance ligand-induced activation, and were initially identified in a subset of gefitinib-responsive NSCLC tumors (48).

Downstream modulators of signaling are also important in determining response to EGFR-targeted therapies. The best-characterized example is that of *KRAS*, encoding a powerful stimulator of the MAPK signaling pathway (43, 45). Activation of Ras by EGFR initiates a phosphorylation cascade leading to increased proliferation and resistance to apoptosis. *KRAS* point mutations in tumors, most commonly found in codons 12, 13, or 61 of the gene, produce a constitutively active protein that signals independently of upstream activation by EGFR or other receptors (45).

Studies in colorectal cancer have shown that, although presence of wild-type *KRAS* is no guarantee of success, *KRAS* mutations virtually eliminate any response to treatment with the anti-EGFR antibodies cetuximab or panitumumab (43, 49). In contrast, these agents are efficacious in either monotherapy or combination for *KRAS*–wild-type metastatic colorectal cancer (50). For this reason, clinical guidelines recommend screening colorectal tumors for *KRAS* mutations prior to administering these very expensive agents; some insurers have made *KRAS* status a mandatory condition to receive coverage for anti-EGFR antibody therapy (51). However, studies in NSCLC are less clear-cut. Meta-analyses of several smaller trials with EGFR inhibitors found significantly poorer response in *KRAS*-mutant tumors, whereas larger studies of single-agent EGFR inhibitors or addition of anti-EGFR antibodies to chemotherapy showed no significant differences based on *KRAS* mutation status (45). Modest responses to anti-EGFR therapy in unselected populations of NSCLC and in pancreatic cancer (where the majority of tumors have KRAS mutations) suggest that the role of KRAS in colorectal cancer may not be universally applicable to other cancers (45).

Other downstream modulators play a role in the efficacy of EGFR-targeted agents as well. Raf is the immediate target of Ras, thus activating mutations in genes encoding Raf proteins would be expected to affect anti-EGFR therapy in a similar fashion to

KRAS mutants (43). Point mutations in *BRAF* tend to cluster at a single codon, resulting in a V600E amino acid change and a constitutively active protein. In colorectal cancer, B-Raf V600E is less common and less well characterized than *KRAS* mutants, yet several studies have demonstrated poor response to EGFR antibodies in colorectal tumors with V600E mutations (43, 47). Mutation of *KRAS* and *BRAF* are largely mutually exclusive in colorectal tumors, supporting the concept that these alterations have similar oncogenic effects and implications for targeted therapy. Treatment with the nonselective Raf inhibitor sorafenib appears to restore sensitivity to anti-EGFR therapies in colorectal cancer, but is ineffective against *BRAF*-mutant melanomas (47, 52). Development of more selective B-Raf inhibitors may provide more effective targeting of this oncogenic pathway (52).

There are several additional effectors and modulators of EGFR signaling that have been investigated for associations with response to therapy. These include PI3K, cyclin D1, and various ErbB ligands (e.g., epidermal growth factor, amphiregulin, and epiregulin), all of which stimulate EGFR-responsive signaling pathways (43, 50). Intriguingly, alongside these potentially oncogenic molecules, the phosphatase and tumor suppressor *PTEN* which inhibits PI3K has been associated with therapeutic success in high-grade gliomas (44). As a powerful tumor suppressor, PTEN expression is often lost in cancers due to somatic mutation or epigenetic regulation. However, wild-type expression of PTEN appears to be a necessary condition for response to erlotinib in glioma; similarly, *PTEN* copy number may be a prognostic factor for response to cetuximab in colorectal cancer (44, 50). *PTEN*, *BRAF*, and a variety of other genes may therefore be targets for future personalization of chemotherapy, but much work remains to characterize their association with response to anti-EGFR agents.

Conclusions

The genetic considerations involved in predicting the success of chemotherapy include analysis of both germline (patient) and somatic (tumor) variations.

Optimizing use of chemotherapeutics, particularly those that are highly toxic or expensive, can improve patient outcome and reduce exposure to unhelpful agents. Currently, the best-understood areas of cancer pharmacogenetics are the polymorphic metabolic enzymes such as CYP2D6 and UGT1A1, and the molecular targets of specific inhibitors such as imatinib and anti-EGFR therapies. However, there are a host of other potential players whose roles are only beginning to be explored, including drug transporters, secondary metabolic pathways, and pharmacodynamic targets. There are also many other drugs whose pharmacogenetics hold promise for optimizing clinical practice, including 5-fluorouracil, doxorubicin, and taxanes (19). The drugs discussed in this chapter are merely the earliest examples of the power of applying pharmacogenetics to chemotherapy, but they represent the first steps on the path towards the eventual goal of selecting a customized regimen of therapeutic agents, tailored for each individual patient's disease.

References

1 Imyanitov, E. N., Moiseyenko, V. M. (2007) Molecular-based choice of cancer therapy: realities and expectations. *Clinica Chimica Acta: International Journal of Clinical Chemistry*, **379**, 1–13.

2 Dawood, S., Leyland-Jones, B. (2009) Pharmacology and pharmacogenetics of chemotherapeutic agents. *Cancer Investigation*, **27**, 482–488.

3 Longo, R., D'Andrea, M., Sarmiento, R., Gasparini, G. (2010) Pharmacogenetics in breast cancer: focus on hormone therapy, taxanes, trastuzumab and bevacizumab. *Expert Opinion on Investigational Drugs*, **19(Suppl. 1)**, S41–S50.

4 Janne, P. A., Gray, N., Settleman, J. (2009) Factors underlying sensitivity of cancers to small-molecule kinase inhibitors. *Nature Reviews*, **8**, 709–723.

5 Sahasranaman, S., Howard, D., Roy, S. (2008) Clinical pharmacology and pharmacogenetics of thiopurines. *European Journal of Clinical Pharmacology*, **64**, 753–767.

6 Wang, L., Weinshilboum, R. (2006) Thiopurine S-methyltransferase pharmacogenetics: insights, challenges and future directions. *Oncogene*, **25**, 1629–1638.

7 Ford, L. T., Berg, J. D. (2009) Thiopurine S-methyltransferase (TPMT) assessment prior to starting

thiopurine drug treatment: a pharmacogenomic test whose time has come. *Journal of Clinical Pathology*, **63**, 288–295.

8 Fakhoury, M., Andreu-Gallien, J., Mahr, A., Medard, Y., Azougagh, S., Vilmer, E., Jacqz-Aigrain, E. (2007) Should TPMT genotype and activity be used to monitor 6-mercaptopurine treatment in children with acute lymphoblastic leukaemia? *Journal of Clinical Pharmacy and Therapeutics*, **32**, 633–639.

9 Payne, K., Newman, W. G., Gurwitz, D., Ibarreta, D., Phillips, K. A. (2009) TPMT testing in azathioprine: a 'cost-effective use of healthcare resources'? *Personalized Medicine*, **6**, 103–113.

10 Al Hadithy, A. F., de Boer, N. K., Derijks, L. J., Escher, J. C., Mulder, C. J., Brouwers, J. R. (2005) Thiopurines in inflammatory bowel disease: pharmacogenetics, therapeutic drug monitoring and clinical recommendations. *Digestive and Liver Disorders*, **37**, 282–297.

11 Marinaki, A. M., Ansari, A., Duley, J. A., Arenas, M., Sumi, S., Lewis, C. M., Shobowale-Bakre el, M., Escuredo, E., Fairbanks, L. D., Sanderson, J. D. (2004) Adverse drug reactions to azathioprine therapy are associated with polymorphism in the gene encoding inosine triphosphate pyrophosphatase (ITPase). *Pharmacogenetics*, **14**, 181–187.

12 Gearry, R. B., Roberts, R. L., Barclay, M. L., Kennedy, M. A. (2004) Lack of association between the ITPA 94C>A polymorphism and adverse effects from azathioprine. *Pharmacogenetics*, **14**, 779–781.

13 Irinotecan hydrochloride (2011) In: *Physicians' Desk Reference*. Thompson Reuters, New York.

14 Kweekel, D., Guchelaar, H. J., Gelderblom, H. (2008) Clinical and pharmacogenetic factors associated with irinotecan toxicity. *Cancer Treatment Reviews*, **34**, 656–669.

15 Perera, M. A., Innocenti, F., Ratain, M. J. (2008) Pharmacogenetic testing for uridine diphosphate glucuronosyltransferase 1A1 polymorphisms: are we there yet? *Pharmacotherapy*, **28**, 755–768.

16 Cecchin, E., Innocenti, F., D'Andrea, M., Corona, G., De Mattia, E., Biason, P., Buonadonna, A., Toffoli, G. (2009) Predictive role of the UGT1A1, UGT1A7, and UGT1A9 genetic variants and their haplotypes on the outcome of metastatic colorectal cancer patients treated with fluorouracil, leucovorin, and irinotecan. *Journal of Clinical Oncology*, **27**, 2457–2465.

17 Zhou, Q., Sparreboom, A., Tan, E. H., Cheung, Y. B., Lee, A., Poon, D., Lee, E. J., Chowbay, B. (2005) Pharmacogenetic profiling across the irinotecan path-

way in Asian patients with cancer. *British Journal of Clinical Pharmacology*, **59**, 415–424.

18 Passon, R. G., Howard, T. A., Zimmerman, S. A., Schultz, W. H., Ware, R. E. (2001) Influence of bilirubin uridine diphosphate-glucuronosyltransferase 1A promoter polymorphisms on serum bilirubin levels and cholelithiasis in children with sickle cell anemia. *Journal of Pediatric Hematology and Oncology*, **23**, 448–451.

19 Ma, B. B., Hui, E. P., Mok, T. S. (2011) Population-based differences in treatment outcome following anticancer drug therapies. *The Lancet Oncology*, **11**, 75–84.

20 Braun, M. S., Richman, S. D., Thompson, L., Daly, C. L., Meade, A. M., Adlard, J. W., Allan, J. M., Parmar, M. K., Quirke, P., Seymour, M. T. (2009) Association of molecular markers with toxicity outcomes in a randomized trial of chemotherapy for advanced colorectal cancer: the FOCUS trial. *Journal of Clinical Oncology*, **27**, 5519–5528.

21 McLeod, H. L., Sargent, D. J., Marsh, S., Green, E. M., King, C. R., Fuchs, C. S., Ramanathan, R. K., Williamson, S. K., Findlay, B. P., Thibodeau, S. N., Grothey, A., Morton, R. F., Goldberg, R. M. (2010) Pharmacogenetic predictors of adverse events and response to chemotherapy in metastatic colorectal cancer: results from North American Gastrointestinal Intergroup Trial N9741. *Journal of Clinical Oncology*, **28**, 3227–3233.

22 Toffoli, G., Cecchin, E., Gasparini, G., D'Andrea, M., Azzarello, G., Basso, U., Mini, E., Pessa, S., De Mattia, E., Lo Re, G., Buonadonna, A., Nobili, S., De Paoli, P., Innocenti, F. (2010) Genotype-driven phase I study of irinotecan administered in combination with fluorouracil/leucovorin in patients with metastatic colorectal cancer. *Journal of Clinical Oncology*, **28**, 866–871.

23 Innocenti, F., Kroetz, D. L., Schuetz, E., Dolan, M. E., Ramirez, J., Relling, M., Chen, P., Das, S., Rosner, G. L., Ratain, M. J. (2009) Comprehensive pharmacogenetic analysis of irinotecan neutropenia and pharmacokinetics. *Journal of Clinical Oncology*, **27**, 2604–2614.

24 Martinez-Balibrea, E., Abad, A., Martinez-Cardus, A., Gines, A., Valladares, M., Navarro, M., Aranda, E., Marcuello, E., Benavides, M., Massuti, B., Carrato, A., Layos, L., Manzano, J. L., Moreno, V. (2011) UGT1A and TYMS genetic variants predict toxicity and response of colorectal cancer patients treated with first-line irinotecan and fluorouracil combination therapy. *British Journal of Cancer*, **103**, 581–589.

25 van der Bol, J. M., Mathijssen, R. H., Creemers, G. J., Planting, A. S., Loos, W. J., Wiemer, E. A., Friberg, L. E., Verweij, J., Sparreboom, A., de Jong, F. A. (2010) A

CYP3A4 phenotype-based dosing algorithm for individualized treatment of irinotecan. *Clinical Cancer Research*, **16**, 736–742.

26 Hoskins, J. M., Carey, L. A., McLeod, H. L. (2009) CYP2D6 and tamoxifen: DNA matters in breast cancer. *Nature Reviews Cancer*, **9**, 576–586.

27 Brauch, H., Jordan, V. C. (2009) Targeting of tamoxifen to enhance antitumour action for the treatment and prevention of breast cancer: the 'personalised' approach? *European Journal of Cancer*, **45**, 2274–2283.

28 Seruga, B., Amir, E. Cytochrome P450 2D6 and outcomes of adjuvant tamoxifen therapy: results of a meta-analysis. *Breast Cancer Research and Treatment*, **122**, 609–617.

29 Sideras, K., Ingle, J. N., Ames, M. M., Loprinzi, C. L., Mrazek, D. P., Black, J. L., Weinshilboum, R. M., Hawse, J. R., Spelsberg, T. C., Goetz, M. P. (2010) Coprescription of tamoxifen and medications that inhibit CYP2D6. *Journal of Clinical Oncology*, **28**, 2768–2776.

30 Schroth, W., Goetz, M. P., Hamann, U., Fasching, P. A., Schmidt, M., Winter, S., Fritz, P., Simon, W., Suman, V. J., Ames, M. M., Safgren, S. L., Kuffel, M. J., Ulmer, H. U., Bolander, J., Strick, R., Beckmann, M. W., Koelbl, H., Weinshilboum, R. M., Ingle, J. N., Eichelbaum, M., Schwab, M., Brauch, H. (2009) Association between CYP2D6 polymorphisms and outcomes among women with early stage breast cancer treated with tamoxifen. *Journal of the American Medical Association*, **302**, 1429–1436.

31 Newman, W. G., Hadfield, K. D., Latif, A., Roberts, S. A., Shenton, A., McHague, C., Lalloo, F., Howell, S., Evans, D. G. (2008) Impaired tamoxifen metabolism reduces survival in familial breast cancer patients. *Clinical Cancer Research*, **14**, 5913–5918.

32 Kiyotani, K., Mushiroda, T., Hosono, N., Tsunoda, T., Kubo, M., Aki, F., Okazaki, Y., Hirata, K., Takatsuka, Y., Okazaki, M., Ohsumi, S., Yamakawa, T., Sasa, M., Nakamura, Y., Zembutsu, H. (2010) Lessons for pharmacogenomics studies: association study between CYP2D6 genotype and tamoxifen response. *Pharmacogenetics and Genomics*, **20**, 565–568.

33 Dezentje, V. O., van Blijderveen, N. J., Gelderblom, H., Putter, H., van Herk-Sukel, M. P., Casparie, M. K., Egberts, A. C., Nortier, J. W., Guchelaar, H. J. (2010) Effect of concomitant CYP2D6 inhibitor use and tamoxifen adherence on breast cancer recurrence in early-stage breast cancer. *Journal of Clinical Oncology*, **28**, 2423–2429.

34 Rae, J. M., Sikora, M. J., Henry, N. L., Li, L., Kim, S., Oesterreich, S., Skaar, T. C., Nguyen, A. T., Desta, Z.,

Storniolo, A. M., Flockhart, D. A., Hayes, D. F., Stearns, V. (2009) Cytochrome P450 2D6 activity predicts discontinuation of tamoxifen therapy in breast cancer patients. *The Pharmacogenomics Journal*, **9**, 258–264.

35 Kelly, C. M., Juurlink, D. N., Gomes, T., Duong-Hua, M., Pritchard, K. I., Austin, P. C., Paszat, L. F. (2009) Selective serotonin reuptake inhibitors and breast cancer mortality in women receiving tamoxifen: a population based cohort study. *British Medical Journal*, **340**. (clinical research ed.), c693.

36 Lash, T. L., Cronin-Fenton, D., Ahern, T. P., Rosenberg, C. L., Lunetta, K. L., Silliman, R. A., Hamilton-Dutoit, S., Garne, J. P., Ewertz, M., Sorensen, H. T., Pedersen, L. (2009) Breast cancer recurrence risk related to concurrent use of SSRI antidepressants and tamoxifen. *Acta Oncologica*, **49**, 305–312.

37 Ahmad, A., Shahabuddin, S., Sheikh, S., Kale, P., Krishnappa, M., Rane, R. C., Ahmad, I. (2010) Endoxifen, a new cornerstone of breast cancer therapy: demonstration of safety, tolerability, and systemic bioavailability in healthy human subjects. *Clinical Pharmacology and Therapeutics*, **88**, 814–817.

38 Stein, B., Smith, B. D. Treatment options for patients with chronic myeloid leukemia who are resistant to or unable to tolerate imatinib. *Clinical Therapeutics*, **32**, 804–820.

39 Bayraktar, U. D., Bayraktar, S., Rocha-Lima, C. M. (2010) Molecular basis and management of gastrointestinal stromal tumors. *World Journal of Gastroenterology*, **16**, 2726–2734.

40 Agrawal, M., Garg, R. J., Kantarjian, H., Cortes, J. (2010) Chronic myeloid leukemia in the tyrosine kinase inhibitor era: what is the "best" therapy? *Current Oncology Reports*, **12**, 302–313.

41 Reynoso, D., Trent, J. C. (2010) Neoadjuvant and adjuvant imatinib treatment in gastrointestinal stromal tumor: current status and recent developments. *Current Opinion in Oncology*, **22**, 330–335.

42 Lasota, J., Miettinen, M. (2008) Clinical significance of oncogenic KIT and PDGFRA mutations in gastrointestinal stromal tumours. *Histopathology*, **53**, 245–266.

43 Saridaki, Z., Georgoulias, V., Souglakos, J. (2010) Mechanisms of resistance to anti-EGFR monoclonal antibody treatment in metastatic colorectal cancer. *World Journal of Gastroenterology*, **16**, 1177–1187.

44 Karpel-Massler, G., Schmidt, U., Unterberg, A., Halatsch, M. E. (2009) Therapeutic inhibition of the epidermal growth factor receptor in high-grade

gliomas: where do we stand? *Molecular Cancer Research*, **7**, 1000–1012.

45 Roberts, P. J., Stinchcombe, T. E., Der, C. J., Socinski, M. A. (2010) Personalized medicine in non-small-cell lung cancer: is KRAS a useful marker in selecting patients for epidermal growth factor receptor-targeted therapy? *Journal of Clinical Oncology*, **28**, 4769–4777.

46 Walther, A., Johnstone, E., Swanton, C., Midgley, R., Tomlinson, I., Kerr, D. (2009) Genetic prognostic and predictive markers in colorectal cancer. *Nature Reviews Cancer*, **9**, 489–499.

47 Lievre, A., Blons, H., Laurent-Puig, P. (2011) Oncogenic mutations as predictive factors in colorectal cancer. *Oncogene*, **29**, 3033–3043.

48 Lynch, T. J., Bell, D. W., Sordella, R., Gurubhagavatula, S., Okimoto, R. A., Brannigan, B. W., Harris, P. L., Haserlat, S. M., Supko, J. G., Haluska, F. G., Louis, D. N., Christiani, D. C., Settleman, J., Haber, D. A. (2004) Activating mutations in the epidermal growth factor receptor underlying responsiveness of non-small-cell lung cancer to gefitinib. *The New England Journal of Medicine*, **350**, 2129–2139.

49 Bhushan, S., McLeod, H., Walko, C. M. (2009) Role of pharmacogenetics as predictive biomarkers of response and/or toxicity in the treatment of colorectal cancer. *Clinical Colorectal Cancer*, **8**, 15–21.

50 Baynes, R. D., Gansert, J. (2009) KRAS mutational status as a predictor of epidermal growth factor receptor inhibitor efficacy in colorectal cancer. *American Journal of Therapeutics*, **16**, 554–561.

51 Lieberman, R. (2009) Personalized medicine enters the US marketplace: KRAS, anti-EGFR monoclonal antibodies, and colon cancer. *American Journal of Therapeutics*, **16**, 477–479.

52 Flaherty, K. T., Hodi, F. S., Bastian, B. C. (2008) Mutation-driven drug development in melanoma. *Current Opinion in Oncology*, **22**, 178–183.

CHAPTER 5

Pharmacogenomic Considerations in Anesthesia and Pain Management

Christine M. Formea, PharmD[1] and Wayne T. Nicholson, MD, PharmD[2]

[1]Department of Pharmacy, College of Medicine, Mayo Clinic, Rochester, Minnesota
[2]Department of Anesthesiology, College of Medicine, Mayo Clinic, Rochester, Minnesota

Introduction

The practice of anesthesiology is often thought of as a medical specialty primarily based in the operating room. However, the practice also encompasses critical care medicine and pain management. Due to the criticality and comorbidities of patients, today's anesthesiology practitioner often is faced with numerous pharmacologic challenges. These include adverse drug reactions due to drug–drug interactions, poor metabolism, and altered drug response due to pathology. These issues may be further complicated by pharmacodynamic or pharmacokinetic alterations caused by genetics.

As of January 1, 2002, there were more than 300 dietary supplements, 600 herbal products, and 3,200 prescription drugs on the market in the United States (1). Adverse drug reactions (ADRs) were estimated to be the cause of 106,000 hospitalized patient deaths in 1994, making these reactions between the fourth and sixth leading cause of death within the United States (2). Drug-related morbidity and mortality were estimated to cost $76.6 billion in the ambulatory setting in the United States, with the greatest component of this cost associated with drug related hospitalizations (3). In hospitalized patients, lengths of stay attributable to adverse drug events were significantly prolonged and were associated with an almost twofold increased risk of death (4). Additionally, during the period of 1998–2005, deaths and serious injuries associated with drug

therapy reported to the U.S. Food and Drug Administration (FDA) showed a marked increase (5). Using these considerations as a background, it would appear that earlier prediction of ADRs would be essential for the ability to decrease drug-induced morbidity and mortality. The hope of employing pharmacogenomics considerations in practice has the potential to assist practitioners by reducing and preventing ADRs (6).

Historical perspective

Heritability of genetic traits has been a subject of human interest for centuries. The practice of plant selection and cultivation was the basis for Gregor Mendel's observations that resulted in his description of rules of heredity in 1866 (6, 7). During the subsequent twentieth century, scientific discoveries exponentially increased with advancement of molecular genetic technologies and expansion of genetic and pharmacologic knowledge. Explosive growth can be measured from William Bateson's new term *genetics*, coined around 1910, to the completion of the first draft of the human genome sequence in 2001 (6–9).

The 1950s was the decade in which pharmacogenetics emerged as a new and respected discipline. The field was first described by Arno Motulsky in 1957, when he wrote "Drug Reactions, Enzymes, and Biochemical Genetics" at the invitation of an

Pharmacogenomics in Clinical Therapeutics, First Edition. Edited by Loralie J. Langman and Amitava Dasgupta.
© 2012 John Wiley & Sons, Ltd. Published 2012 by John Wiley & Sons, Ltd.

American Medical Association committee and posited that genetic inheritance might contribute to variability in drug efficacy and toxicity (6, 10, 11). The field of pharmacogenetics was born and was formally coined in 1959 by Frederick Vogel, and in 1962 Werner Kalow's monograph firmly established pharmacogenetics as a discipline (6, 10). Anesthesiology was one of the first areas of medicine to demonstrate variability in drug response due to underlying genetic variations in enzymatic activity and contribute to the emergence of *pharmacogenetics*, the melding of pharmacology and genetics. Key anesthesiology examples include elucidation of pseudocholinesterase enzyme deficiency, malignant hyperthermia, and opioid metabolism in pain syndromes.

In 1953, Watson and Crick described the double helical nature of deoxyribonucleic acid (DNA) (12). In 1956, succinylcholine was identified as the drug responsible for an unanticipated drug response of prolonged apnea in some patients due to genetic variability in plasma cholinesterase (butyrylcholinesterase) enzyme activity (6, 7, 13). Succinylcholine was used as an adjunct to anesthesia as a short-acting paralytic agent used to facilitate mechanical ventilation during surgery and in psychiatry to prevent muscular contractions resulting from electroshock therapy. Due to the rapid drug destruction by plasma cholinesterase in most patients, the effect of succinylcholine would last a few minutes; however, some patients would experience paralysis for an hour or more (13).

A suspected familial link between general anesthetics and hyperthermia was first described by reports in 1960 and 1962 (14, 15). Further elucidation followed, and *malignant hyperthermia* was the term eventually given to the condition of hyperthermia, muscle contracture and rigidity, and myolysis after exposure to succinylcholine and/or halothane (13, 16, 17). Since the initial identification of a potential familial disorder in the early 1960s, there have been nearly 200 genetic variants identified in the RYR1 gene that control the skeletal muscle sarcoplasmic reticulum calcium channel using molecular genetic techniques and technologies (18).

Scientific advancements in molecular genetics advanced pharmacogenetics in the following dec-

ades. In the 1970s, an important genetic polymorphism was inadvertently identified when it impacted the metabolism of debrisoquine/sparteine, resulting in unexpected side effects to pharmacokinetics study volunteers. This genetic variation was finally attributed to CYP2D6 in the 1980s (6, 19). This oxidative Phase I metabolism system affects clearance of many drugs including opioids, antidepressants, and antiarrhythmics. Opioid drugs including codeine, dihydrocodeine, hydrocodone, oxycodone, and tramadol require activation by CYP2D6; however, individuals with slower CYP2D6 enzyme activity have incomplete conversion to active metabolites, resulting in reduced clinical efficacy producing large interindividual variability in opioid response (6, 17, 18, 20). Presently, research continues at the level of the mu-opioid receptor to elucidate the relationships between gene expression and variability in morphine analgesic response.

During the last 50 years of advancements in anesthesiology, from the identification and characterization of pseudocholinesterase deficiency to molecular investigations involving mu-opioid receptors, the importance of genetic factors has been recognized in contributing to wide interindividual variability in drug response. Advances in molecular genetics, biomedical technology, and the completion of the Human Genome Project continue to move the practice toward the future of individualized medicine.

Pharmacogenetics or pharmacogenomics?

Pharmacogenetics is the discipline of evaluating inherited differences in individual drug response that originally stemmed from collaborative work in pharmacology and genetics beginning 50 years ago (6, 10). With the increasing importance of a whole genome approach to drug response, pharmacogenetics has evolved into pharmacogenomics. Often the two terms are used interchangeably. Pharmacogenomics aims to evaluate the relationship of whole genome relationships to phenotypic drug responses and has been made possible because of successful mapping of the human genome and improved molecular biology and pharmacology techniques (6, 10, 18).

Drug metabolism

The liver is the organ primarily responsible for bio-transforming endogenous compounds and exogenous lipophilic chemicals into water-soluble substances that are more easily eliminated from the body. The process of drug biotransformation is accomplished by two categories of reactions: phase I and phase II. Phase I reactions involve oxidation, reduction, or hydrolysis. Phase II biosynthetic conjugation reactions involve glucuronidation, sulfation, acetylation, methylation, glutathione conjugation, or amino acid conjugation to endogenous substrates or phase I metabolic products. Collectively, both phase I and phase II reactions result in increased metabolite polarity and hydrophilicity, resulting in enhanced renal elimination from the body (21).

Pharmacokinetics
Drug-metabolizing enzymes
Genetic variability of enzymes and biosynthetic conjugations involved with phase I and phase II drug metabolism can impact the rate and extent of drug action and can have important clinical consequences (17, 19, 22). This variability is especially important for drugs used in anesthesia and pain management (19). Individuals with a poor or slow metabolizer phenotype have deficient metabolism and likely require reductions in drug doses to prevent toxicities and to obtain a therapeutic drug response (17, 19). In contrast, individuals with a rapid or extensive metabolizer phenotype have higher levels of metabolism and likely require increased drug doses to prevent therapeutic failure (17, 19).

Phase I enzymes
CYP P450
In order to appropriately identify cytochrome P450 metabolic enzymes, a standardized nomenclature has been developed for cytochrome isoenzymes. Cytochrome "CYP" root is followed by an Arabic number designating the enzyme family (i.e., CYP2),

which is followed by the subfamily letter (i.e., CYP2D). An Arabic number is the final identifier for the individual gene of interest (i.e., CYP2D6) (19, 23).

Cytochrome P450 enzymes compose an important superfamily of enzymes of which families 1–3 are responsible for 70–80% of phase I oxidative drug metabolism (24). The CYP superfamily of enzymes metabolizes endogenous biological substances such as lipids and steroids and exogenous compounds such as drugs. CYP P450 enzymes are contained in the greatest amount in the liver; however, CYP P450 enzymes are located throughout the human body in areas including the intestines, kidneys, lungs, and brain (23, 25). CYP P450 activity is influenced by numerous factors including age, sex, concomitant drugs, disease states, genetics, surgery, nutritional status, and environment (17, 19, 23).

Of the 57 identified CYP450 genes in humans, contributions from the CYP1, CYP2, and CYP3 enzyme families appear to be the most active in the metabolism of drugs (17, 23, 26). The most important CYP450 enzymes to anesthesia providers include the CYP2C, CYP2D, and CYP3A subfamilies. While CYP2E1 contributes to an estimated 1% of the total drugs metabolized, and its clinically relevant drug substrates include halothane, isoflurane, enflurane, sevoflurane, methoxyflurane, and acetaminophen, no clinically relevant genetic variants have been associated with this enzyme (17, 23, 25).

CYP2C
CYP2C enzymes of interest to anesthesia providers include CYP2C9 and CYP2C19. The estimated CYP2C enzymatic contribution to the total percentage of drugs metabolized is about 18% (23). Important CYP2C9 drug substrates include phenytoin, warfarin, oral hypoglycemics, and nonsteroidal anti-inflammatory drugs (NSAIDs) such as ibuprofen, naproxen, and diclofenac (23, 25). Clinically important relationships have been identified between CYP2C9 genetic polymorphisms and narrow therapeutic window drugs phenytoin and warfarin, leading to CYP2C9 genetic testing to aid identification of individuals with impaired metabolism (23–25). Further study is needed to understand the clinical impact of CYP2C9 genetic variants on

other drugs metabolized by this pathway (23). Important drug substrates of CYP2C19 include clopidogrel, diazepam, barbiturates, phenytoin, citalopram, amitriptyline, and proton pump inhibitors (27, 28). Clinically important relationships have been identified in poor CYP2C19 poor metabolizers with drugs such as diazepam. Diazepam is a drug used for sedation that demonstrates twice the elimination half-life in CYP2C19 poor metabolizers as compared to extensive metabolizers, resulting in prolonged sedation (19, 29).

CYP2D6

CYP2D6 is another important drug metabolizing enzyme that is highly polymorphic with 100 variant genes identified (18, 20). Four main CYP2D phenotypes have been characterized: poor, intermediate, extensive, and ultra-rapid metabolizers. Poor metabolizers lack enzyme activity; intermediate metabolizers have one allele lacking enzymatic activity or two alleles with reduced enzyme activity; extensive metabolizers have two normal enzymatic activity alleles; and ultra-rapid metabolizers have three or more copies of enzymatic genes, resulting in high enzymatic activity (24).

CYP2D6 is responsible for around 25% of total phase I drug biotransformation reactions of drugs, including antidepressants, antiarrhythmics, betablockers, neuroleptics, antiemetics, and anesthetic agents (17, 23). Important anesthesia drugs impacted by CYP2D6 metabolism include codeine, tramadol, oxycodone, hydrocodone, methadone, ondansetron, and granisteron (17–19, 23). Individuals who are CYP2D6 poor metabolizers are not able to convert codeine to morphine by CYP2D6-mediated demethylation, and as a result, these individuals do not experience morphine's potent analgesic effects but are likely to experience parent drug side effects (17, 19, 25). Conversely, individuals who are CYP2D6 ultra-rapid metabolizers rapidly and effectively convert codeine to morphine, and as a result, these individuals are more likely to experience excessive morphine effects and toxicities from the effects of the metabolite (17, 19, 25). Observable postoperative drug effects of opioid analgesics and anti-emetics may be attributable to CYP2D6 genetic variability. Although increasing CYP2D6 genotype testing is occurring for patients undergoing treatment for breast cancer and psychiatric diagnoses, CYP2D6 genotype testing is not routinely performed in patients undergoing surgery and anesthesia.

CYP3A

CYP3A enzymes are abundantly expressed in the intestinal epithelium and liver and are responsible for metabolizing more than 60% of commonly used medications including opioid analgesics (e.g., fentanyl), benzodiazepines (e.g., midazolam), local anesthetics (e.g., lidocaine), immunosuppressants (e.g., tacrolimus), calcium antagonists (e.g., diltiazem), antiarrhythmics (e.g., quinidine), antimicrobials (e.g., erythromycin), antiretrovirals (e.g., indinivir), and HMG CoA-reductase inhibitors (e.g., atorvastatin) (23, 25, 28). As a result, CYP3A is vital to first-pass metabolism of medications. The CYP3A family includes CYP3A4 and CYP3A5. While CYP3A4 and CYP3A5 demonstrate similar substrate specificity, CYP3A4 is more abundantly expressed and is clinically more important (23, 26). While CYP3A5 demonstrates genetic variability and generally slower metabolism compared to CYP3A4, genetic variations have not been shown to result in clinically meaningful changes in CYP3A activity requiring medication dose alterations (23, 25). For this reason, CYP3A genotype testing is not routinely performed in patients undergoing surgery and anesthesia.

Phase II-conjugation enzymes
UGT-glucuronosyltransferase

Generally, phase II conjugation enzymes are located in microsomal cytosol with the exception of uridine diphosphate glucuronosyltransferases (UGTs), which is located on the endoplasmic reticulum (25). Most drugs that undergo phase II metabolism are glucuronidated by UGTs. Although found mainly in the liver, UGTs are found throughout the body in the kidney, colon, prostate, stomach, and small intestine (25). Genetic polymorphisms exist in phase II enzymes, including UGTs, N-acetyltransferases (NATs), glutathione-S-transferases (GSTs), and sulfotransferases (STs). Wide interpatient variability in postsurgical opioid use has been observed, and contributing factors have been investigated including genetic variation of UGTs' glucuronidation of opioids (17, 19, 22, 25).

While glucuronidation generally reduces pharmacological activity, in the case of morphine, the glucuronidated product known as morphine 6-glucuronide has higher analgesic potency than morphine (25, 30). Surgical patients with two copies of UGT variant genes have been shown to glucuronidate morphine faster than patients with one copy of the variant gene or no variant genes (22, 31). Conflicting results of pharmacogenomics studies suggest that polymorphic UGTs impact opioid glucuronidation and result in altered metabolism of opiates; however, the clinical relevance remains to be elucidated (18, 20, 22, 30).

Polymorphisms in drug transport proteins
P-glycoprotein

Drug transport proteins mediate drug absorption across biological membranes in the intestines, kidneys, liver, and blood–brain barrier (17, 18). Uptake and efflux activities of transporters ultimately impact the bioavailability of oral drug absorption, distribution, and elimination (20). P-glycoprotein (P-gp) functions as an ATP-dependent efflux pump for many classes of substrates including analgesics (morphine, fentanyl, methadone, and sufentanil), antiarrhythmics (e.g., amiodarone), and antiemetics (e.g., ondansetron) (18, 19, 25). As an important result of P-gp localization at the blood–brain barrier, opioids may have variable distribution into the CNS to reach their primary site of action (18, 20, 22). Thus, variable genetic expression of P-gp in the blood–brain barrier may impact the clinical efficacy of analgesia by enhancing or preventing morphine and other opiates from entering the brain (17).

P-gp is under the control of the polymorphic multidrug resistance (MDR1) gene and results in widely variable expression of P-gp proteins among individuals. In healthy individuals, hepatic P-gp protein levels may vary 20–50-fold, while intestinal P-gp protein levels may vary two- to 10-fold (20, 32–34). Although more than 100 polymorphisms have been identified in MDR1, association studies involving opioids have yielded inconsistent results that were potentially confounded by ethnicity, diet, and xenobiotics (18–20). The clinical relevance of P-gp genetic variability remains to be elucidated.

Pharmacodynamics
Polymorphisms of drug receptors and targets

As protein products of genetic expression, drug receptors and targets may be influenced by genetic polymorphisms. Genetic variability of receptors and targets may result in wide differences in response and sensitivity to anesthetic and analgesic drugs between individuals.

Ryanodine receptors

Malignant hyperthermia is a rare hypermetabolic disorder of skeletal muscle that has been associated with genetic variants of the ryanodine receptor (RYR1) gene and exposure to specific anesthetic drugs (18). Briefly, when susceptible patients are exposed to volatile anesthetics (e.g., halothane and isoflurane) and/or intravenous depolarizing muscle relaxants (i.e., succinylcholine), they may experience hyperthermia, hyperkalemia, acidosis, rhabdomyolysis, and multi-organ failure as a result of uncontrolled calcium release from skeletal muscle cells (18, 22). While nearly 200 mutations of RYR1 exist, only about 50% of MHS cases have been associated with genetic mutations of the RYR1 gene (17–19, 22). Increasing evidence suggests that in addition to RYR1 genetic variants, MHS results from additional complex genetic interactions (18).

Opioid receptors

Morphine and other opioid analgesics are used in the treatment of acute and chronic pain syndromes and bind to mu-opioid receptors located in the central nervous system (CNS). In increasing doses, physiologic effects of opioid drugs include pain relief, sedation, and respiratory depression. Genetic variability has been investigated as one factor contributing to wide interindividual sensitivity to pain and variable analgesic dosing requirements (18). The polymorphic OPRM1 gene encodes mu-opioid receptors, and approximately 100 genetic variants have been identified in OPRM1 (18, 20). To date, clinical studies have yielded conflicting results but suggest that patients have genetically mediated opioid requirements and pain sensitivity (18–20).

Emerging drug receptor and targets

Investigations continue into wide interpatient variability in anesthetic and analgesic drug response. Many factors may influence and contribute to variable human pain sensitivity and associated drug response including pain physiology pathways, environment, and culture (20). Active areas of molecular genetic and phenotypic association studies include catechol-O-methyltransferase (COMT), γ-aminobutyric acid type A (GABA$_A$) receptor, N-methyl-D-aspartate (NMDA) receptor, and serotonin transporter (5-HTT) (17–20, 35, 36).

Additional considerations

Pseudocholinesterase deficiency

One of the earliest pharmacogenetic discoveries was prolonged apnea and muscle relaxation following the administration of succinylcholine (suxamethonium).[15] This adverse drug effect is due to decreased metabolism of succinylcholine by the plasma cholinesterase enzyme. Plasma cholinesterase is also commonly described in the literature as pseudocholinesterase and frequently as butyrylcholinesterase, since it hydrolyzes butyryl acetylcholine better than acetylcholine (37, 38). Although presentation of this condition is rare, the routine use of succinylcholine makes pseudocholinesterase function a consideration for potential clinical adverse effects.

Under normal conditions, pseudocholinesterase causes hydrolysis of the majority of the administered succinylcholine dose prior to the interaction with the neuromuscular junction (39). This hydrolysis accounts for approximately 90% to 95% of the dose administered (40). The remaining succinylcholine acts as receptor agonist at the neuromuscular junction, causing prolonged depolarization of skeletal muscle (40). Following initial depolarization skeletal muscle paralysis occurs. Inadequate hydrolysis of succinylcholine due to poor enzyme metabolism leads to a higher availability, resulting in increased duration of paralysis (40).

Currently, succinylcholine is the only depolarizing neuromuscular blocking agent available. It has been in clinical use since the early 1950s, and it remains a mainstay due to its pharmacologic effects resulting in quick onset and duration. Following administration, the onset of skeletal muscle relaxation occurs rapidly usually within 30–60 seconds, which facilitates conditions for endotracheal intubation. In addition to the rapid onset the short duration of action of 3 to 5 minutes allows for quick recovery (39). It is unlikely that decreased succinylcholine metabolism would be noted clinically until pseudocholinesterase metabolism is reduced to less than 75% of normal (39, 40). Although the pharmacologic profile of succinylcholine is beneficial, the adverse effect profile is less than ideal. These ADRs include cardiac dysrhythmias, muscle fasciculations, hyperkalemia, and prolonged neuromuscular blockade that may result in respiratory compromise. Due to the potential for adverse effects, research for new neuromuscular blocking agents has been performed by the pharmaceutical industry. However, the pharmacologic profile exhibited by succinylcholine has not been reproduced by currently available nondepolarizing agents, and it remains in clinical use.

Additionally, other medications undergo ester hydrolysis by pseudocholinesterase. Prolonged paralysis has also been seen with the nondepolarizing neuromuscular junction blocker mivacurium in individuals with pseudocholinesterase deficiency. Mivacurium induced neuromuscular blockade can be prolonged up to 6 to 8 hours from a normal duration of 30 minutes in individuals homozygous for the atypical or silent genetic variants (41). However, the manufacturer has discontinued mivacurium production, and it is no longer used in current practice. Cocaine, procaine, and tetracaine are ester local anesthetics that undergo hydrolysis by pseudocholinesterase (40, 42).

Genetic variations for altered metabolism by pseudocholinesterase are associated with chromosome 3 and are more common in individuals of European descent (40). Homozygotes for the U type (usual) or wild type have a phenotype demonstrating an enzyme of normal concentration and activity. It is estimated that approximately 96% of the population is homozygous for the U type (40). Inadequate metabolism by this enzyme is rare, and only a limited number of the population is homozygous or heterozygous for atypical alleles resulting in adverse clinical outcomes. These allelic variants involved with inadequate metabolism include the A, F, S, H, J, and K subtypes. Three of these variants have altered hydrolyzing ability (A, F, and S) and the remaining three subtypes (H, J, and K) are associated with decreased concentration but normal activity (43). The A or atypical variant is dibucaine resistant and along with the fluoride-resistant or F variant both demonstrate reduced metabolic activity. The S or silent variant is associated with no enzyme activity. S-variant homozygotes have the greatest reduction in metabolism and succinylcholine action may be increased as much as 8 hours (40). Reduction in concentration is associated with H, J, or K variants and leads to approximately a 10, 33, or 66% reduced pseudocholinesterase enzyme concentration, respectively (43). Some of these variants may not produce clinically significant apnea with succinylcholine since the duration of the surgery is longer than the apneic period (39).

In addition to genetic causes, atypical metabolism involving lowered plasma pseudocholinesterase may be related to physiological alterations, pathological conditions, and medications. Drugs that inhibit pseudocholinesterase include acetylcholinesterase inhibitors, pancuronium, procaine, and organophosphate pesticides, whereas chemotherapeutic drugs and steroids may decrease synthesis (39). Additionally, pathology (e.g., hepatic disease) or physiologic changes (e.g., pregnancy) alter concentrations of pseudocholinesterase. It is likely these considerations gain a greater importance in the presence of genetic reductions of pseudocholinesterase.

There are several methods for testing pseudocholinesterase deficiency. Determination of total serum cholinesterase, a dibucaine number, and a fluoride number are laboratory analyses that may be performed. When considering a dibucaine number, homozygous typical individuals demonstrate 70–80% pseudocholinesterase inhibition by dibucaine (39). A 50–60% inhibition would be indicative of a heterozygous presentation (39). Atypical homozygotes demonstrate less than 30% inhibition by dibucaine. (39). A test of pseudocholinesterase enzyme activity can be also be performed using the Acholest test paper. This test elicits a color change over time. The amount of time required to change the color

from green to yellow is inversely proportional to the pseudocholinesterase enzyme activity in the plasma sample (40). Additionally, molecular genetic techniques such as polymerase chain reaction (PCR) amplification with allele-specific oligonucleotide probes for identifying abnormal pseudocholinesterase genotypes may also be performed at some institutions (40).

Malignant hyperthermia

Malignant hyperthermia (MH) or malignant hyperthermia syndrome (MHS) is a life threatening, hypermetabolic state that occurs after exposure to anesthesia with MH-triggering agents such as volatile halogenated anesthesia agents and/or succinylcholine (44). Examples of volatile agents that cause MH include halothane, isoflurane, desflurane, and sevoflurane. Although these triggering agents are commonly found within the practice of anesthesiology, there are many agents for anesthetic use that are known to be safe for MH patients. These include, barbiturates, benzodiazepines, opioids, and nondepolarizing neuromuscular junction blockers (45) (Table 5.1). MH is a rare condition with an estimated incidence of 1:5,000 to 1:50,000 in adults and 1:15,000 in children (46, 47).

This pharmacogenetic clinical syndrome is autosomal dominant in inheritance. Susceptible MH patients present as phenotypically normal and display the clinical sequelae of MH only after exposure to a triggering agent. The most common genetic mutation occurs in a gene on chromosome 19q13.1.for the ryanodine receptor (RYR1) (48). Past analysis of MH patients in the United Kingdom

Table 5.1 Anesthetic Considerations with Malignant Hyperthermia (45)

Known Triggers of MH	Example of Anesthesia Agents Safe for MH Patients	
Succinylcholine	Diazepam	Fentanyl
Desflurane	Etomidate	Hydromorphone
Enflurane	Ketamine	Morphine
Halothane	Midazolam	Meperidine
Isoflurane	Propofol	Cisatracurium
Methoxyflurane	Thiopental	Vecuronium
Sevoflurane	Nitrous Oxide	Rocuronium

has indicated that mutations in the RYR1 gene are responsible for approximately 50% of MH cases; however, technological advances in sequencing suggest mutations involving this gene may be more in the order of 70% of MH cases (49). In addition to the mutations in the RYR1 gene, other genetic associations have also been identified. Two mutations in the dihydropyridine receptor DHP have been implicated, 7q21–q22, the site of coding for the $alpha_2$/delta subunit of the dihydropyridine receptor and 1q32, associated with the gene encoding the $alpha_1$ subunit of the dihydropyridine receptor (50, 51). Additionally, a mutation on chromosome 17q11.2–q24, which is associated with the voltage-dependent sodium channel of the skeletal muscle membrane, has been studied (52, 53). Other loci have also been described in the literature (54). These multiple loci associations cause genetic testing sensitivity to be an issue.

When considering the mechanism of this syndrome, ryanodine receptors, dihydropyridine receptors, and voltage-regulated channels are involved with the maintenance of calcium between the sarcoplasmic reticulum and the sarcoplasm. In an MH-susceptible patient following exposure to a triggering agent, a rapid release of calcium from the sarcoplasmic reticulum occurs. This results in sustained muscle cell contraction, a high metabolic state, and cellular ATP depletion. If this process continues untreated, this leads to muscle cell destruction (rhabdomyolysis), multiple organ failure, and eventual fatality.

Several clinical signs and laboratory findings are present with MH (44, 48). Early signs seen include the increased end tidal concentration of carbon dioxide or masseter muscle rigidity after succinylcholine administration. Generalized muscle rigidity and hyperthermia, often considered the hallmark of this syndrome, may not be noted until later. Red-brown colored urine due to myoglobin present in the urine following rhabdomyolysis and arrhythmias secondary to intracellular potassium release may also occur. Nonspecific signs of MH include tachycardia, tachypnea, and hypertension. Alterations in laboratory findings include increased PCO_2, acidosis, hyperkalemia, increased creatinine kinase, and abnormal coagulation tests.

Early recognition and treatment have decreased mortality from 80% 30 years ago to less than 5% today (47) Currently, the skeletal muscle relaxant dantrolene sodium is the only available pharmacologic therapy of the MH syndrome in humans (55). Dantrolene acts on the ryanodine receptor, causing it to favor the closed state, thereby reversing the uninhibited flow of calcium into the sarcoplasm (48). This decreases the imbalance of calcium and exaggerated excitation–contraction coupling in skeletal muscle (55). Other supportive treatment of MH includes discontinuation of the triggering agent, hyperventilatation with 100% oxygen, and cooling the patient with temperatures $>39\,°C$. As this syndrome progresses, prompt treatment of metabolic acidosis, hyperkalemia, and cardiac dysrhythmias is essential. Although standard therapy is administered for these accompanying conditions, it is important to note that calcium channel blockers are not to be used in therapy of dysrhythmias since they may cause hyperkalemia or cardiac arrest in the presence of dantrolene (56).

When testing susceptibility in an individual with suspected MH, the common method for determination is the caffeine–halothane contracture test (CHCT) (57). The CHCT will require approximately 2 grams of skeletal muscle, usually from the patient's thigh. In a laboratory setting, the force of muscle contraction is measured by two separate measurements following exposure to caffeine and halothane. The goal of CHCT is to compare the strength of contracture with established standards resulting in the determination of MH susceptibility. The sensitivity of the CHCT is approximately 97%; however, the specificity is somewhat lower, 78%, leading to a false positive diagnosis in some patients (58). As the expense of this test may exceed US$5,000, this test is only performed on patients with a suspected MH episode or family members of known MH patients. Currently, testing is offered at limited sites within the United States and Canada, including Maryland, California, Minnesota, North Carolina, and Ontario.

Due to the invasive procedure involved with the CHCT, molecular genetic testing would be an attractive alternative. However, as suggested earlier, although the genetic test is very specific, it is not highly sensitive (25–30%) due to numerous mutations that may occur (59). Since a negative genetic result does not ensure a diagnosis of MH, it is important to explain to a patient the need for CHCT in case of a negative genetic test result (60). The Malignant Hyperthermia Association of the United States (MHAUS) has identified several types of individuals who may benefit from molecular genetic testing (59). These include patients who have tested CHCT positive or relatives of those who have been tested positive by CHCT. In addition, genetic testing could be considered for relatives of those with a known mutation for malignant hyperthermia and individuals with a very high likelihood of having experienced an MH episode. A meeting of geneticists and MH researchers concluded that even with a sensitivity of 23% in the small population of North American patients studied, examination of a limited number of RYR1 exons is practical (61). Currently, clinical molecular genetic testing is available at two sites in the United States, in Pennsylvania and Wisconsin.

Postoperative nausea and vomiting

Postoperative nausea and vomiting (PONV) is a widely recognized complication of anesthesia and surgery that may occur in 20% to 30% of general surgical patients or up to 80% in high-risk surgical patients (62–64). PONV may result in additional postoperative morbidity, including surgical site dehiscence, bleeding, dehydration, electrolyte abnormalities, hypertension, and airway compromise (65). Four risk factors have been identified that predict PONV, including female sex, nonsmoking status, postoperative opioid use, and a history of motion sickness or PONV. The presence of three or four of these risk factors correlated with a 61% and 79% incidence of PONV, respectively (63). Other PONV risk factors may include age, type of surgery, use of volatile anesthetics, duration of anesthesia, and anesthesia type (e.g., general versus regional) (64).

In PONV, serotonin binds 5-hydroxytryptamine type 3 (5-HT_3) receptors that are located centrally in the chemoreceptor trigger zone and peripherally in vagal nerve terminals (66, 67). Stimulation of the central 5-HT_3 receptors initiates the vomiting reflex through activation of the vomiting center located in the medulla oblongata, while peripheral 5-HT_3 receptor stimulation results in activation of the vomiting center through the nucleus tractus solitarius (66, 67). Other neurotransmitters are believed to contribute to PONV, including acetylcholine, dopamine, histamine, muscarine, neurokinin-1, and opioids (67). In order to prevent emetogenic signals from reaching the vomiting center, 5-HT_3 receptor antagonists were developed to selectively and competitively bind serotonin receptors both centrally and peripherally. Drug receptor affinity and selectivity vary between agents and may impact clinical efficacy. Five 5-HT_3 receptor antagonists are used to treatment PONV in the United States and Europe, including ondansetron, granisetron, dolasetron, palonosetron, and tropisetron (66). Interestingly, use of 5-HT_3 receptor antagonists has reduced but not completely eliminated the risk of PONV. Therapeutic failure may be explained by variability in drug metabolism, which provides an opportunity for exploring the potential role of pharmacogenomics in individual drug response.

All of the 5-HT_3 receptor antagonists are metabolized by hepatic cytochrome (CYP) P450 isoenzymes. The CYP P450 system oxidizes endogenous substances such as steroids and fatty acids and exogenous drug compounds by various isoenzymes including 1A2, 2C9, 2C19, 2D6, 2E1, and 3A4 (62). CYP2D6 is responsible for metabolism of approximately 25% of drugs used clinically, including 5-HT_3 receptor antagonists (67). Ondansetron, dolasetron, palonosetron, and tropisetron are metabolized by CYP2D6 to varying extents. Ondansetron is metabolized by CYP2D6, CYP3A4, CYP1A2, and CYP2E1. Dolasetron is activated to its active metabolite hydrodolasetron by carbonyl reductase, which is then degraded by CYP2D6 and CYP3A4. Palonosetron is metabolized by CYP2D6, CYP3A4, and CY1A1/2. Tropisetron is degraded by CYP2D6 and CYP3A4 (62). In contrast to the other four agents, granisetron is metabolized primarily by CYP3A4 and is not metabolized by the CYP2D6 pathway (62). The impact of genetic polymorphisms in CYP2D6 has not been fully elucidated in clinical practice; however, pharmacogenomics studies conducted to date suggest that a relationship exists between CYP2D6 genotype and 5-HT3 receptor antagonists and that PONV antiemetic therapy might be individualized based upon the CYP2D6 genotype (62, 68, 69). Prospective gene–association studies are needed to further elucidate pharmacogenomics relationships in PONV.

Analgesics

Pain is one leading reason that an individual will seek medical attention (70, 71). When comparing the incidence of pain to other major conditions, it is estimated that pain affects more Americans than diabetes, heart disease, and cancer combined (72). Analgesics are subject to genomic variation and have been of great interest due to their adverse event profile and widespread use. Commonly used analgesics both in the surgical and outpatient areas include opioids and nonsteroidal anti-inflammatory drugs. Additionally, tricyclic antidepressants are often used for neuropathic pain.

Opioids have been the mainstay for pain management due to their ability to mimic endogenous pain-reducing substances (e.g., endorphins) at the mu receptor. However, limitations may include physical dependence, tolerance, sedation, respiratory depression, and nausea or vomiting. Opioids are classified by chemical structure. *Opiates* are derived from the poppy *Papaver somniferum*, include the natural compounds (e.g., morphine and codeine), and are in the phenanthrene class. *Opioids* include all of the agents (natural and synthetic) that have morphine-like properties. The phenylpiperidines meperidine and fentanyl are examples of purely synthetic opioids.

Opioids demonstrate variability in both pharmacokinetics and pharmacodynamics. Some of this interpatient variability is attributable to disease states, physiologic changes, and environmental factors (20). In addition to these factors, pharmacodynamic variability can cause genetic differences. The *OPRM1* gene responsible for the mu receptor has over 100 identified variants (73). The most common variant is the substitution of adenine (A) to guanine (G) at position 118. The frequency of occurrence appears to be greater in the Asian population.

There have been numerous studies examining the *OPRM1* A118G polymorphism in the literature. Although no functional association has been demonstrated conclusively with drug dependence, there

appears to be a requirement for increased doses needed for analgesia (20). Patients undergoing laparoscopic abdominal surgery receiving fentanyl analgesia demonstrated a decreased analgesic response and decreased time to awakening and extubation, but no clinically significant effect on the incidence of respiratory depression (74). In a study of colorectal surgery patients, there was no effect of the A118G polymorphism on morphine dose requirements or side effects; however, there was a trend for higher doses in those with the G variant allele (20, 75). The higher dose requirements were also demonstrated in a postoperative pain study of Asian patients. Morphine PCA requirements were greater in participants with the homozygous variant of A118G than the heterozygous or the wild-type presentation (76).

Opioid pharmacokinetics can demonstrate variability by alteration of distribution by transporters or metabolism. P-glycoprotein (P-gp) is an efflux transporter which acts to decrease concentrations of drugs by actively pumping substrates out of tissues (77). P-gp is present in many tissues including the gastrointestinal tract and the central nervous system. The multidrug resistance gene *ABCB1* (adenosine triphosphate-binding cassette, subfamily B, member 1) encodes for P-gp and with over 100 SNPs previously identified, and may cause alteration of P-gp expression or function (20, 75). These alterations potentially allow greater concentrations of opioids to enter into the CNS following distribution across the blood–brain barrier. The most studied polymorphism for *ABCB1* and opioid effects is the C3435T polymorphism, where it would be expected that T-variant homozygotes would have increased analgesia and adverse effect profile due to an ineffective efflux pump (20, 78).

Functional studies of the C3435T polymorphism demonstrate somewhat mixed outcomes and might be more predictive of adverse drug reactions. In surgical patients receiving morphine, there was no significant association between the C3435T polymorphism and postoperative morphine dose requirements; however, there was an association with the requirement for nausea and vomiting therapy (75). Fentanyl-induced respiratory depression was associated with *ABCB1* polymorphisms; however, there was no significant correlation between *ABCB1* gene polymorphisms and a sedative effect (77). In contrast, chronic pain patients receiving morphine displayed a statistically significant functional effect of the C3435T polymorphism on morphine pain relief and predictability of response, and had an increased significance when correlated with the A118G SNP in the *OPRM1* gene (78). Additionally, haplotype analysis for *ABCB1* gene may be more predictive for dose requirement. In therapy of opioid dependence with methadone, patients carrying two copies of the wild-type haplotype required higher methadone doses when compared with one or both variants (79). Outcome differences in these studies may be due to additional population variation or sample size; however, it appears that haplotype or multiple-gene analysis may provide an interpretative advantage for prediction of analgesia and adverse effects related to *ABCB1* variants.

In addition to distributional changes via transporter polymorphisms, opioid pharmacokinetics may be altered by genomic differences in metabolism (Table 5.2) (70, 80, 81). The CYP2D6 gene is highly polymorphic, with 100 allelic variants identified (20). The CYP2D6 enzyme metabolizes the codeine to the more active compound morphine via O-demethylation. Morphine has 200-fold greater affinity for the mu receptor compared with codeine (82). Individuals deficient of CYP2D6 activity (poor metabolizer) will not convert codeine to morphine, and postoperative pain management with codeine-containing drugs will have limited effect (83).

The codeine derivatives oxycodone and hydrocodone are also transformed by CYP2D6 to the more potent active metabolites oxymorphone and hydromorphone, respectively. Although, CYP3A-mediated N-demethylation is the principal metabolic pathway of oxycodone in humans, O-demethylation to oxymorphone by CYP2D6 has been reported to account for 11% of oxycodone dose (20, 84). Additionally, five- to 10-fold higher plasma hydromorphone concentrations have been reported in extensive metabolizers compared with poor metabolizers following hydrocodone administration establishing the importance of CYP2D6 in this metabolic pathway (20, 85). Although hydrocodone and oxycodone undergo metabolism to active metabolites which may provide analgesia, unlike codeine,

Table 5.2 Examples of Opioid Metabolism and Active Metabolites Providing Analgesia (70, 80, 81)

Drug	Enzyme	Metabolite
Phase I		
Codeine	CYP2D6	Morphine
Hydrocodone	CYP2D6	Hydromorphone
Oxycodone	CYP2D6	Oxymorphone
	CYP3A4	Noroxycodone
Tramadol	CYP2D6	O-desmethyltramadol
	CYP3A4	
Fentanyl	CYP3A4	
Meperidine	CYP3A4	
	CYP2B6	
	CYP2C19	
Methadone	CYP3A4	
	CYP2B6	
	CYP2C8	
	CYP2C19	
	CYP2D6	
	CYP2C9	
Phase II		
Morphine	UGT2B7	morphine-6-G glucuronide
Hydromorphone	UGT2B7	
Oxymorphone	UGT2B7	

UGT2B7 = uridine diphosphate glucuronosyltransferase 2B7.

the parent compounds possess a greater inherent activity and therefore, a lower dependence on CYP2D6 for efficacy.

Morphine toxicity may occur in individuals with ultra-rapid CYP2D6 metabolism following codeine administration. Normally, O-demethylation of codeine into the metabolite morphine by CYP2D6 accounts for a minor amount (0–15%) of codeine metabolism (82). Ultra-rapid metabolizers have multiple copies of the CYP2D6 gene, and enhanced conversion of codeine to morphine may result in adverse sedative and respiratory depressive effects (30). In addition, ultra-rapid CYP2D6 metabolism has been associated with infant toxicity from breastfeeding during maternal codeine therapy (86, 87).

Similar to codeine, tramadol also undergoes O-demethylation by CYP2D6 to the more active metabolite (M1). The affinity of O-desmethyltramadol for the mu receptor is approximately 200 times greater than that of the parent compound, suggesting the main analgesic activity after tramadol administration is due to the metabolite (81). Clinically, analysis of tramadol and O-desmethyltramadol were performed in patients recovering from major abdominal surgery; nonresponse rates to pain medication increased fourfold in the CYP2D6 poor metabolizers (88).

Methadone is metabolized by several CYP450 enzymes and can be somewhat influenced by genetic polymorphisms in metabolism, leading to variability of clinical response. CYP3A4 and CYP2B6 have been identified as the main isoforms involved in methadone metabolism (89). The polymorphic CYP2B6 contributes to (S)- and (R)-methadone metabolism; however, it appears a major influence of the CYP2B6 genotype on metabolism is unlikely (90). CYP2D6 genetic variability may explain some of the individual variability seen in the steady-state concentrations of (R)- and (S)-methadone, with differences demonstrated between poor metabolizers and ultra-rapid metabolizers (20, 91). In contrast, CYP2C9 and CYP2C19 genotypes do not appear to influence methadone plasma concentrations (90). Since the pharmacokinetics of methadone are complex, interpatient variability is not easily explained by a single polymorphic pathway.

Metabolism via glucuronidation of the phenanthrenes is mediated by uridine diphosphate glucuronosyltransferase 2B7 (UGT2B7). UGT2B7 is responsible for glucuronidation of morphine to morphine-3-glucuronide (M3G) and morphine-6-glucuronide (M6G) (80). M3G possesses no analgesic activity but is believed to cause neuroexcitatory effects (70, 92). M6G has analgesic effects similar to morphine; however, it may have a lower association with respiratory depression due to a lower affinity for the mu 2 subtype receptor (93). Hydromorphone metabolism by UGT2B7 produces the hydromorphone-3-glucuronide, which has neuroexcitatory activity without analgesic properties (92).

The UGT2B7 gene is also polymorphic, for example the variant UGT2B7*2, caused by T802C SNP of the UGT2B7 coding region (94). In surgical patients receiving morphine, there was no significant association UGT2B7*2 variant and postoperative morphine dose requirements (75). Other studies of UGT2B7 polymorphisms in individuals receiving morphine have demonstrated morphine-6-glucuronide to morphine ratios of mixed results (31, 95). Although the UGT2B7 polymorphism may contribute to some variability, based on current data, the impact of this polymorphism on morphine analgesia may be of little importance clinically (20).

In addition to opioids, NSAIDs are commonly used for analgesia. NSAIDs are substrates for metabolism primarily by CYP2C9. Agents metabolized by this pathway include diclofenac, ibuprofen, meloxicam, piroxicam, S-naproxen, and celecoxib (28). Individuals with poor CYP2C9 metabolism may have a reduction in clearance with the potential of increased adverse effects (96). Compared to the wild-type CYP2C9*1/*1, the CYP2C9*1/*3 and CYP2C9*1/*2 genotypes were significantly associated with a higher risk of gastrointestinal bleeding (97). In addition to reduced metabolism by CYP2C9, there appears to be a contribution of CYP2C8 polymorphisms. Individuals homozygous or double-heterozygous for CYP2C8*3 and CYP2C9*3 variant alleles had extremely low ibuprofen clearance rates (98). Additionally, the combined presence of both CYP2C8*3 and CYP2C9*2 is a relevant determinant in the risk of development of gastrointestinal bleeding in patients receiving NSAIDs that are CYP2C8/9 substrates (99).

Conclusion

Although anesthesiology is one of the first areas of medicine to consider genetic variability in drug response, routine testing is not commonplace. Consideration for testing usually relies on a drug event or family genetic history of a serious drug reaction (e.g., malignant hyperthermia). There are therapeutic areas, including oncology and psychiatry, that have demonstrated some clinical utility; however, currently pharmacogenomics has had limited impact on the clinical practice of anesthesiology (100).

There are several considerations for implementation of this emerging information into practice. Genomic testing for many conditions is not currently available to the degree it can be implemented. Future development of high-throughput assays with sufficient sensitivity and specificity for issues common in anesthesiology may allow this to move forward. This future assay development might also assist with the expense associated with testing. Currently, it would be cost-prohibitive to test every surgical candidate for pseudocholinesterase deficiency by laboratory analysis with polymerase chain reaction amplification.

As pharmacogenomics is a newer consideration, education for current practitioners would need to be developed. Additionally, many pharmacogenetic clinical considerations still need to be studied. For example, drug toxicity seen with poor metabolizers may not be a toxicity issue for individuals that present with intermediate metabolism. However, with the addition of other patient factors (e.g., comorbidities, or drug–drug interactions), the intermediate metabolism may now have an increased clinical relevance. So as new pharmacogenomic information becomes available, the clinician will need to incorporate emerging pharmacogenomic information with established pharmacokinetic and pharmacodynamic considerations. With an improved understanding of the clinical implications of pharmacogenomics, anesthesia providers in the future may have an increased potential to individualize therapy and reduce drug toxicity (101).

References

1 Prybys, K.M. (2004) Deadly drug interactions in emergency medicine. *Emerg Med Clin North Am.*, **22**(**4**), 845–863.

2 Lazarou, J., Pomeranz, B.H., Corey, P.N. (1998) Incidence of adverse drug reactions in hospitalized patients: a meta-analysis of prospective studies. *JAMA*, **279**(**15**), 1200–1205.

3 Johnson, J.A., Bootman, J.L. (1995) Drug-related morbidity and mortality: a cost-of-illness model. *Arch Intern Med.* **155**(**18**), 1949–1956.

4 Classen, D.C., Pestotnik, S.L., Evans, R.S., Lloyd, J.F., Burke, J.P. (1997) Adverse drug events in hospitalized patients: excess length of stay, extra costs, and attributable mortality. *JAMA*, **277**(**4**), 301–306.

5 Moore, T.J., Cohen, M.R., Furberg, C.D. (2007) Serious adverse drug events reported to the Food and Drug Administration, 1998–2005. *Arch Intern Med.* **167**(**16**), 1752–1759.

6 Meyer, U.A. (2005) Pharmacogenetics: five decades of therapeutic lessons from genetic diversity. *Nat Rev Genet.*, **5**(**9**), 669–676.

7 Lorentz, C.P., Wieben, E.D., Tefferi, A., Whiteman, D.A., Dewald, G.W. (2002) Primer on medical genomics part I: History of genetics and sequencing of the human genome. *Mayo Clin Proc.*, **77**(**8**), 773–782.

8 Streetman, D.S. (2007) Emergence and evolution of pharmacogenetics and pharmacogenomics in clinical pharmacy over the past 40 years. *Ann Pharmacother.*, **41**(**12**), 2038–2041.

9 Lander, E.S., Linton, L.M., Birren, B., *et al.* (2001) Initial sequencing and analysis of the human genome. *Nature*, **409**(**6822**), 860–921.

10 Motulsky, A.G. (2002) From pharmacogenetics and ecogenetics to pharmacogenomlcs. *Med Secoll.*, **14**(**3**), 683–705.

11 Motulsky, A.G. (1957) Drug reactions enzymes, and biochemical genetics. *J Am Med Assoc.*, **165**(**7**), 835–837.

12 Watson, J.D., Crick, F.H. (1953) The structure of DNA. *Cold Spring Harb Symp Quant Biol.*, **18**,123–131.

13 Kalow, W. (2004) Pharmacogenetics: a historical perspective. In: W. Allen, J. Johnson,and D. Knoell (eds.), *Pharmacogenomics: Applications to Patient Care*. American College of Clinical Pharmacy, Kansas Clty, MO.

14 Denborough M.A., Lovell, R.R. (1960) Anaesthetic deaths in a family. *Lancet*, **276**,45.

15 Denborough M.A., Forster, J.F., Lovell, R.R., Maplestone, P.A., Villiers, J.D. (1962) Anaesthetic deaths in a family. *Br J Anaesth*, **34**,395–396.

16 Kalow, W. (1964) Pharmacogenetics and anesthesia. *Anesthesiology*, **25**,377–387.

17 Iohom, G., Fitzgerald, D., Cunningham. A.J. (2004) Principles of pharmacogenetics: implications for the anaesthetist. *Br J Anaesth*, **93**(**3**), 440–450.

18 Searle, R., Hopkins, P.M. (2009) Pharmacogenomic variability and anaesthesia. *Br J Anaesth*, **103**(**1**), 14–25.

19 Galley, H.F., Mahdy, A., Lowes, D.A. (2005) Pharmacogenetics and anesthesiologists. *Pharmacogenomics*, **6**(**8**), 849–856.

20 Somogyi, A.A., Barratt, D.T., Coller, J.K. (2007) Pharmacogenetics of opioids. *Clin Pharmacol Ther*, **81**(**3**), 429–444.

21 Kashuba, A., Park, J., Persky, A., Brouwer, K. (2006) Drug metabolism, transport, and the influence of hepatic disease. In: M. Burton, L. Shaw, J. Schentag,

and W. Evans (eds.), *Applied Pharmacokinetics and Pharmacodynamics: Principles of Therapeutic Drug Monitoring.* Lippincott Williams & Wilkins, Philadelphia, PA.

22 Palmer, S.N., Giesecke, N.M., Body, S.C., Shernan, S.K., Fox, A.A., Collard, C.D. (2005) Pharmacogenetics of anesthetic and analgesic agents. *Anesthesiology,* **102**(3), 663–671.

23 Frye, R. (2004) Pharmacogenetics of oxidative drug metabolism and its clinical applications. In: W. Allen, J. Johnson, and D. Knoell (eds.), *Pharmacogenomics: Applications to Patient Care.* American College of Clinical Pharmacy, Kansas City, MO.

24 Ingelman-Sundberg, M. (2004) Pharmacogenetics of cytochrome P450 and its applications in drug therapy: the past, present and future. *Trends Pharmacol Sci,* **25**(4), 193–200.

25 Burton, M., Shaw, L., Schentag, J., Evans, W. (eds.) (2006) *Applied Pharmacokinetics and Pharmacodynamics: Principles of Therapeutic Drug Monitoring.* Lippincott Williams & Wilkins, Philadelphia, PA.

26 Wilkinson, G.R. (2005) Drug metabolism and variability among patients in drug response. *N Engl J Med,* **352**(21), 2211–2221.

27 Simon, T., Verstuyft, C., Mary–Krause, M., *et al.* (2009) Genetic determinants of response to clopidogrel and cardiovascular events. *N Engl J Med,* **360**(4), 363–375.

28 Flockhart, D.A. (2001) *Drug interactions: Cytochrome P450 drug interaction table* [WWW document]. URL http://medicine.iupui.edu/flockhart/table.htm [accessed on 28 June 2011]

29 Blaisdell, J., Mohrenweiser, H., Jackson, J., *et al.* (2002) Identification and functional characterization of new potentially defective alleles of human CYP2C19. *Pharmacogenetics,* **12**(9), 703–711.

30 Gasche, Y., Daali, Y., Fathi, M., *et al.* (2004) Codeine intoxication associated with ultrarapid CYP2D6 metabolism. *N Engl J Med,* **351**(27), 2827–2831.

31 Sawyer, M.B., Innocenti, F., Das, S., *et al.* (2003) A pharmacogenetic study of uridine diphosphate–glucuronosyltransferase 2B7 in patients receiving morphine. *Clin Pharmacol Ther,* **73**(6), 566–574.

32 Owen, A., Goldring, C., Morgan, P., Chadwick, D., Park, B.K., Pirmohamed, M. (2005) Relationship between the C3435T and G2677T(A) polymorphisms in the ABCB1 gene and P-glycoprotein expression in human liver. *Br J Clin Pharmacol,* **59**(3), 365–370.

33 Meier, Y., Pauli-Magnus, C., Zanger, U.M., *et al.* (2006) Interindividual variability of canalicular ATP-binding-cassette (ABC)-transporter expression in human liver. *Hepatology,* **44**(1), 62–74.

34 Thorn, M., Finnstrom, N., Lundgren, S., Rane, A., Loof, L. (2005) Cytochromes P450 and MDR1 mRNA expression along the human gastrointestinal tract. *Br J Clin Pharmacol,* **60**(1), 54–60.

35 Szilagyi, A., Boor, K., Orosz, I., *et al.* (2006) Contribution of serotonin transporter gene polymorphisms to pediatric migraine. *Headache,* **46**(3), 478–485.

36 Kosek, E., Jensen, K.B., Lonsdorf, T.B., Schalling, M., Ingvar, M. (2009) Genetic variation in the serotonin transporter gene (5-HTTLPR, rs25531) influences the analgesic response to the short acting opioid Remifentanil in humans. *Mol Pain,* **5**,37.

37 Pantuck, E.J. (1993) Plasma cholinesterase: gene and variations. *Anesth Analg,* **77**(2), 380–386.

38 Imerman, B., Caruso, L.J., Zori, R.T. (2001) Prolonged neuromuscular block in a patient undergoing renal transplantation. *J Clin Anesth,* **13**(7), 540–544.

39 Faust, R.J. (2002) Prolongation of succinylcholine effect. In: R. Faust, R. Cucchiara, S. Rose, T. Spackman, D. Wedel, C. Wass (eds.), *Anesthesiology Review,* 3rd ed., Churchill Livingstone, Philadelphia, PA, 137–138.

40 Alexander, D.R. (2006) *Pseudocholinesterase deficiency* [WWW document]. *Emedicine,* 17 July, updated 1 May 2009, 1–9. URL http://www.emedicine.com/med/topic1935.htm [accessed on 28 June 2011]

41 Petersen, R.S., Bailey, P.L., Kalameghan, R., Ashwood, E.R. (1993) Prolonged neuromuscular block after mivacurium. *Anesth Analg,* **76**(1), 194–196.

42 Whyte, A.J., Wang, H.E. (2007) Prehospital airway management complicated by reported pseudocholinesterase deficiency. *Prehosp Emerg Care,* **11**(3), 343–345.

43 Levano, S., Ginz, H., Siegemund, M., *et al.* (2005) Genotyping the butyrylcholinesterase in patients with prolonged neuromuscular block after succinylcholine. *Anesthesiology,* **102**(3), 531–535.

44 Denborough, M. (1998) Malignant hyperthermia. *Lancet,* **352**(9134), 1131–1136.

45 Malignant Hyperthermia Association of the United States (2001) *Anesthetic list for MH-susceptible patients* [WWW document]. URL http://medical.mhaus.org/index.cfm/fuseaction/Content.Display/PagePK/AnestheticList.cfm [accessed on 28 June 2011]

46 Greenbaum, I., Weigl, Y., Pras, E. (2007) The genetic basis of malignant hyperthermia. *Isr Med Assoc J,* **9**(1), 39–41.

47 Rosenberg, H., Davis, M., James, D., Pollock, N., Stowell, K. (2007) Malignant hyperthermia. *Orphanet J Rare Dis*, **2**,21.

48 Litman, R.S., Rosenberg, H. (2005) Malignant hyperthermia: update on susceptibility testing. *JAMA*, **293** (**23**), 2918–2924.

49 Robinson, R., Carpenter, D., Shaw, M.A., Halsall, J., Hopkins, P. (2006) Mutations in RYR1 in malignant hyperthermia and central core disease. *Hum Mutat*, **27** (**10**), 977–989.

50 Iles, D.E., Lehmann-Horn, F., Scherer, S.W., *et al.* (1995) Localization of the gene encoding the alpha 2/delta-subunits of the L-type voltage-dependent calcium channel to chromosome 7q and analysis of the segregation of flanking markers in malignant hyperthermia susceptible families. *Hum Mol Genet*, **3**(**6**), 969–975.

51 Monnier, N., Procaccio, V., Stieglitz, P., Lunardi, J. (1997) Malignant-hyperthermia susceptibility is associated with a mutation of the alpha 1-subunit of the human dihydropyridine-sensitive L-type voltage-dependent calcium-channel receptor in skeletal muscle. *Am J Hum Genet*, **60**(**B**),1316–1325.

52 Levitt, R.C., Olckers, A., Meyers, S., *et al.* (1992) Evidence for the localization of a malignant hyperthermia susceptibility locus (MHS2) to human chromosome 17q. *Genomics*, **14**(**3**), 562–566.

53 Olckers, A., Meyers, D.A., Meyers, S., *et al.* (1992) Adult muscle sodium channel alpha-subunit is a gene candidate for malignant hyperthermia susceptibility. *Genomics*, **14**(**3**), 829–831.

54 Sudbrak, R., Procaccio, V., Klausnitzer, M., *et al.* 2011. Mapping of a further malignant hyperthermia susceptibility locus to chromosome 3q13.1. *Am J Hum Genet*, **56**(**3**), 684–691.

55 Krause, T., Gerbershagen, M.U., Fiege, M., Weisshorn, R., Wappler, F. (2004) Dantrolene: a review of its pharmacology, therapeutic use and new developments. *Anaesthesia*, **59**(**4**), 364–373.

56 Malignant Hyperthermia Association of the United States (2008) *Emergency therapy of MH 2008* [WWW document]. URL http://medical.mhaus.org/PubData/PDFs/treatmentposter.pdf [accessed on 28 June 2011]

57 Rosenberg, H., Antognini, J.F., Muldoon, S. (2002) Testing for malignant hyperthermia. *Anesthesiology*, **96** (**1**), 232–237.

58 Allen, G.C., Larach, M.G., Kunselman, A.R. (1998) The sensitivity and specificity of the caffeine-halothane contracture test: a report from the North American Malignant Hyperthermia Registry of MHAUS. *Anesthesiology*, **88**(**3**), 579–588.

59 Malignant Hyperthermia Association of the United States (2011) Testing for susceptibility to MH: muscle contracture or molecular genetics? [WWW document]. URL http://medical.mhaus.org/index.cfm/fuseaction/OnlineBrochures.Display/BrochurePK/71A5AFFC-1BC7-4A36-970C6FDB27999FE5.cfm [accessed on 28 June 2011]

60 Girard, T., Treves, S., Voronkov, E., Siegemund, M., Urwyler, A. (2004) Molecular genetic testing for malignant hyperthermia susceptibility. *Anesthesiology*, **100**(**5**), 1076–1080.

61 Brandom, B.W., Muldoon, S.M. (2005) The practicality and need for genetic testing for malignant hyperthermia. *Anesthesiology*, **103**(**5**), 1100, author reply 1101.

62 Janicki, P.K. (2005) Cytochrome P450 2D6 metabolism and 5-hydroxytryptamine type 3 receptor antagonists for postoperative nausea and vomiting. *Med Sci Monit*, **11**(**10**), RA322–RA328.

63 Apfel, C.C., Laara, E., Koivuranta, M., Greim, C.A., Roewer, N. (1991) A simplified risk score for predicting postoperative nausea and vomiting: conclusions from cross-validations between two centers. *Anesthesiology*, **91**(**3**), 693–700.

64 Gan, T.J., Meyer, T.A., Apfel, C.C., *et al.* (2007) Society for Ambulatory Anesthesia guidelines for the management of postoperative nausea and vomiting. *Anesth Analg*, **105**(**6**), 1615–1628, table of contents.

65 Gan, T.J. (2006) Risk factors for postoperative nausea and vomiting. *Anesth Analg*, **102**(**6**), 1884–1898.

66 Ho, K.Y., Gan, T.J. (2006) Pharmacology, pharmacogenetics, and clinical efficacy of 5-hydroxytryptamine type 3 receptor antagonists for postoperative nausea and vomiting. *Curr Opin Anaesthesiol*, **19**(**6**), 606–611.

67 Nielsen, M., Olsen, N.V. (2008) Genetic polymorphisms in the cytochrome P450 system and efficacy of 5-hydroxytryptamine type 3 receptor antagonists for postoperative nausea and vomiting. *Br J Anaesth*, **101** (**4**), 441–445.

68 Candiotti, K.A., Birnbach, D.J., Lubarsky, D.A., *et al.* (2005) The impact of pharmacogenomics on postoperative nausea and vomiting: do CYP2D6 allele copy number and polymorphisms affect the success or failure of ondansetron prophylaxis? *Anesthesiology*, **102**(**3**), 543–549.

69 Janicki, P.K., Schuler, H.G., Jarzembowski, T.M., Rossi, M. II. (2006) Prevention of postoperative nausea and

vomiting with granisetron and dolasetron in relation to CYP2D6 genotype. *Anesth Analg*, **102**(**4**), 1127–1133.

70 Nagar, S., Raffa, R.B. (2008) Looking beyond the administered drug: metabolites of opioid analgesics. *J Fam Pract*, **57**(**Suppl. 6**), S25–S32.

71 Pletcher, M.J., Kertesz, S.G., Kohn, M.A., Gonzales, R. (2008) Trends in opioid prescribing by race/ethnicity for patients seeking care in US emergency departments. *JAMA*, **299**(**1**), 70–78.

72 American Pain Foundation (2011) *Pain facts & figures* [WWW document]. URL http://www.painfoundation.org/archive/newsroom/reporter-resources/pain-facts-figures.html [accessed on 28 June 2011]

73 Ikeda, K., Ide, S., Han, W., Hayashida, M., Uhl, G.R., Sora, I. (2005) How individual sensitivity to opiates can be predicted by gene analyses. *Trends Pharmacol Sci*, **26**(**6**), 311–317.

74 Wu, W.D., Wang, Y., Fang, Y.M., Zhou, H.Y. (2009) Polymorphism of the micro-opioid receptor gene (OPRM1 118A>G) affects fentanyl-induced analgesia during anesthesia and recovery. *Mol Diagn Ther*, **13**(**5**), 331–337.

75 Coulbault, L., Beaussier, M., Verstuyft, C., *et al.* (2006) Environmental and genetic factors associated with morphine response in the postoperative period. *Clin Pharmacol Ther*, **79**(**4**), 316–324.

76 Tan, E.C., Lim, E.C., Teo, Y.Y., Lim, Y., Law, H.Y., Sia, A.T. (2009) Ethnicity and OPRM variant independently predict pain perception and patient-controlled analgesia usage for post-operative pain. *Mol Pain*, **5**,32.

77 Park, H.J., Shinn, H.K., Ryu, S.H., Lee, H.S., Park, C.S., Kang, J.H. (2007) Genetic polymorphisms in the ABCB1 gene and the effects of fentanyl in Koreans. *Clin Pharmacol Ther*, **81**(**4**), 539–546.

78 Campa, D., Gioia, A., Tomei, A., Poli, P., Barale, R. (2008) Association of ABCB1/MDR1 and OPRM1 gene polymorphisms with morphine pain relief. *Clin Pharmacol Ther*, **83**(**4**), 559–566.

79 Coller, J.K., Barratt, D.T., Dahlen, K., Loennechen, M.H., Somogyi, A.A. (2006) ABCB1 genetic variability and methadone dosage requirements in opioid-dependent individuals. *Clin Pharmacol Ther*, **80**(**6**), 682–690.

80 Smith, H.S. (2009) Opioid metabolism. *Mayo Clin Proc*, **84**(**7**), 613–624.

81 Mikus, G., Weiss, J. (2005) Influence of CYP2D6 genetics on opioid kinetics, metabolism and response. *Current Pharmacogenomics*, **3**,43–52.

82 Thorn, C.F., Klein, T.E., Altman, R.B. (2009) Codeine and morphine pathway. *Pharmacogenet Genomics*, **19**(**7**), 556–558.

83 Fagerlund, T.H., Braaten, O. (2001) No pain relief from codeine...? An introduction to pharmacogenomics. *Acta Anaesthesiol Scand*, **45**(**2**), 140–149.

84 Lalovic, B., Kharasch, E., Hoffer, C., Risler, L., Liu-Chen, L.Y., Shen, D.D. (2006) Pharmacokinetics and pharmacodynamics of oral oxycodone in healthy human subjects: role of circulating active metabolites. *Clin Pharmacol Ther*, **79**(**5**), 461–479.

85 Otton, S.V., Schadel, M., Cheung, S.W., Kaplan, H.L., Busto, U.E., Sellers, E.M. (1993) CYP2D6 phenotype determines the metabolic conversion of hydrocodone to hydromorphone. *Clin Pharmacol Ther*, **54** (**5**),463–472.

86 Berlin, C.M., Jr., Paul, I.M., Vesell, E.S. (2009) Safety issues of maternal drug therapy during breastfeeding. *Clin Pharmacol Ther*, **85**(**1**), 20–22.

87 Madadi, P., Ross, C.J., Hayden, M.R., *et al.* (2009) Pharmacogenetics of neonatal opioid toxicity following maternal use of codeine during breastfeeding: a case-control study. *Clin Pharmacol Ther*, **85**(**1**), 31–35.

88 Stamer, U.M., Lehnen, K., Hothker, F., *et al.* (2003) Impact of CYP2D6 genotype on postoperative tramadol analgesia. *Pain*, **105**(**1–2**), 231–238.

89 Li, Y., Kantelip, J.P., Gerritsen-van Schieveen, P., Davani, S. (2008) Interindividual variability of methadone response: impact of genetic polymorphism. *Mol Diagn Ther*, **12**(**2**), 109–124.

90 Crettol, S., Deglon, J.J., Besson, J., *et al.* (2005) Methadone enantiomer plasma levels, CYP2B6, CYP2C19, and CYP2C9 genotypes, and response to treatment. *Clin Pharmacol Ther*, **78**(**6**), 593–604.

91 Eap, C.B., Broly, F., Mino, A., *et al.* (2001) Cytochrome P450 2D6 genotype and methadone steady-state concentrations. *J Clin Psychopharmacol*, **21**(**2**), 229–234.

92 Smith, M.T. (2000) Neuroexcitatory effects of morphine and hydromorphone: evidence implicating the 3-glucuronide metabolites. *Clin Exp Pharmacol Physiol*, **27**(**7**), 524–528.

93 Hucks, D., Thompson, P.I., McLoughlin, L., *et al.* (1992) Explanation at the opioid receptor level for differing toxicity of morphine and morphine 6-glucuronide. *Br J Cancer*, **65**(**1**), 122–126.

94 Bhasker, C.R., McKinnon, W., Stone, A., *et al.* (2000) Genetic polymorphism of UDP-glucuronosyltransferase 2B7 (UGT2B7) at amino acid 268: ethnic diversity

of alleles and potential clinical significance. *Pharmacogenetics*, **10**(**8**), 679–685.

95 Holthe, M., Klepstad, P., Zahlsen, K., *et al.* (2002) Morphine glucuronide-to-morphine plasma ratios are unaffected by the UGT2B7 H268Y and UGT1A1*28 polymorphisms in cancer patients on chronic morphine therapy. *Eur J Clin Pharmacol*, **58** (**5**), 353–356.

96 Rollason, V., Samer, C., Piguet, V., Dayer, P., Desmeules, J. (2008) Pharmacogenetics of analgesics: toward the individualization of prescription. *Pharmacogenomics*, **9**(**7**), 905–933.

97 Pilotto, A., Seripa, D., Franceschi, M., *et al.* (2007) Genetic susceptibility to nonsteroidal anti-inflammatory drug-related gastroduodenal bleeding: role of cytochrome P450 2C9 polymorphisms. *Gastroenterology*, **133**(**2**), 465–471.

98 Garcia-Martin, E., Martinez, C., Tabares, B., Frias, J., Agundez, J.A. (2004) Interindividual variability in ibuprofen pharmacokinetics is related to interaction of cytochrome P450 2C8 and 2C9 amino acid polymorphisms. *Clin Pharmacol Ther*, **76**(**2**), 119–127.

99 Blanco, G., Martinez, C., Ladero, J.M., *et al.* (2008) Interaction of CYP2C8 and CYP2C9 genotypes modifies the risk for nonsteroidal anti-inflammatory drugs-related acute gastrointestinal bleeding. *Pharmacogenet Genomics*, **18**(**1**), 37–43.

100 Candiotti, K. (2009) Anesthesia and pharmacogenomics: not ready for prime time. *Anesth Analg*, **109**(**5**), 1377–1378.

101 Ama, T., Bounmythavong, S., Blaze, J., Weismann, M., Marienau, M.S., Nicholson, W.T. (2010) Implications of pharmacogenomics for anesthesia providers. *AANA J*, **78**(**5**), 393–399.

CHAPTER 6

Pharmacogenomics of Immunosuppressants

Nicolas Picard, PharmD, PhD and Pierre Marquet, MD, PhD
Université de Limoges, Centre Hospitalier Universitaire (CHU) de Limoges, Institut National de la Santé et de la Recherche Médicale (Inserm), Limoges, France

Introduction

Immunosuppressants are drugs with high interindividual pharmacokinetic variability and narrow therapeutic ranges that have been rapidly identified as good candidates for pharmacogenomic research. The aim of such research is dual: to understand the sources of this variability, and then to use genotyping to try to limit this variability. In this second aspect, pharmacogenetics can be regarded as one of the available tools for treatment personalization, in addition to, or sometimes as a replacement for, therapeutic drug monitoring.

In most cases, in vitro studies supported the hypothesis that polymorphisms in genes involved in their disposition pathways (metabolic enzymes, or influx or efflux transporters) could affect their dose–concentration relationships, hence their pharmacokinetic variability.

Another potential source of variability of clinical outcome on immunosuppressive drugs is the pharmacogenetic variability of the proteins involved in the pharmacodynamics of immunosuppressants and the immune response. However, the pharmacogenetic variability of drug target proteins in general is currently less well known and understood, and the study of such pharmacogenetic–pharmacodynamic associations requires different and more complex approaches than pharmacogenetic–pharmacokinetic associations, both in vitro and in vivo.

Also, one has to keep in mind that transplantation is a special condition in that the transplanted organ, often involved in drug metabolism (liver), elimination (liver, kidney), distribution (heart), or even absorption (small bowel), carries a different genome than that of the donor. Hence, pharmacogenetic studies or pharmacogenetic treatment personalization may require analyzing the donor, or both the donor and recipient DNA, which renders matters more complex technically and ethically.

In any case, the genome alone cannot account for interindividual variability, as environmental factors, including the patients' medical history, food or the associated drugs can interact with genotype–phenotype relationships.

This book chapter is a literature review of the impact of genetic polymorphisms of the metabolic enzymes, efflux and influx transporters, and therapeutic targets of the main immunosuppressants (mycophenolic acid, calcineurin, and mTOR inhibitors), with a particular focus on the influence of the donor's genome. In addition to summarizing current knowledge, it will try to critically appraise the current level of evidence in favor of pharmacogenetics as an immunosuppressive treatment individualization tool in organ transplant recipients.

Mycophenolic acid (MPA)

Two different pharmaceutical formulations of MPA currently exist: mycophenolate mofetil (MMF) (the 2-morpholinoethyl ester of MPA) and a sodium-salt

Pharmacogenomics in Clinical Therapeutics, First Edition. Edited by Loralie J. Langman and Amitava Dasgupta.
© 2012 John Wiley & Sons, Ltd. Published 2012 by John Wiley & Sons, Ltd.

of MPA, formulated as delayed-release tablets. Carboxylesterase (CES) 1 and CES2 catalyze MMF hydrolysis in the intestine and the liver respectively, while acetylcholinesterase may be responsible for hydrolysis in blood (1, 2). However, an in vitro study has suggested that the hydrolysis of MMF to MPA occurs principally in the intestine and in the liver, rather than in blood (1).

Pharmacogenetic–pharmacokinetic associations
Metabolism and transport pathways of MPA
MPA is mainly metabolized by glucuronidation to its inactive hydroxy-β-glucuronide (MPA-phenyl-glucuronide; MPAG) (3). The reaction is catalyzed by several members of the UDP-glucuronosyltransferase 1A family (UGT1A1, UGT1A7, 1A8, 1A9, 1A10) (4–8), with a predominant role of UGT1A9 (highly expressed in human kidney and liver) (9) and UGT1A8 (exclusively expressed in intestinal cells) (5, 7). It was estimated using chemical inhibition experiments with human microsomes that UGT1A9 is responsible for at least 55%, 75%, and 50% of MPAG production by the liver, kidney, and intestinal mucosa, respectively (7). A carboxyl-linked glucuronide (acyl-MPA-glucuronide; AcMPAG) produced by UGT2B7 was also described (7, 10). It inhibits inosine-monophosphate dehydrogenase activity with the same uncompetitive mechanism as MPA and exerts additional inhibitory effects on lymphocyte proliferation (11). However, AcMPAG only accounts for 1.3% of MPA in vitro hepatic glucuronidation (7). It has low plasma concentrations (2.9–11.8 % of those of parent drug) and reduced capacity to cross cell membranes as compared to the parent drug (7, 12, 13). Any significant contribution of this metabolite to MPA clinical effect is thus very unlikely. Other minor metabolites of MPA include two phase II metabolites (an ether- and a carboxyl-linked glucosides) and one phase I metabolite (6-O-desmethyl-MPA) produced by the cytochromes P450 (CYP) 3A and 2C8 (14, 15).

Significant amounts of the glucuronides produced in hepatocytes are excreted into bile (3), but the glucuronides may also be transported back into the blood sinusoids by active transporters, to be further eliminated by the kidneys. The major disposition pathway for MPA is indeed tubular secretion in urine as MPAG (3). This involves an active uptake of the metabolite by the organic anion transporter 3 (OAT3; SLC22A8), located at the basolateral side of the proximal tubule (16, 17), followed by an apically-directed efflux in urine, presumably by the multidrug resistance-associated protein 2 (MRP2). MPA itself is not a substrate of OAT3 (16), which explains why negligible amounts of unchanged MPA (<1%) are excreted in urine (18).

The biliary excretion of MPAG is mediated by MRP2, while that of AcMPAG involves not only MRP2 but also another unidentified canalicular transporter, at least in Wistar rats (19). MPAG is a substrate for the organic anion transporting polypeptides (OATP) 1B1 and 1B3, two uptake transporters located on the sinusoidal side of the hepatocytes (20). Circulating MPAG may thus partly be taken up by hepatocytes to be eliminated through the bile. MPA itself is a weak substrate for MRP2 (21) and is not transported by OATP1B1 and OATP1B3 (20). This may explain why unchanged MPA is not significantly excreted in bile (3). MPAG contributes to mycophenolic acid enterohepatic circulation after deglucuronidation in the gut. This feature accounts for 10% to 61% of total MPA exposure and is reflected as a second increase in the MPA time concentration curve, occurring 6 to 12 hours after oral dosing (3).

Based on this data, the genes listed in Table 6.1 have been highlighted as candidates for the pharmacogenetics of MPA.

Effects of genetic polymorphisms on MPA disposition
Polymorphisms in carboxylesterase
Given that MMF hydrolysis is the initial step in MPA pharmacokinetics, genetic variability in this pathway might possibly contribute to MPA interindividual pharmacokinetic variability. MMF hydrolysis is mainly catalyzed by CES1, predominantly expressed in the liver. CES2 is responsible for MMF hydrolysis in the intestine, but it is less active than CES1 (1, 2). *CES1* and *CES2* genes are located on chromosome 16q22.2 and 16q22.1, respectively. Numerous polymorphisms have been described in both genes (22, 23). To the best of our knowledge, the

Table 6.1 Candidate Genes for MPA Pharmacogenetics

Protein	Role	Gene Symbol
Carboxylesterases 1 and 2	MMF hydrolysis	*CES1; CES2*
UGT1A9	MPA intestinal, hepatic, and renal metabolism to MPAG	*UGT1A9*
UGT1A8	MPA intestinal metabolism to MPAG and AcMPAG	*UGT1A8*
UGT2B7	MPA intestinal, hepatic, and renal metabolism to AcMPAG	*UGT2B7*
MRP2	MPAG and AcMPAG efflux from hepatocytes to bile	*ABCC2*
OATP1B1/OATP1B3	MPAG uptake in hepatocytes	*SLCO1B1; SLCO1B3*
IMPDH2 (IMPDH1)	MPA cellular target	*IMPDH2 (IMPDH1)*

consequence of genetic polymorphisms in *CES1* on MMF pharmacokinetics has not been explored. The effect of three *CES2* polymorphisms known to affect enzyme activity has been studied in 80 Japanese renal transplant patients. These SNPs are located in the *CES2* 5'UTR ($-1548A > G$: rs3890213) and intronic regions (IVS2b-152A > G: rs2303218; IVS10a-108C > T: rs2241409) (2). The authors found no difference in MPA pharmacokinetics (MPA T_{max}, C_{max}/dose, AUC_{0-12h}/dose, MPAG AUC_{0-12h}/dose) between carriers and noncarriers of these SNPs. No association with the incidence of acute rejection or diarrhea was found either.

Polymorphisms in UDP-glucuronosyltransferase

The UGT superfamily comprises two families (UGT1 and UGT2) and three subfamilies (UGT1A, UGT2A, and UGT2B). The UGT1A family members are all encoded by a single locus of approximately 200 kb, mapped to chromosome 2q37 (the *UGT1A* gene locus). This locus consists of 13 unique exons at the 5' end, which are alternatively spliced to four consecutive exons (exons 2–5) at the 3' end to form individual UGT1A transcripts. The constant exons 2–5 encode a carboxy terminal portion of 280 amino acids identical for all UGT1A proteins. Each individual exon 1 is preceded by its own promoter and encodes a divergent amino terminal portion of approximately 250 amino acids. UGT2 family members are encoded by unique genes of six exons located on chromosomes 4q13 and 4q28 (24). An international nomenclature committee compiles and updates the current nomenclature of the UGT

supergene family and the genetic variants. For more details, we refer the reader to the nomenclature home page, http://www.pharmacogenomics.pha. ulaval.ca/sgc/ugt_alleles/.

Functional polymorphisms have been reported in all the UGT isoforms involved in MPA glucuronidation but most studies focused on the major isoforms involved (UGT1A9, 1A8, and UGT2B7). The consequence of functional variations in UGT1A1, 1A7, and 1A10 for MPA pharmacokinetics is expected to be weak and not clinically relevant and will not be addressed in this chapter.

UGT1A9: genetic polymorphisms and their functional consequences

At least 11 single nucleotide polymorphisms (SNP) have been reported in the proximal promoter region of *UGT1A9* (25). Two of them were associated with increased UGT1A9 protein content in human liver microsomes (25). These SNPs are located 275 and 2152 bases upstream the adenine ($+1$) of the ATG initiation codon and are referred to as -275T > A (rs6714486) and $-2152C > T$ (rs17868320). They are in complete linkage disequilibrium and have a variant allele frequency of 6% in Caucasians (25). Four other UGT1A9 promoter SNPs have been shown to have a functional impact on UGT1A9 catalytic activity in vitro: a T to C transition at position -440 (rs2741045) in complete linkage with a C to T transition at position -331 (rs2741046); a C to T transition at -665 (rs10176246) and a T to G transition at -1887 (rs6731242). Although none of them significantly affected UGT1A9 protein levels in human liver, all were reported to significantly increase MPAG production, and for two of them, propofol glucuronidation ($-665C > T$ and $-1887T > G$), by human liver microsomes (25).

Six SNPs within the first exon of UGT1A9 have been published (26–28). Two of them are synonymous ($153G > A$: R51R; $588G > T$: G196G). Three lead to aminoacid changes with variable consequences on enzyme activity (Table 6.2). The last one produces a termination TAG codon, which results in a truncated protein, most likely nonfunctional since it lacks more than 50 % of its structure (27) (Table 6.2). These variants are rare and their frequency is dependent on ethnicity (Table 6.2): only the UGT1A9*3 was reported in Caucasians, with an allele frequency of 1.5 %. It was found to have a lower affinity for MPA as compared to UGT1A9*1, which resulted in a 1.7-fold lower intrinsic clearance of MPAG formation by microsomes prepared from UGT-transfected human embryonic kidney 293 cells (5).

A number of SNPs in the UGT1A9 intron 1 have also been reported, one of which has been particularly studied (IVS1 + 399, rs2741049) because it was found to be associated in vitro with increased protein expression and 7-ethyl-10-hydroxycamptothecin (i.e., SN-38; irinotecan metabolite) glucuronidation in the liver (29).

Given the high expression of UGT1A9 in the liver and the kidney, and its major role in MPAG formation, genetic polymorphisms in this enzyme are expected to influence MPA total clearance. A change in MPAG production may also indirectly affect MPA pharmacokinetics, both by increasing its disposition and by modifying the extent of its enterohepatic cycling.

The UGT1A9 SNPs which were studied in relation to MPA pharmacokinetics are the promoter $-275T > A/-2152C > T$, $-1887T > G$ and $-440C > T/-331T > C$ SNPs, the $98T > C$ coding SNP, and the IVS1 + 399 intronic SNP.

The intronic SNP (IVS1 + 399) may not have any actual influence on MPA clinical pharmacokinetics since two different studies of large population size ($n = 80$ and 338) found no difference in MPA exposure between carriers and noncarriers (30).

Three different studies reported an increase of MPA dose-normalized AUC_{0-12h}, ranging from 30% to 54%, in individuals carrying the UGT1A9*3 allele (31–33). This is consistent with experimental evidence that this SNP decreases enzyme activity (Table 6.1). Nonetheless, UGT1A9*3 is a very rare allele, and the above-mentioned studies did not have a sufficient statistical power to formally conclude. In addition, the clinical relevance of a variation occurring in 3% or less of the population is very limited, in particular when considering pharmacokinetic parameters influenced by numerous other factors.

The effect of the two common SNPs in the UGT1A9 promoter ($-275T > A$ and $-2152C > T$) is probably more clinically pertinent, but the exact mechanism associated with the change in MPA pharmacokinetics in unclear. In a study conducted in 32 kidney transplant recipients given MMF with tacrolimus, it was reported that patients carrying one or both of these SNPs had significantly lower MPA AUC_{0-12h} as compared to noncarriers. However, this effect was only observed in patients given 2g/day of the drug and not in those given 1g/day (31). Another study conducted in 100 renal allograft recipients cotreated with tacrolimus suggested that the $-275T > A$ and/or $-2152C > T$ SNP may be important in MPA therapeutic drug monitoring (34). The authors reported that a significantly higher proportion of MPA AUC_{0-12h} (measured over 5 years) was below the recommended target range (30–60 mg.h/l) in patients carrying one or both of these SNPs. In a subgroup of 163 tacrolimus-treated patients from the FDCC study, UGT1A9 $-275T > A$ and/or $-2152C > T$ carriers displayed a 20% lower MPA AUC_{0-12h} ($P = 0.012$) (33). A fourth study similarly conducted in kidney transplant patients cotreated with tacrolimus also showed a decrease in MPA AUC_{0-12h} in carriers of the $-275T > A$ and/or $-2152C > T$ SNP (35). In two of these studies, the decrease in MPA exposure was mainly due to lower AUC_{6-12h}, consistent with an increased metabolic rate or a reduction of enterohepatic recirculation. A similar decrease in MPA AUC_{6-12h} was also observed in a study comparing 17 healthy volunteers carrying these two SNPs to 17 wild-type controls (32). However, there was no association between these SNPs and MPAG plasma levels in the study conducted in healthy volunteers, as well as in a study in 70 renal transplant patients cotreated with tacrolimus or sirolimus, where none of the UGT1A9 SNPs tested ($-440C > T$, $-275T > A/-2152T > C$, $98T > C$)

Table 6.2 Frequencies and Functional Consequences of UGT1A9 Nonsynonymous SNPs

SNP (rs Number)	Allele	Amino acid Change	Functional Change	Allelic Frequency	Reference
8G > A (no rs)	UGT1A9*2	C^3Y	No change in flavopiridol and SN-38 glucuronidation. **No change in MPAG production.**	0 (Caucasians); 0.125 (African Americans)	(5, 28)
98T > C (rs72551330)	UGT1A9*3	$M^{33}T$	Decreased activity for SN-38; Similar activity for flavopiridol; **Decreased affinity for MPA.**	0.015 (Caucasians)	(5, 28)
726T > G (rs66915469)	UGT1A9*4	$Y^{242}X$	No activity (truncated protein). **MPA not studied.**	0 (Caucasians); 0.005 (Japanese)	(27)
766G > A (rs58597806)	UGT1A9*5	$D^{256}N$	Decreased activity for SN-38. **MPA not studied.**	0 (Caucasians); 0.008 (Japanese)	(26, 155)

SN-38: 7-ethyl-10-hydroxycamptothecin; MPA: mycophenolic acid.

significantly influenced MPAG (or MPA) pharmacokinetics (20).

This piece of data was missing in all the other above-mentioned clinical trials. One hypothesis is that the effect observed might result from an increase in intestinal UGT1A9 activity.

Whether the comedication influences this genetic effect is unclear. In most studies, the effect of UGT1A9 −275T > A and −2152C > T SNPs on MPA pharmacokinetics was observed in patients on tacrolimus (31, 33–35). No such association with these two SNPs was observed in three other studies in kidney transplant patients on cyclosporine, in 163 (33), 40 (36), and 115 (20) patients. At odds with these studies, Johnson et al. reported significantly lower MPA dose-normalized trough levels in kidney and/or pancreas transplant recipients cotreated with cyclosporine (n = 55), but not in those cotreated with tacrolimus (n = 40) or receiving MMF alone (n = 22) (37). The low number of patients studied may explain this discrepancy.

One of these studies, which also investigated the effects of UGT1A9 promoter SNPs at positions −1887, −665, and −440/−331 found that patients homozygous for the variant haplotype (−440T/−331C) had lower dose-normalized MPA AUC_{0-12h} as compared to heterozygotes or noncarriers (MPAG levels unaffected) (36), while UGT1A9 −440C > T had no significant influence in a larger one (20).

Only a few studies have investigated the consequence of UGT1A9 SNPs on patients' outcome. In the initial study from Kuypers et al., reduced MPA exposure in carriers of UGT1A9 −275T > A and −2152C > T SNPs was not associated with acute graft rejection (31). Conversely, using a logistic regression model which simultaneously took into account other factors (e.g., tacrolimus levels, CYP3A5 genotypes, HLA mismatches, age, and so on), van Schaik et al. found that these SNPs significantly predicted acute rejection in patients on tacrolimus randomized in the MMF fixed-dose group of the FDCC trial (OR = 13.3, 95%CI 1.1–162.3; P < 0.05) (33).

UGT1A8: genetic polymorphisms and their functional consequences

The initial analysis of UGT1A8 genetic variations has led to the description of two variant alleles

(UGT1A8*2 and UGT1A8*3), each bearing a missense SNP at nucleotides 518 (C > G; $A^{173}G$) and 830 (G > A; $C^{277}Y$), respectively [38]. UGT1A8*3 is rare (e.g., 1.2% in Caucasians) but leads to a severely reduced enzyme activity (10, 38). UGT1A8*2 is frequent (e.g., 23.8 % in Caucasians), but its impact on enzyme activity is unclear and may depend on the substrate [10,38]. Eleven additional UGT1A8 SNPs have been identified, including four missense mutations in Caucasians and two in African Americans. This led to the description of additional variants (UGT1A8*1a-d; *2a-b, *4-9) with allelic frequencies ranging from 0.2 to 22 % (10). Experiments with HEK293 cells stably expressing each of the different UGT variants predicted a reduced production of MPAG for UGT1A8*3, *5 (G^{173}-A^{240}), *7 (T^{231}), *8 (L^{43}), and *9 (G^{53}). All these variants also showed reduced production of AcMPAG (10). The reduced catalytic activity of UGT1A8*3 toward MPAG was confirmed with human intestinal microsomes (5).

Because UGT1A8 expression is limited to the small intestine, genetic polymorphisms in this isoform might theoretically affect the presystemic intestinal metabolism of MPA, as well as limit MPA enterohepatic cycling by reducing MPA reabsorption after deglucuronidation in the gut. This isoform might also influence local exposure of intestinal cells to MPA metabolites, which was put forward as a putative cause of gastrointestinal tract toxicity.

Although there is robust evidence that the UGT1A8*3 allele decreases enzyme activity (see above), at least three clinical studies reported no effect on MPA pharmacokinetics. The first study was conducted in healthy volunteers given a single 1.5 g dose of MMF; no difference was found in MPA and MPAG AUC_{0-12h} between UGT1A8*3 heterozygous carriers (n = 4) and noncarriers (n = 17) (32). The other two studies were conducted in kidney and/or pancreas transplant recipients and reported no effect of UGT1A8*3 on MPA dose-standardized AUC_{0-12h} (33) or trough levels (37). Given the low frequency of UGT1A8*3, it is likely that these different studies did not have the power to detect any significant effect. If any, the impact of UGT1A8*3 may not be clinically relevant.

The effect of the common allele UGT1A8*2 on the pharmacokinetics of MPA is unclear. In healthy volunteers administered a single 1.5 g dose, no difference in MPA, MPAG, and AcMPAG, AUC_{0-12h} was observed between UGT1A8*2 carriers (n = 9) and noncarriers (n = 17) (32). In addition, two studies in renal transplant recipients reported no effect of the UGT1A8*2 allele on MPA exposure and/or dose normalized exposure. The first study was conducted in 72 Japanese patients receiving 1-2g MMF, tacrolimus and corticosteroids (39), while the second was conducted in 115 patients, mostly of European descent, receiving MMF, cyclosporine, and corticosteroids (20). This latter study also includes a group of 70 patients co-treated with tacrolimus or sirolimus. Unexpectedly, a trend toward a lower dose-normalized MPA exposure was observed in patients homozygous carriers of UGT1A8*2 (n = 4). However, this association did not reach a significant p-value after correction for multiple testing and can probably be attributed to the low number of patient studied (20).

In another study conducted in kidney and/or pancreas transplant recipients given MMF alone (n = 22) or in combination with tacrolimus (n = 40) or cyclosporine (n = 55), the SNP was associated with a 60 % increase in MPA dose-corrected trough levels (p < 0.01) in the tacrolimus, but not in the cyclosporine, subgroup (37). The authors hypothesized a genotype-dependent inhibition of UGT1A8, whereby the enzyme would be more potently inhibited by tacrolimus in UGT1A8*2 carriers than in noncarriers. Tacrolimus was indeed described as an inhibitor of the UGT-catalyzed metabolism of MPA (40) and the amino acid change resulting from UGT1A8*2 can possibly modify the sensitivity of UGT1A8 to tacrolimus. Strangely enough, the opposite was observed in another study conducted in kidney transplant recipients: the UGT1A8*2 allele was associated with significantly higher MPA AUC_{0-12h} (+ 18%) in cyclosporine, but not in tacrolimus, co-treated patients (33). The hypothesis of a genotype-dependent interaction of tacrolimus with UGT1A8 is thus uncertain.

As an intestinal MPA metabolizing enzyme, UGT1A8 was identified as a candidate gene to influence MMF digestive adverse events. In a long-term cohort of renal transplants, UGT1A8*2 (but not UGT1A8*3) was associated with a reduced incidence of diarrhea. A second independent factor associated with a lower risk of diarrhea identified in this study was the administration of cyclosporine (as opposed to tacrolimus or sirolimus). These results suggest that a possible inhibition of the biliary excretion of MPA metabolites by cyclosporine and a decreased intestinal production of these metabolites in UGT1A8*2 carriers may be protective factors against MMF-induced diarrhea (41).

UGT2B7: genetic polymorphisms and their functional consequences

Several SNPs have been identified in UGT2B7. Among them, the nonsynonymous 802C > T SNP (rs7439366; UGT2B7*2) in exon 2 results in a histidine to tyrosine substitution at codon 268. The functional impact of this SNP is controversial. In a clinical study of reasonable size (n = 99 patients), the 802T variant was associated with increased glucuronidation of morphine (42). However, several other studies reported no significant effect of this variant regarding blood levels of morphine glucuronides in cancer patients (n = 175) (43) or UGT2B7 catalytic activity toward selective substrates in human liver microsomes or HEK293 transfected cells (43–45). Bernard et al. studied the production of AcMPAG by the wild-type and mutated variants and found that the protein encoded by UGT2B7*2 had very similar affinity and catalytic efficiency to that encoded by UGT2B7*1 (10).

At least six other SNPs have been identified, in the UGT2B7 promoter region (−1248A > G, −1241T > C, −1054T > C, −842G > A, −268A > G, and −102T > C) (46). All these SNPs are in complete linkage disequilibrium with the 802C > T exonic SNP (42). A significant influence of two UGT2B7 SNPs (−842G > A and 802C > T) on the production of AcMPAG by human liver microsomes was reported (47). AcMPAG production velocity rate was significantly increased in microsomes carrying an adenosine at position -842 (i.e., wild type for the 802C > T SNP) as compared to those carrying a guanine (i.e., mutated at position 802). There was no substantial change in apparent affinity. Added to the fact that the 802C > T coding SNP is most likely nonfunctional, these results strongly suggest that the pharmacogenetic effect is due to the −842G > A promoter SNP. An additional evidence was provided by Duguay et al., who observed a twofold increase in the transcriptional activity of hepatic and colon cell lines carrying the variant haplotype of the promoter region compared with the wild-type promoter (46).

As highlighted before, UGT2B7 only catalyzes the production of AcMPAG, a minor MPA metabolic pathway. Any substantial effect of *UGT2B7* polymorphisms on MPA pharmacokinetics is thus very unlikely. Accordingly, four studies in kidney transplant recipients of different origin (Caucasian, Chinese, and Japanese) reported no effect of the *UGT2B7*2* or −842G > A polymorphisms on MPA dose-normalized AUC_{0-12h} (33, 36, 39, 48).

Three other studies investigated the effect of UGT2B7 genetic polymorphisms (*UGT2B7*2* or *UGT2B7* −840G > A) on the pharmacokinetics of AcMPAG. Two of these found no significant association (48, 49) and one reported that the *UGT2B7* −842G > A SNP resulted in a significantly higher AcMPAG AUC_{0-9h} at 1 and 3 months post transplant in 40 kidney transplant recipients co-treated with sirolimus (47). No effect was observed in patients co-treated with tacrolimus (n = 24) or cyclosporine (n = 28), but the small number of patients studied did not allow a definitive conclusion.

In only one study was the *UGT2B7*2* allele found to be associated with higher free and total MPA AUC_{0-12h} in 52 healthy volunteers given a single dose of MMF (32). This result is surprising because the carriers of *UGT2B7*2* had no significant difference in AcMPAG levels as compared to noncarriers.

Finally, the association between *UGT2B7* polymorphisms and MMF-related digestive side effects was investigated. A study conducted in 67 renal transplant recipients of different ethnicities (Caucasian, African American, Hispanic, and others) suggests that patients with the *UGT2B7*2* variant genotype are protected from the gastrointestinal side effects of MPA regardless of the formulation used or concurrent calcineurin inhibitors administered. This study was based on a self-administered questionnaire, the Gastrointestinal Symptom Rating Scale (50). In the specific case of diarrhea, the scale score was, however, not associated with patient genotypes for *UGT2B7*. At least two other studies have reported no association between *UGT2B7* −842G > A and the occurrence of MMF related-diarrhea in renal transplant recipients (41, 49). In the study from van Agteren *et al.*, AcMPAG levels were included in the analysis, and no association was found either. The role of the UGT2B7-catalyzed formation of AcMPAG in the digestive side effects of MPA remains thus unclear.

Polymorphisms in transporters

MRP2: genetic polymorphisms and their functional consequences

MRP2 is encoded by *ABCC2*, a gene of 32 exon/s mapped on chromosome 10q24. Some very rare mutations result in almost complete loss of function and are causative of the Dubin-Johnson syndrome (a recessive liver disorder characterized by chronic conjugated hyperbilirubinemia) (51). In addition, 68 SNPs have been reported in *ABCC2* in different ethnic groups during the resequencing phase of the UCSF Pharmacogenomics of Membrane Transporters project (database at http://pharmacogenetics. ucsf.edu). Approximately half of these SNPs are in the coding region of *ABCC2*, with 19 causing an amino acid change in MRP2. Fourteen are located in the *ABCC2* proximal promoter or 5′-untranslated regions. In most ethnic groups, the more frequent SNPs are located 1549 (G > A; rs1885301), 1410 (A > G; rs1885301), 1023 (G > A; rs7910642), 1019 (A > G; rs2804402), and 24 (C > T; rs717620) bases upstream the ATG initiation codon, or in exon 10 (1249G > A; rs2273697) and exon 28 (3972C > T; rs3740066).

There is no experimental evidence that the SNPs in the noncoding region are functional, except for the −24C > T polymorphism. In a reporter gene assay in HepG2 cells, the *ABCC2* -24T construct showed an 18.7% reduced activity (p = 0.003). In addition, the SNP was associated with a decrease in *ABCC2* mRNA in human kidney tissues (52). The 1249G > A SNP in exon 10 leads to a valine-to-isoleucine substitution at position 417. It was associated with a reduced expression of MRP2 in preterm placentas (53). However, no effect of this SNP was found in vitro on MRP2 expression or activity (54). The 3972 C > T SNP in exon 28 is synonymous ($I^{1324}I$) and is not expected to be functional. However, this SNP is in linkage disequilibrium with the −24C > T SNP, which may explain certain indirect associations.

Seven studies investigated the effect of the *ABCC2* −24C > T SNP on MPA exposure (20, 33, 36, 48, 55, 56) with only one reporting a positive result. This study in 95 renal transplants on tacrolimus showed that the MRP2 C-24T SNP was associated with significantly higher dose-corrected MPA trough levels between day 42 and 1 year, but not at day 7 post transplantation. It was also noted that mild liver dysfunction was associated with significantly lower MPA dose–interval exposure and higher MPA oral clearance at day 7, except in patients with the MRP2 C-24T variant. However, the number of patients with the different combinations was very small (between 7 and 45) and the p values reported in this study were apparently not corrected for multiple analyses (56). The 3972T variant was also associated with a higher MPA C0/dose at day 42, which could be explained by the linkage disequilibrium between the two SNPs. However, the p value was not convincing (see above) and there was no such association at the other posttransplantation periods.

It was suggested that the absence of pharmacogenetic–pharmacokinetic association in other studies was due to the potent inhibitory effect of cyclosporine on MRP2. However, at least three of the negative studies were in renal transplant patients cotreated with tacrolimus.

Given that MRP2 contributes to the biliary excretion of, and thus the intestinal exposure to MPA metabolites, it was hypothesized that genetic variations in this transporter could be associated with MPA-related diarrhea. The above-mentioned study by Naesens *et al.* reported that, in addition to changes in MPA pharmacokinetics, the −24C > T SNP was associated with a higher incidence of diarrhea within the first-year post-transplantation (29% vs. 13%; p = 0.049 – without correction for multiple tests) (56). However, three other studies found no such association (41, 50, 55), including two that concomitantly investigated the effects of the −24C > T SNP and MPAG levels (20, 57).

OATP1B1 and OATP1B3
OATP1B1 (formerly known as OATP2 or OATP-C) and OATP1B3 (formerly known as OATP8) are encoded by *SLCO1B1* and *SLCO1B3*, respectively.

Genetic polymorphisms and their functional consequences
A number of SNPs have been described in *SLCO1B1*. We refer the reader to the UCSF Pharmacogenomics of Membrane Transporters project database (available at http://pharmacogenetics.ucsf.edu). Among these, the nonsynonymous 521T > C ($V^{174}A$) SNP is associated with a markedly reduced transport activity of several model substrates (e.g., estrone-3-sulphate, 17-β-glucuronosyl estradiol, statins ...). The 388A > G ($N^{130}D$) is another *SLCO1B1* SNP associated with altered transport activity. These two SNPs are in linkage disequilibrium and form different haplotypes designated as *SLCO1B1*1A* (388A/521T), *SLCO1B1*1B* (388G-521T), *SLCO1B1*5* (388A-521C), and *SLCO1B1*15* (388G-521C) (58).

The most frequent SNPs in *SLCO1B3* are a T > G inversion at position 334 and a G > A inversion at position 699, both of which result in an aminoacid change: $S^{112}A$ and $M^{233}I$, respectively (59). These two SNPs were reported to be in complete linkage disequilibrium (20). The first in vitro study investigating the functional consequences of *SLCO1B3* polymorphisms showed that variant OATP1B3 proteins resulting from either of the two coding nonsynonymous SNPs had similar basolateral membrane localization with the reference protein in MDCKII and HEK293 cells. They did not find differences in uptake activities between these proteins using several model substrates (estrone-3-sulfate, bromosulfophthalein, and 17-β-glucuronosyl estradiol) (59). Hamada *et al.* investigated the functional consequence of the combined amino acid substitutions and found that COS-7 cells transfected with the variant *SLCO1B3* haplotype (334G-699A) had a significantly reduced ability to uptake testosterone as compared to cells transfected with the reference *SLCO1B3* gene or with a sequence containing either the 334G or the 699A SNP (60).

We recently reported that the pharmacokinetics of MPA was significantly influenced by the *SLCO1B3* 334T > G polymorphism in 70 renal transplant patients receiving MMF in a cyclosporine-free immunosuppressive regimen, while no significant effect was observed in 115 patients coadministered cyclosporine (20). Reduced transport of MPAG was observed in HEK293T-cells expressing this particular

OATP1B3 variant, which is consistent with the trend toward a gene–dose decrease in MPAG exposure with the number of variant alleles observed in these patients. Carriers of the 334G allele had a significant decrease of MPA dose-normalized exposure. Based on the in vitro findings and on the change in MPAG exposure in patients, we suggested that this was secondary to reduced MPAG hepatic uptake, hence reduced reabsorption of MPA via the entero-hepatic cycle (20). A study conducted in Japanese patients reported, in accordance with our hypothesis, that patients homozygous for the *SLCO1B3* 334G-699A allele had significantly higher MPAG dose-normalized AUC_{0-12h} than patients heterozygous or homozygous for the reference allele (57).

Conversely, Miura el al. described higher MPA dose-normalized AUC_{6-12} (regarded a marker of MPA recirculation) in patients carrying the 334GG (or 699AA) genotype as compared to carriers of the 334TT genotype (55). Based on this pharmacokinetic observation, the authors proposed that MPA uptake into hepatocytes and excretion into bile might be increased in patients with the *SLCO1B3* 334GG genotype. However, this is in contradiction with in vitro evidence showing that MPA is not a substrate for OATP1B3 and that the 334G allele reduces OATP1B3 activity (20, 60).

No association was found between the *SLCO1B3* 334T > G and 699G > A SNPs and the incidence of diarrhea in a study conducted in 87 Japanese kidney transplant recipients coadministered tacrolimus (55). OATP1B1 in vitro activity with respect to MPAG was found to be relatively modest as compared to that of OATP1B3, suggesting limited implication in MPAG uptake in vivo as compared to the latter (20). The finding that none of the *SLCO1B1* SNPs or haplotypes tested in two different studies was significantly associated with MPA or MPAG pharmacokinetics supports this hypothesis (14, 55).

Pharmacogenetics of MPA target proteins

The immunosuppressive effect of MPA is essentially attributed to the inhibition of inosine monophosphate dehydrogenase (IMPDH), a rate-limiting enzyme involved in de novo purine synthesis (61). Lymphocytes are devoid of the salvage pathway that allows most other cells to recycle guanine nucleotides and are therefore dependent on IMPDH for DNA synthesis. Two different isoforms of IMPDH are encoded by *IMPDH1* and *IMPDH2*. *IMPDH2* is located on chromosome 3p21.2 and is approximately 5.2 kb in length. It comprised 14 exons encoding a 1.7 kb mRNA (NM_000884.2) leading to a 514 amino-acid protein of 56 kDa (NP_000875.2) (62). This protein shares 84% homology with the type 1 isoform, which is encoded by a different gene of approximately 18 kb on chromosome 7q31.3. MPA is a fivefold more potent inhibitor of IMPDH2, which is expressed in activated lymphocytes as compared to IMPDH2, which is expressed in most cell types (61).

IMPDH2: genetic polymorphisms and their functional consequences

Seventy-two SNPs within *IMPDH2* gene regions (including 3′ and 5′ UTRs, introns, and exons) have been referenced in the NCBI SNP database (http://www.ncbi.nlm.nih.gov/projects/SNP/; gene ID: 3615). However, these SNPs have inconstantly been confirmed in resequencing projects (63, 64). A reason for this may be the wide variation in SNP allele frequencies within ethnic groups. For instance, Wu *et al.* identified 25 *IMPDH2* SNPs: 12 in African Americans, 9 in Caucasian Americans, and 4 in Han Chinese Americans. Only one of these SNPs was observed in all three populations (64). Functional data are available for two *IMPDH2* SNPs. The nonsynonymous SNP located in *IMPDH2* exon 7 (787C > T; $L^{263}F$) was reported to dramatically decrease the catalytic activity of the enzyme in vitro (65) through accelerated protein degradation (64). The −95C > T promoter SNP, located in a transcription factor binding site CRE(A) (cyclic adenosine monophosphate [cAMP] response element), was found to decrease luciferase activity in two different cell lines (66).

Consequences of IMPDH2 polymorphisms on MPA clinical effects

No clinical association study has been published so far regarding the two *IMPDH2* functional SNPs (−95C > T and 787C > T). Given their extremely low allelic frequency (<1%) (65, 66), any clinically relevant contribution to interpatient variability in MPA effects is unlikely.

A SNP located in *IMPDH2* intron 7 (IVS7 + 10T > C; rs11706052) has been extensively studied. Two different studies suggest that it may be associated with a poorer response to MPA. The first study, conducted in 80 renal transplanted patient treated with MMF, reported an increased IMPDH activity in carriers of the variant allele as compared to noncarriers (67). The second study was conducted in human healthy volunteers. The presence of the rs11706052 polymorphism was found to reduce the antiproliferative effect of MPA on lymphocytes by approximately 50% (n = 8 carriers of rs11706052 *versus* 12 noncarriers) (68). Given the intronic localisation of this SNP, the exact molecular mechanism involved is unclear. This particular SNP was also associated with a higher risk of acute rejection in renal transplant recipients in a cohort of 237 renal transplant recipients (69). However, two other studies similarly conducted in large groups of renal transplant recipients (191 and 456 patients) were unable to confirm the association of this particular SNP with acute rejection (63, 70).

IMPDH1: genetic polymorphisms and their functional consequences

Seventy-three SNPs have been identified in *IMPDH1*, including four nonsynonymous SNPs (64). These SNPs vary widely depending on the ethnic origins of individuals. Among the four nonsynonymous *IMPDH1* SNPs, the 824C > T SNP in exon 8 (S^{275}L) was found to be associated with a drastic decrease in enzyme activity in vitro (< 25% of the wild-type enzyme), caused by accelerated protein degradation (64). Molecular modeling showed that the amino acid substitution resulting from this SNP might compromise protein folding, tetramerization, and thus stability (64).

No study has examined the influence of the *IMPDH1* 824C > T SNP (S^{275}L) on MPA clinical effects. Two other SNPs within *IMPDH1* intron 7 (rs2278293 and rs2278294) were reported to be associated with a decreased risk of biopsy-proven acute rejection (BPAR) over the first year after renal transplantation (70). In another study in renal transplant recipients, the protective effect of the rs2278294 variant allele regarding BPAR was confirmed (Odds Ratio: 0.54 95% CI [0.34–0.85]; p = 0.0075), while no association

between BPAR and rs2278293 was found (63). In this study, the rs2278294 variant allele carriers also had a 1.6-fold increased risk of leucopenia. The fact that BPAR and leucopenia were inversely associated to the same SNP reinforces the pertinence of this finding: the rs2278294 may protect patients from developing an immunological reaction against the allograft by favoring low lymphocyte levels (i.e., leucopenia).

A third study conducted in 82 Japanese renal transplant recipients has investigated the association of these two SNPs with the incidence of subclinical acute rejection diagnosed by a biopsy examination 29 days after transplantation (71). Daytime and nighttime MPA pharmacokinetic data obtained within 24 h of the biopsy (day 28) was included in the analysis. The rs2278293 or rs2278294 SNPs were not found to be associated with the incidence of subclinical acute rejection. However, when the authors stratified their analysis based on the AUC range of MPA during day- and nighttime periods, a significant influence of the rs2278293 genotype on the incidence of subclinical acute rejection was found in patients with high nighttime exposure to MPA ($>60\,\mu g.h.l^{-1}$), while a similar trend was observed in patients with high daytime exposure to MPA. The authors mentioned in their discussion the limitations of their study, which include the unique period of AUC measurement at day 28 and the lack of statistical power due to the small sample size. One can also regret that exposure data and genotypes were not tested simultaneously rather than in stratified analyses.

Potential and limits of MPA pharmacogenetics in treatment selection and therapeutic drug monitoring

In summary, based on current knowledge, the following hypotheses can be raised:

– Genotyping *UGT1A9* may help avoid underexposure to MPA in carriers of the −275T > A, −2152C > T, and, to a lesser extent, −440C > T and −331T > C SNPs, although this effect is inconstant across studies and depends on the associated calcineurin inhibitor. Genotyping the first two may even help reduce the acute rejection rate in kidney transplant recipients, whether on cyclosporine or tacrolimus, provided mycophenolate is not dose adjusted. Indeed, MPA AUC monitoring is expected to compensate for differences in exposure and abolish this pharmacogenetic-outcome association.

– Genotyping *SLCO1B3* 334T > G may also help identify patients at risk of (slight) underexposure to MPA.

– Genotyping *UGT1A8* might be useful to either avoid giving MPA in *UGT1A8*2* carriers, or to combine MPA with cyclosporine rather than tacrolimus or mTOR inhibitors in these patients, in order to lower the risk of severe diarrhea, which in turn may lead to drastic MPA dose decreases or to drug discontinuation

– Genotyping *IMPDH I* may help select a lower mycophenolate dose, or a lower target exposure in carriers of the rs2278294 SNP, and possibly also of the rs2278293 SNP.

However, none of these hypotheses have been tested prospectively in randomized clinical trials, so the level of evidence in favor of these pharmacogenetic tests is currently at the lowest. Ideally, a three-arm randomized trial should compare the clinical outcome of organ transplant recipients on mycophenolate therapy at fixed dose, receiving dose-individualized MMF based on therapeutic drug monitoring or with treatment personalization based on UGT1A9, UGT1A8 and IMPDH genotyping.

Calcineurin inhibitors

Pharmacogenetic–pharmacokinetic associations
Metabolism and transport pathways

Cyclosporine is subject to extensive phase 1 metabolism with approximately 90% of the oral dose eliminated through the bile as metabolites and only 1% as unchanged cyclosporine. Renal elimination only accounts for 6% of the administered dose with as low as 0.1% of unchanged cyclosporine found in urine (72). At least 30 hydroxylated, demethylated or cyclic metabolites have been reported (73). The metabolites are referred to as the two letters *AM* (A for cyclosporine A; M for metabolite), followed by Arabic numbers to locate the modified amino acid.

Table 6.3 Catalytic Activity of the Human Recombinant Cytochrome P450 (rhCYP) 3A5 Relatively to rhCYP3A4

	CYP3A5 Catalytic Activity (Relatively to CYP3A4)	Reference
Cyclosporine	0.43	(75)
Tacrolimus	2.00 (2.16)	(81, 151)
Sirolimus	0.27	(143)
Everolimus	0.16	(151)

The letters *n* or *c* are added to denote demethylated or cyclic metabolites, respectively. AM1, AM4n, and AM9 are the major metabolites. Only AM1 and AM9 are active, but they may only contribute to 10–20% of the cyclosporine immunosuppressive effect. Cyclosporine is metabolized by CYP3A4 and CYP3A5 (74). The three primary metabolites are produced by CYP3A4, whereas CYP3A5 apparently shows regioselectivity and produces only AM9 (75). CYP3A5 also has a fivefold higher K_m than CYP3A4 for AM9 production, which results in lower intrinsic clearance estimated from total metabolite formation rates (75) (Table 6.3). Consequently, the total metabolic clearance of cyclosporine in vivo may be only modestly affected by CYP3A5 activity.

Cyclosporine is a substrate for the P-glycoprotein (permeability glycoprotein, abbreviated as P-gp). P-gp is a member of the ATP-binding cassette (ABC) transporters family. It is expressed in enterocytes, hepatocytes, renal proximal tubular cells, adrenal glands, and capillary endothelial cells comprising the blood–brain and bloodvtestis barrier. At the intestinal level, the protein forms a cooperative barrier with CYP3A by pumping the drug out of enterocytes. The process results in repeated exposure of the drug to CYP3A and also tends to keep the intracellular drug concentration in the linear range of enzyme-metabolizing capacity (76). P-gp, as well as MRP2, another membrane transporter (77), may also contribute to the biliary excretion of cyclosporine or its metabolites.

In addition to being substrate, cyclosporine inhibits both P-gp and MRP2. Cyclosporine is also known as a potent inhibitor of OATPs, but has not been directly shown to be substrate of these influx transporters (78).

Tacrolimus is almost completely metabolized by intestinal and hepatic CYP3A prior to elimination: only 0.5% of the dose is found unchanged in urine or feces (79, 80). At least 15 metabolites of first or second generation have been identified. The primary metabolites are 13-O-desmethyl-tacrolimus (M-I), 15-O-desmethyl-tracrolimus (M-III), 31-O-desmethyl-tacrolimus (M-II) and 12-hydroxy-tacrolimus (M-VI) (81). Only M-II is active with a pharmacological activity similar to that of tacrolimus (82). Given its low blood concentration, it may not contribute to tacrolimus therapeutic effect. In contrast to cyclosporine, the in vitro intrinsic clearance of tacrolimus is approximately twofold higher with CYP3A5 than CYP3A4 (81) (Table 6.3). Tacrolimus is a substrate (and a weak inhibitor) of P-gp, which influences both its intestinal absorption and hepatic clearance (83, 84). In contrast to cyclosporine, tacrolimus is neither a substrate, nor a potent inhibitor of MRP2 or OATPs (21, 85).

Effects of genetic polymorphisms on the pharmacokinetics of calcineurin inhibitors

Polymorphisms in CYP3A

A substantial number of variant CYP3A4 alleles have been described, with several bearing nonsynonymous SNPs (see the CYP alleles database at http://www.cypalleles.ki.se). No polymorphism that would result in the absence of CYP3A4 activity has been described, and SNPs giving rise to alterations in catalytic activity are seen at low population frequencies.

A number of SNPs in the promoter region of CYP3A4 have also been reported with one being common (−392A > G; the *CYP3A4*1B* allele). The functional consequence of this SNP is very controversial. It was reported to be associated with an increased transcription of the *CYP3A4* gene in vitro (86). A later study found no such effect in vitro, and the authors hypothesized that the effect noted in the first study was an artifact of the expression system used (87). Most studies have not attributed any functional significance to this SNP with regard to the in vitro or in vivo metabolism of typical CYP3A probes (e.g., erythromycin, nifedipine, and midazolam) (88, 89).

CYP3A5 gene expression is another factor affecting CYP3A overall metabolism. CYP3A5 is expressed in only approximately 10 % of Caucasians as a result of a frequent mutation of adenosine to guanosine at position 6986 within intron 3 of the CYP3A5 gene (rs776746) (89). This SNP creates a cryptic splice site that results in the incorporation of an intron sequence in the mature mRNA. The aberrant *CYP3A5*3* mRNA encodes an inactive protein, truncated at amino acid 102 (89). Therefore, only individuals with at least one *CYP3A5*1* allele actually express the CYP3A5 protein at a significant level, with large differences in prevalence across ethnicities (5–30% CYP3A5 expressers in Caucasians, and 50–80% in African Americans and Chinese) (90).

Other CYP3A5 variants allele with functional consequence include *CYP3A5*6* (rs10264272), which also results in abnormal splicing and protein truncation, and *CYP3A5*7*, which results in a shift in reading frame introducing a premature termination codon. These are relatively frequent in African Americans (10–22%) and very rare or absent in Caucasians (91).

CYP3A polymorphisms and cyclosporine

Several studies conducted in adult (92, 93) or pediatric renal transplant recipients (94) found no influence of the *CYP3A4*1B* allele on cyclosporine pharmacokinetics. In contrast, in one study conducted in 14 healthy volunteers, higher dose-normalized AUC of cyclosporine (+83% on average) were observed in homozygous carriers of the wild-type genotype (−392AA; n = 4) as compared to homozygous carriers of the variant genotype (−392GG; n = 4). There were no differences between the AA and AG or AG and GG groups (95). In this study, 11 African American subjects were included, which increased the power of the study given the high prevalence of *CYP3A4*1B* in this population. The finding seems to be consistent with a higher CYP3A4 metabolic activity in patients with the variant allele, as well as with the ethnic differences of cyclosporine pharmacokinetics. However, the *CYP3A5* variant alleles which also influence CYP3A activity (*CYP3A5*3*; *CYP3A5*6*) and which are highly frequent in African Americans were not investigated and may be confounding factors. Also, the functional allele of

CYP3A5 (CYP3A5*1) is in linkage disequilibrium with CYP3A4*1B. This might indirectly explain the association observed. In another study conducted in 151 kidney and heart transplant recipients of mixed ethnic origins (White: 83.4%, Asian: 8.6%, and Black: 8%), a small but significant increase in the apparent clearance of cyclosporine (Cl/F; +9%; 95% CI: 1–17%; p<0.05) was observed in CYP3A4*1B carriers (96). This effect was not dependent of CYP3A5 genotypes and patient ethnicity.

At least 16 clinical studies have been performed to analyze the association between the CYP3A5*3 allele and cyclosporine exposure. Most of these studies were conducted in renal transplant recipients. The CYP3A5*3 allele was found to result in lower dose-standardized exposure to cyclosporine in both healthy volunteers (97) and renal transplant patients of Caucasian (98), Chinese (99–103), or Indian (104) origins. However, at least seven studies found no association (92, 105–110). Recently, two meta-analyses (111, 112) concluded that the CYP3A5*3 allele could be associated, to a moderate extent, with increased cyclosporine C_0/dose or C_2/dose and reduced mean daily doses. The second meta-analysis also studied the association of the variant with the incidence of acute rejection and found no such association. The consequence of CYP3A5*3 on cyclosporine pharmacokinetics remains thus uncertain and may not be of major extent. A reason for this can be the limited catalytic efficiency of CYP3A5 as compared to CYP3A4 regarding cyclosporine (75). The absence of clinical impact can also be explained by routine monitoring and dose adjustment, compensating at least in part for exposure variability.

CYP3A polymorphisms and tacrolimus

Hesselink et al. reported significantly lower dose-standardized trough levels of tacrolimus in renal transplant patients carrying at least one CYP3A4*1B allele (n = 10) than in noncarriers (n = 54) (92). However, when the analysis was restricted to Caucasians, the association was lost. As described above, the functional consequence of this SNP is controversial. The association described might be an artifact of different ethnic population distributions or a consequence of the linkage with the CYP3A5 6986A > G SNP (CYP3A5*1/*3).

A strong association between CYP3A5*1/*3 and tacrolimus pharmacokinetics has been demonstrated in multiple studies conducted in renal (92, 98, 104, 107, 110, 113–116) or lung transplant patients (117). The dose required to achieve the therapeutic range in renal transplantation was estimated to be twice as much in carriers of at least one active CYP3A5 allele than in noncarriers (98, 113, 118, 119). In liver transplant patients, the mean tacrolimus C_0/dose was lower in recipients engrafted with a liver carrying the CYP3A5*1/*1 genotype (120). These findings are consistent with experimental evidence that CYP3A5 contributes significantly to the metabolic clearance of tacrolimus in the liver and kidney (81). In 2009, a European Consensus Conference acknowledged that there is a significant impact of CYP3A5 polymorphisms on tacrolimus disposition, but concluded that the clinical role of any pharmacogenetic intervention remained unclear, and that further large-scale trials were needed before reaching relevant recommendations (121). Thervet et al. recently provided an important piece of information by conducting a prospective multicenter clinical trial named TACTICS (dose individualization of TACrolimus in renal transplantation through pharmacogeneTICS) (122). Renal transplant patients (n = 280) were randomly assigned to receive tacrolimus at an initial dose either based on the CYP3A5 genotype or according to the recommended daily regimen. Further dose adjustments based on tacrolimus C_0 were allowed in both arms. After six doses, a significantly higher proportion of patients had reached the therapeutic range in the adapted than in the control group (43.2% vs. 29.1%, p = 0.030). In addition, the number of dose modifications was significantly less in the adapted group (280 vs. 420 over 3 months; p=0.004). Nonetheless, there was no difference in the rate of biopsy-proven acute rejection in relation to CYP3A5 genotype.

Polymorphisms in the P-glycoprotein

At least 60 SNPs have been described within the ABCB1 promoter, exons, or introns (http://pharmacogenetics.ucsf.edu). Three of these SNPs have been more intensively studied: the 1236C > T SNP in exon 12 (rs1128503), the 2677G > A/T SNP in exon

21 (rs2032582), and the 3435C > T SNP in exon 26 (rs1048642). Of these, only the second leads to an amino acid change in the protein sequence ($A^{893}S/T$), while the other two are silent. The first association studies concerning digoxin or immunosuppressive drugs only involved the silent 3435C > T SNP, generally leading to conflicting results. However, experimental arguments are in favor of an altered P-gp conformation as a result of this silent mutation, the rarity of the corresponding codon affecting the timing of co-translational folding and insertion of P-gp into the membrane (123).

P-gp polymorphisms and cyclosporine pharmacokinetics

The influence of *ABCB1* SNPs on cyclosporine pharmacokinetics remains uncertain. As recently described in a review by Staatz *et al.*, more than 10 independent studies, mainly conducted in renal transplant patients, have failed to find associations between the *ABCB1* 1236C > T, 3435C > T, or 2677G > T SNPs and the pharmacokinetics of cyclosporine (124). Conversely, a few studies have shown significant associations, although with conflicting results. Most of these studies concerned the 3435C > T SNP. The variant allele at position 3435 was associated with decreased exposure to cyclosporine in 75 Caucasian renal transplant recipients, which is not consistent with the hypothesis of a lower functional activity of the mutant protein. In this study, a gene–dose effect was found with approximately a 15% decrease in dose-normalized AUC_{0-4h} per allele (125). Conversely, the same SNP was associated with significantly higher dose-normalized cyclosporine exposure in at least two other studies, one in liver (n = 44) (126) and the other in renal transplant patients (73). The authors of the first study reported that, one month after transplantation, patients with the 3435TT genotype required approximately 50% lower weight-adjusted cyclosporine dose than wild-type patients (126). A recent meta-analysis involving 1,036 individuals (healthy volunteers or renal transplant patients) from 14 different studies attempted to solve the discrepancy (127). It failed to demonstrate a definitive association between the 3435C > T SNP and cyclosporine pharmacokinetics. No significant influence of the SNP on cyclosporine

AUC_{0-4h}/dose, CL/F, C_{max}/dose, or C_0/dose could be found, but the wild-type genotype carriers had lower AUC_{0-12h} than patients with at least one 3435T allele. The authors suggested that the inter-dose exposure might better reflect P-gp influence (on both absorption and elimination) than other exposure indices. However, the fact that cyclosporine is a potent inhibitor of P-gp may limit or suppress the influence of genetic polymorphisms and presumably explain part of the discrepancy reported.

P-gp polymorphisms and tacrolimus pharmacokinetics

Similarly, the influence of P-gp 1236C > T, 3435C > T, and 2677G > T/A polymorphisms on tacrolimus pharmacokinetics is uncertain. In a recent review, Staatz *et al.* identified 21 studies, mainly conducted in renal transplant patients, which failed to find an association between the 3435C > T SNP and tacrolimus pharmacokinetics. Nine and 15 negative studies concerning the 1236C > T and the 2677G > T/A SNPs were also listed (124). Conversely, a few studies demonstrated a higher C_0/dose or dose requirement in patients with the *ABCB1* 3435TT variant genotype. Interestingly, one of these studies, conducted in 136 renal transplant recipients over 1 year post transplantation, estimated using a linear mixed model the relative variability in tacrolimus dose requirement attributable to different genotypes (*ABCB1* 3435C > T, *CYP3A5* 6986A > G [*CYP3A5*1/*3*], and CYP3A4 −392A > G [*CYP3A4*1B*]). Tacrolimus overall dose requirement was 19% ($CI_{95\%}$: 3–33%, p = 0.023) higher in carriers of the 3435TT than in carriers of the wild-type genotype. This is to be compared with the 68% ($CI_{95\%}$: 27–123%, p < 0.001) higher dose requirement in expressers of CYP3A5 (i.e., *CYP3A5*1/*3* or *1/*1* genotypes) as compared to nonexpressers (116). Similarly, higher C_0/dose were also reported in patients with at least one variant allele at positions 1236 or 2677 in the context of renal (128, 129) or lung transplantation (117). One of these studies reported a small but significant association of the variant haplotype (3435T-2677T/A-1236T) with dose requirement in 236 renal transplant patients (129). However, the association was lost when patients were sub-classified as expressers or nonexpressers of CYP3A5. It arose from these different studies that P-gp polymorphisms might only have a limited influence on tacrolimus pharmacokinetics.

P-gp polymorphisms and the clinical effects of calcineurin inhibitors

There have been few studies investigating the relations between *ABCB1* polymorphisms and the efficacy or toxicity of calcineurin inhibitors. Crettol *et al.* described higher cyclosporine concentrations in the lymphocytes of carriers of the *ABCB1* 3435C > T SNP (130), suggesting that cyclosporine activity may be affected by this polymorphism independently of its effect on the drug bioavailability or clearance. In a very large-scale study involving 832 renal transplant recipients, it was found that the recipient's *ABCB1* haplotype gathering the exon 12, 21, and 26 alleles predicted acute graft rejection (131). In liver transplantation, one study showed that the interindividual variability of the *ABCB1* mRNA intestinal level was associated with the occurence of acute cellular rejection, presumably through a lower tacrolimus blood level (132). Another study in liver transplant patients showed that *ABCB1* 2677C > T and 1199G > A were associated with lower tacrolimus concentrations in the hepatic tissue, which might themselves influence graft outcome (133).

In addition, P-gp activity in the kidney graft, which carries the donor's and not the recipient's genome, may contribute to the nephrotoxicity of calcineurin inhibitors. This was initially shown by Hauser *et al.* (n = 97), who found that the donor but not the recipient *ABCB1* 3435 variant genotype was associated with cyclosporin nephrotoxicity (OR = 13.4; CI95%, 1.2–148, p = 0.034) (134).

Recently, in a long-term follow-up of a cohort of 259 renal transplant patients on cyclosporine, we found that the *ABCB1* 1236T, 2677T, and 3435T variant alleles and the corresponding (1236T-2677T-3435T) variant haplotype in graft donors were associated with a higher risk of graft loss, visible beyond the fourth year post transplantation on the survival curves. Among several clinical characteristics, only this haplotype and previous episodes of acute rejection were identified as significant predictors of long-term graft survival. The decrease in renal function over the follow-up period (estimated as

delta creatinine clearance per year) was also more pronounced when the donor was carrier of the *ABCB1* TTT haplotype (135).

A recent study in renal transplant patients treated with tacrolimus showed that a higher IF/TA grade was found over the first 3 years post transplantation when both the donor and the recipient were homozygous for the *ABCB1* 3435C > T SNP (OR = 3.9; CI95% 2.0–7.6, p < 0.001), while there was no association with tacrolimus exposure (136). Degradation of the renal graft function was also quicker when the donor, the recipient and above all both were carriers of the 3435T variant. Finally, the only significant determinants of graft survival were acute T cell-mediated and antibody-mediated rejections. The authors proposed that P-gp in tubular epithelial cells influences local tacrolimus accumulation and, in addition, suggested that the recipient *ABCB1* polymorphisms might also contribute to graft injury because of the high prevalence of epithelial chimerism after kidney transplantation.

Pharmacogenetics of the calcineurin pharmacodynamic pathway

Calcineurin is a calmodulin-regulated protein phosphatase which plays an important role in signal transduction. In resting cells, it is an inactive heterodimer composed of a calmodulin-binding catalytic subunit (calcineurin A; CNA) and a $Ca2^+$-binding regulatory subunit (calcineurin B; CNB). After activation, the $Ca2^+$/calmodulin complex binds to CNA resulting in the active heterotrimeric phosphatase. Finally, calcineurin regulates the nuclear import of NF-AT (nuclear factors of activated T-cells), required for expression of the genes involved in T-cells activation (IL-2, mainly). Cyclosporine or tacrolimus inhibit calcineurin after association with intracellular binding proteins called immunophillins (i.e., cyclophilin A and FK506 Binding Protein-12: FKBP-12, respectively). Theoretically, polymorphisms in each of these different proteins may affect the cellular response to calcineurin inhibitors. For instance, it was shown that mutations generated by site-directed mutagenesis in the CNB subunit of calcineurin were associated with a lower phosphatase activity (137), while other mutations seemed to block the binding of cyclophillin A-cyclosporine or FKBP-12-tacrolimus complexes and thereby conferred cell resistance to the effect of the drugs, as demonstrated in vitro (138). In humans, two SNPs were described in the cyclophilin A gene using single strand conformation analysis PCR and sequencing: one located on the first exon (c.36A > G) and the second on the gene promoter (c.-11C>G). No correlation between those SNPs and acute rejection was found, whereas the SNP -11C>G was associated with an increased risk of nephrotoxicity (OR = 3.5; CI95% 1.5–8.2, p = 0.006) (139). Numerous SNPs were described in the different proteins involved in the cellular effect of calcineurine inhibitors through the international HapMap project (www.hapmap.org). However, to the best of our knowledge, none of them were studied in the context of cyclosporine or tacrolimus effect.

Potential and limits of pharmacogenetics in treatment selection and therapeutic drug monitoring of the calcineurin inhibitors

The results of association studies suggest that genotyping for *CYP3A4*1B* and *CYP3A5*3* may help detect patients at risk of cyclosporine or tacrolimus overexposure, although this is most probably compensated for by routine drug monitoring, as shown by the absence of genotype-outcome association. It is clearer that genotyping for the *ABCB1 1236T/2677T/3435T* haplotype, and maybe for the immunophilin A -11C > G SNP, should help detect patients with an increased risk of cyclosporine nephrotoxicity and hence avoid this drug, provided the other immunosuppressants are devoid of such associations, which remains to be investigated. There are already hints that tacrolimus nephrotoxicity may also be enhanced by the donor and recipient ABCB1 polymorphisms. In any case, comparative clinical trials will be necessary to ascertain the relevance of treatment personalization based on these pharmacogenetic tests. The level of evidence is currently too low to employ any of these tests in the clinics.

mTOR inhibitors

Metabolism and transport pathways

Sirolimus (rapamycin) is metabolized by the intestinal (140) and hepatic CYP3A enzymes (141). At least 12 first-, second-, and third-generation metabolites have been isolated from various biologic sources or in vitro experiments (142). None contributes significantly to the pharmacological activity of sirolimus. Experiments using recombinant P450 showed that CYP3A4 is a more efficient catalyzt of sirolimus metabolism than CYP3A5 (intrinsic clearance of sirolimus depletion: 2.34 vs. 0.66 µl/min/pmol P450) (143) (Table 6.3). CYP2C8, which is only expressed in hepatocytes, is also involved in the formation of some metabolites (144) but has a very limited role in sirolimus overall metabolism (143).

Everolimus is a 40-O-(2-hydroxyethyl) derivative of sirolimus. Like sirolimus, it gives rise to mono-, di-hydroxylated, demethylated, ring-open metabolites, as well as a specific dehydroxyethylated derivative, all produced by the CYP3A and/or CYP2C8. As for sirolimus, experiments using recombinant P450 suggest that CYP3A4 play a more dominant role than CYP3A5 in the metabolism of everolimus (Table), and that CYP2C8 accounts for less than 10% of everolimus hepatic metabolism (unpublished personal data). Although structurally similar, everolimus and sirolimus are not metabolized at the same extent. It was shown that the 40-O-2-hydroxyethyl group on everolimus inhibits the 39-O-demethylation of the molecule and also decreases two major hydroxylation pathways, which results in an overall decrease of the intrinsic clearance of metabolite formation in human liver microsomes (144).

Everolimus and sirolimus are substrates for the P-glycoprotein (P-gp) (145), which may limit their intestinal absorption (145). The primary elimination route of sirolimus and everolimus is through the bile. Hepatic extraction may not involve active transporters (146), so much so that everolimus and sirolimus have very low affinities for OATP1B1 and 1B3 (personal data). Canalicular excretion of these two drugs or their metabolites probably involves P-gp. There is currently no evidence that other canalicular transporters such as MRP2 are involved. In the kidney, P-gp is constitutively expressed on the brush border of the proximal tubular cells and on the distal tubule. It is not expected to play a significant role in the pharmacokinetics of mTOR inhibitors since renal elimination is not their primary disposition pathway. However, P-gp inhibition by sirolimus enhances the nephrotoxicity of cyclosporine when the two drugs are coadministered (147).

Genetic polymorphism effects on the pharmacokinetics of mTOR inhibitors
CYP3A polymorphisms

The association between the CYP3A4*1B and CYP3A5*3 alleles and sirolimus dose requirement was investigated in 149 renal transplant recipients, mostly of European descent (148). The authors only found significant associations between both alleles and sirolimus trough levels standardized by the dose in the subgroup of 69 patients undergoing a sirolimus-based rescue therapy with low-dose corticosteroids (3.5 to 239.9 months after transplantation) and taking no calcineurin inhibitor. These pharmacogenetic effects may be abrogated by pharmacokinetic drug–drug interactions, since no association was found in patients on cyclosporine or tacrolimus. Acute rejection, anemia, dyslipidemia, thrombocytopenia, and graft function were not significantly influenced by these polymorphisms.

However, patients had to be on sirolimus for 3 months before being enrolled, which means that patients in whom sirolimus had to be interrupted because of side effects (if any) were not studied.

Another study was conducted in 85 renal transplant recipients on sirolimus, of whom 38 received sirolimus as de novo therapy and 47 were switched from a calcineurin inhibitor to sirolimus, mainly for chronic allograft nephropathy or neoplasia (113). No association between CYP3A5*3 and sirolimus C_{trough}/dose was found, neither in the whole population nor in the subgroups.

We also conducted a prospective study in 47 renal transplant recipients on sirolimus and mycophenolate mofetil, without calcineurin inhibitor (149). In all patients, a detailed pharmacokinetic profile was collected over the first nine hours post-dose, at 3 months or more after transplantation. Of the 47 patients, 4 (8.5%) were heterozygous carriers and none was homozygous for the CYP3A4*1B allele.

Although there was a slight tendency toward lower dose-standardized area under the concentration–time curve (AUC) in carriers of the CYP3A4*1B allele, no significant association was found, possibly because of the low frequency of this SNP. In contrast, lower AUC_{0-9h}/dose, C_{trough}/dose, and C_{max}/dose values were found in CYP3A5 expressers (p = 0.008, 0.01, and 0.02, respectively). These significant differences between CYP3A5 genotypes were still obtained when normalizing sirolimus concentrations for hemoglobin levels (owing to the high affinity of sirolimus for red blood cells) and even when only the CYP3A4*1 homozygous carriers were considered, that is when the effect of the linkage disequilibrium between the two SNPs was cancelled. However, we found no association between the CYP3A5 genotype and clinical findings, except for a trend toward a higher leucopenia incidence in nonexpressers.

In 21 of these 47 patients, full profiles were also obtained at weeks 1 and 2 and at month 1. These patients received a loading dose of 15 mg sirolimus on days 1 and 2, followed by 10 mg/day for 7 days, and the dose was then titrated to maintain sirolimus trough blood levels between 10 and 15 ng/mL until month 3 after transplantation. Dose adjustment was performed with a maximal step of 2 mg/day once a week. In this subgroup, significantly lower AUC/dose, C_{trough}/dose, and C_{max}/dose values were also found for the CYP3A5 expressers at all posttransplantation periods. Interestingly, sirolimus AUC_{0-9h} was twice lower in expressers at W1 when a standard dose was given to all patients (p = 0.009), C_{trough} was lower than the protocol target range of 10–15 ng/mL for up to 1 month in most CYP3A5 expressers, and above this range for as long as 1 to 3 months in a considerable number of nonexpressers despite weekly dose adjustments starting as early as days 8 to 11 (149).

Finally, an association study was conducted in 47 Chinese kidney transplant recipients (CYP3A5*3 allele frequency: 71%) on sirolimus with no CNI, showing a significantly higher dose-standardized C_{trough} ratio in nonexpressers (397 vs. 318 ng/ml per mg/kg, p < 0.05) (150).

In summary, these in vivo results suggest that the CYP3A5*3 genotype has a strong influence on sirolimus bioavailability in both de novo and stable renal transplant patients, provided they are not combined with calcineurin inhibitors, which may abolish this effect (although this still needs to be confirmed). They also advocate for the determination of this genotype for a priori dose adjustment of sirolimus, given the long half-life of this drug (149).

Although less data are currently available regarding everolimus, it seems that the *CYP3A5*3* genotype has no marked influence on everolimus pharmacokinetics. Only one study has been reported to date, showing no association between the genotype and everolimus blood levels or dose requirement in 30 adult cardiac transplants (115). We recently investigated such an association in 28 stable renal transplants and similarly found that the *CYP3A5*3* polymorphism did not influence everolimus dose requirement, exposure, or dose-normalized exposure (151). In both studies, patients were not cotreated with calcineurin inhibitors, which ensures that enzyme inhibition cannot have interacted with the pharmacogenetic association.

Further experimental studies demonstrated that CYP3A4 is more active than CYP3A5 in everolimus metabolism and confirmed, using genotyped HLM, that the *CYP3A5*3* polymorphism has no significant influence on the metabolism of everolimus (151). The fact that CYP3A4 is a better catalyzt of everolimus metabolism than CYP3A5 (Table 6.3) provides a first explanation to the fact that CYP3A5 expression does not significantly influence everolimus metabolism.

Polymorphisms in the P-glycoprotein

In 47 Chinese renal transplant recipients on sirolimus, low-dose steroids, and no CNI, the *ABCB1* $3435C > T$ SNP showed no significant association with sirolimus C_{trough}/dose (150). Although this SNP is differentially expressed across ethnicities (68% of African Americans, 24% of Caucasians (152), and 22% of Chinese (150) are homozygous wild-type carriers of the C genotype), the same result was found in 149 renal transplant patients (mostly Caucasians) on sirolimus for more than 3 months; the *ABCB1* exon 12, and exon 21 SNPs were not associated with sirolimus C_{trough}/dose either, whether in the 51 patients undergoing a de novo sirolimus-

based therapy (3.0 to 3.2 months after transplantation), in the 29 patients who were coadministered cyclosporine or tacrolimus, or in the 69 patients undergoing sirolimus-based rescue therapy with low-dose corticosteroids (3.5 to 239.9 months after transplantation) and taking no CNI. Also, there was no association between these three polymorphisms and any clinical outcome (acute rejection, anemia, dyslipidemia, thrombocytopenia, or graft function) (148).

As the three abovementioned SNPs are in significant linkage disequilibrium, haplotype analysis was proposed as a more reliable genetic marker than any of these three SNPs alone (153). However, in a study in 85 renal transplant recipients on sirolimus, of whom 24 were also receiving tacrolimus, no association was found between sirolimus C_{trough}/dose and any of the *ABCB1* exon 12, exon 21, and exon 26 SNPs, nor with their haplotype (113).

In summary, there does not seem to be any *ABCB1* pharmacogenetic effect on sirolimus pharmacokinetics or effects in vivo when administered without a CNI, although P-gp may limit its intracellular passage, as suggested by in vitro experiments. Other experimental data suggest that cyclosporine or another strong P-gp inhibitor such as verapamil might unveil the influence of the $3435C > T$ SNP on sirolimus pharmacokinetics or intracellular transport, owing to altered P-gp folding in the membrane (123). Hence, association studies in patients coadministered sirolimus and cyclosporine might yield more interesting results.

To the best of our knowledge, no study of the consequences of genetic polymorphisms in *ABCB1* regarding everolimus pharmacokinetics has been reported.

Pharmacogenetics of the mTOR pharmacodynamic pathway

The target of sirolimus or everolimus is the mTOR, also known as the FRAP (FKBP–rapamycin-associated) protein. mTOR regulates protein synthesis through the phosphorylation and inactivation of the repressor of m-RNA translation "eukaryotic initiation factor 4E binding protein," and through the phosphorylation and activation of the phosphatidylinositol 3-kinase-p70 ribosomal S6 protein kinase (p70s6K). In particular, p70s6K regulates the cellular response to IL-2. mTOR forms a stoichiometric complex with RAPTOR, which has a positive role in signaling to the downstream effector p70sS6K, maintenance of cell size, and mTOR protein expression. The association of RAPTOR with mTOR also negatively regulates the mTOR kinase activity. Finally, mTOR inhibitors act by forming an inhibitory complex with the intracellular receptor FK-BP12 which subsequently binds a region in the C-terminus of m-TOR protein termed FRB (FKBP12-Rapamycin Binding). This causes dephosphorylation and inactivation of the p70s6 kinase activity.

Mutations of the gene encoding mTOR (especially the FRB domain) and others involved in the everolimus or sirolimus signaling pathway (FK-BP12, P70s6K, RAPTOR) might confer a resistant phenotype to these drugs as was demonstrated in mammalian cell lines (154). However, to our knowledge no association study between such polymorphisms and sirolimus or everolimus effects has been published so far.

Potential and limits of pharmacogenetics in treatment selection and therapeutic drug monitoring of the mTOR inhibitors

The *CYP3A5*3* polymorphisms significantly affect sirolimus pharmacokinetics, provided the drug is not associated with cyclosporine, whose interaction with sirolimus metabolism abolish this association. A similar effect of *CYP3A4*1B* is unlikely, or at most weak, while there is no association with *ABCB1* polymorphisms. Despite prolonged underexposure in CYP3A5 expressers and prolonged overexposure in nonexpressers after treatment initiation at the standard dose (due to the drug very long half-life), no association with sirolimus effects was found, whether in terms of efficacy or adverse effects. However, these studies were not powered to investigate such associations in de novo patients. Clinical trials comparing usual dose adjustment based on SRL trough levels to a priori dose adjustment based on the CYP3A5 genotype followed by TDM would be useful to elucidate the clinical impact of this strong pharmacogenetic–pharmacokinetic association. Currently, the level of clinical evidence for using this polymorphism to dose-adjust patients is very low.

The *CYP3A5*3* SNP has apparently no association with everolimus pharmacokinetics, owing to the minor involvement of this isoform in the drug metabolism. The influence of *CYP3A4*1B* and *ABCB1* polymorphisms has not been investigated so far.

The influence on sirolimus or everolimus efficacy or side effects of polymorphisms in the proteins of the mTOR pathway has not been investigated either.

Conclusion

Most studies published so far have been exploratory, from bedside to bench and sometimes comforted by in vitro experiments. They have investigated the impact of polymorphisms in metabolic enzymes and transport proteins involved in the pharmacokinetics or the tissue distribution of immunosuppressive drugs. They have evidenced only a few (statistically) significant pharmacogenetic–pharmacokinetic, and even less pharmacogenetic–outcome, associations. However, they have provided other benefits, such as improving basic knowledge and our understanding of the actual impact of variations in the genome on the variability of the dose–concentration relationship, showing in some instances the relevance of the donor genome, and revealing that drug–drug interactions may abolish the impact of certain pharmacogenetic variations. In this respect, the sources of the pharmacokinetic variability of the newer mTOR inhibitors, particularly everolimus, should be further investigated.

Very few pharmacogenetic studies concerned drug targets, whose polymorphisms might have a greater impact of patient outcome, in particular for drugs routinely dose adjusted based on exposure (i.e., whose pharmacokinetic variability is partly compensated for).

Also, genome-wide associations studies (GWAS) may help find genetic factors involved in the response of, or tolerance to, immunosuppressive drugs and that may be coding for proteins involved in the regulation of the immunological response at large, which should also be regarded as pharmacogenetics.

For the pharmacogenetics of immunosuppressive drugs to come to the clinics now, the second phase (i. e., from bench to bedside) should be undertaken. Indeed, only comparative, randomized clinical trials evaluating the impact on patient outcome of treatment personalization, or at least dose individualization based on the significant pharmacogenetic tests identified at the previous step versus standard of care, can demonstrate their clinical relevance and convince physicians caring for the patients to prescribe them – and regulatory agencies to allow them when necessary.

Then, a number of practical issues will have to be addressed. First, as a written consent has to be obtained from the patient prior to the pharmacogenetic tests, at least in Europe, it could be wise to obtain it before transplantation, once the patient has been registered on the waiting list, hence permitting the best choice of drugs or drug doses immediately after transplantation. Second, pharmacogenetic tests in the donor (if their pertinence is confirmed) using donor cells or a graft biopsy before transplantation to extract DNA, may pose legal problems in some countries. Third, it should be made clear to the transplantation community that, contrary to what many think, pharmacogenetic tests are not expensive as compared to many other laboratory tests, and that they never need to be repeated. Pharmacoeconomic studies might be useful to demonstrate their cost-efficacy. Finally, the respective merits and use of pharmacogenetic tests and therapeutic drug monitoring, not mentioning biomarkers, will have to be clearly evaluated and recommendations issued. There may still be a long way to go, but immunosuppressive drugs may be one of the first therapeutic classes to actually benefit from a full range of treatment individualization tools.

References

1 Fujiyama, N., Miura, M., Kato, S., *et al.* (2010) Involvement of carboxylesterase 1 and 2 in the hydrolysis of mycophenolate mofetil. *Drug Metab Dispos*, **38**(**12**),2210–2217.

2 Fujiyama, N., Miura, M., Satoh, S., *et al.* (2009) Influence of carboxylesterase 2 genetic polymorphisms on mycophenolic acid pharmacokinetics in Japanese renal transplant recipients. *Xenobiotica*, **39**(**5**), 407–414.

3 Bullingham, R.E., Nicholls, A.J., Kamm, B.R. (1998) Clinical pharmacokinetics of mycophenolate mofetil. *Clin Pharmacokinet*, **34**(**6**), 429–455.

4 Basu, N.K., Kole, L., Kubota, S., *et al.* (2004) Human UDP-glucuronosyltransferases show atypical metabolism of mycophenolic acid and inhibition by curcumin. *Drug Metab Dispos*, **32**(**7**), 768–773.

5 Bernard, O., Guillemette, C. (2004) The main role of UGT1A9 in the hepatic metabolism of mycophenolic acid and the effects of naturally occurring variants. *Drug Metab Dispos*, **32**(**8**), 775–778.

6 Mackenzie, P.I. (2000) Identification of uridine diphosphate glucuronosyltransferases involved in the metabolism and clearance of mycophenolic acid. *Ther Drug Monit*, **22**(**1**), 10–13.

7 Picard, N., Ratanasavanh, D., Premaud, A., *et al.* (2005) Identification of the UDP-glucuronosyltransferase isoforms involved in mycophenolic acid phase II metabolism. *Drug Metab Dispos*, **33**(**1**), 139–146.

8 Mojarrabi, B., Mackenzie, P.I. (1997) The human UDP glucuronosyltransferase, UGT1A10, glucuronidates mycophenolic acid. *Biochem Biophys Res Commun*, **238**(**3**), 775–778.

9 Albert, C., Vallee, M., Beaudry, G., *et al.* (1999) The monkey and human uridine diphosphate-glucuronosyltransferase UGT1A9, expressed in steroid target tissues, are estrogen-conjugating enzymes. *Endocrinology*, **140**(**7**), 3292–3302.

10 Bernard, O., Tojcic, J., Journault, K., *et al.* (2006) Influence of nonsynonymous polymorphisms of UGT1A8 and UGT2B7 metabolizing enzymes on the formation of phenolic and acyl glucuronides of mycophenolic acid. *Drug Metab Dispos*, **34**(**9**), 1539–1545.

11 Shipkova, M., Wieland, E., Schutz, E., *et al.* (2001) The acyl glucuronide metabolite of mycophenolic acid inhibits the proliferation of human mononuclear leukocytes. *Transplant Proc*, **33**(**1–2**), 1080–1081.

12 Picard, N., Premaud, A., Rousseau, A., *et al.* (2006) A comparison of the effect of ciclosporin and sirolimus on the pharmokinetics of mycophenolate in renal transplant patients. *Br J Clin Pharmacol*, **62**(**4**), 477–484.

13 Gensburger, O., Picard, N.,and Marquet, P. (2009) Effect of mycophenolate acyl-glucuronide on human recombinant type 2 inosine monophosphate dehydrogenase. *Clin Chem*, **55**(**5**), 986–993.

14 Picard, N., Cresteil, T., Premaud, A., *et al.* (2004) Characterization of a phase 1 metabolite of mycophenolic acid produced by CYP3A4/5. *Ther Drug Monit*, **26** (**6**), 600–608.

15 Shipkova, M., Armstrong, V.W., Wieland, E., *et al.* (1999) Identification of glucoside and carboxyl-linked glucuronide conjugates of mycophenolic acid in plasma of transplant recipients treated with mycophenolate mofetil. *Br J Pharmacol*, **126**(**5**), 1075–1082.

16 Uwai, Y., Motohashi, H., Tsuji, Y., *et al.* (2007) Interaction and transport characteristics of mycophenolic acid and its glucuronide via human organic anion transporters hOAT1 and hOAT3. *Biochem Pharmacol*, **74**(**1**), 161–168.

17 Wolff, N.A., Burckhardt, B.C., Burckhardt, G., *et al.* (2007) Mycophenolic acid (MPA) and its glucuronide metabolites interact with transport systems responsible for excretion of organic anions in the basolateral membrane of the human kidney. *Nephrol Dial Transplant*, **22**(**9**), 2497–2503.

18 Bullingham, R., Monroe, S., Nicholls, A., *et al.* (1996) Pharmacokinetics and bioavailability of mycophenolate mofetil in healthy subjects after single-dose oral and intravenous administration. *J Clin Pharmacol*, **36** (**4**), 315–324.

19 Westley, I.S., Brogan, L.R., Morris, R.G., *et al.* (2006) Role of Mrp2 in the hepatic disposition of mycophenolic acid and its glucuronide metabolites: effect of cyclosporine. *Drug Metab Dispos*, **34**(**2**), 261–266.

20 Picard, N., Yee, S.W., Woillard, J.B., *et al.* (2010) The role of organic anion-transporting polypeptides and their common genetic variants in mycophenolic acid pharmacokinetics. *Clin Pharmacol Ther*, **87**(**1**), 100–108.

21 Kobayashi, M., Saitoh, H., Kobayashi, M., *et al.* (2004) Cyclosporin A, but not tacrolimus, inhibits the biliary excretion of mycophenolic acid glucuronide possibly mediated by multidrug resistance-associated protein 2 in rats. *J Pharmacol Exp Ther*, **309**(**3**), 1029–1035.

22 Wu, M.H., Chen, P., Wu, X., *et al.* (2004) Determination and analysis of single nucleotide polymorphisms and haplotype structure of the human carboxylesterase 2 gene. *Pharmacogenetics*, **14**(**9**), 595–605.

23 Yamada, S., Richardson, K., Tang, M., *et al.* (2010) Genetic variation in carboxylesterase genes and susceptibility to isoniazid-induced hepatotoxicity. *Pharmacogenomics J*, **10**, 524–536.

24 Strassburg, C.P., Kalthoff, S., Ehmer, U. (2008) Variability and function of family 1 uridine-5′-diphosphate glucuronosyltransferases (UGT1A). *Crit Rev Clin Lab Sci*, **45**(**6**), 485–530.

25 Girard, H., Court, M.H., Bernard, O., *et al.* (2004) Identification of common polymorphisms in the promoter of the UGT1A9 gene: evidence that UGT1A9 protein and activity levels are strongly genetically controlled in the liver. *Pharmacogenetics*, **14**(**8**), 501–515.

26 Jinno, H., Saeki, M., Saito, Y., *et al.* (2003) Functional characterization of human UDP-glucuronosyltransferase 1A9 variant, D256N, found in Japanese cancer patients. *J Pharmacol Exp Ther*, **306**(**2**), 688–693.

27 Saeki, M., Saito, Y., Jinno, H., *et al.* (2003) Three novel single nucleotide polymorphisms in UGT1A9. *Drug Metab Pharmacokinet*, **18**(**2**), 146–149.

28 Villeneuve, L., Girard, H., Fortier, L.C., *et al.* (2003) Novel functional polymorphisms in the UGT1A7 and UGT1A9 glucuronidating enzymes in Caucasian and African American subjects and their impact on the metabolism of 7-ethyl-10-hydroxycamptothecin and flavopiridol anticancer drugs. *J Pharmacol Exp Ther*, **307**(**1**), 117–128.

29 Girard, H., Villeneuve, L., Court, M.H., *et al.* (2006) The novel UGT1A9 intronic I399 polymorphism appears as a predictor of 7-ethyl-10-hydroxycamptothecin glucuronidation levels in the liver. *Drug Metab Dispos*, **34**(**7**), 1220–1228.

30 Inoue, K., Miura, M., Satoh, S., *et al.* (2007) Influence of UGT1A7 and UGT1A9 intronic I399 genetic polymorphisms on mycophenolic acid pharmacokinetics in Japanese renal transplant recipients. *Ther Drug Monit*, **29**(**3**), 299–304.

31 Kuypers, D.R., Naesens, M., Vermeire, S., *et al.* (2005) The impact of uridine diphosphate-glucuronosyltransferase 1A9 (UGT1A9) gene promoter region single-nucleotide polymorphisms T-275A and C-2152T on early mycophenolic acid dose-interval exposure in de novo renal allograft recipients. *Clin Pharmacol Ther*, **78**(**4**), 351–361.

32 Levesque, E., Delage, R., Benoit-Biancamano, M.O., *et al.* (2007) The impact of UGT1A8, UGT1A9, and UGT2B7 genetic polymorphisms on the pharmacokinetic profile of mycophenolic acid after a single oral dose in healthy volunteers. *Clin Pharmacol Ther*, **81**(**3**), 392–400.

33 van Schaik, R.H., van Agteren, M., de Fijter, J.W., *et al.* (2009) UGT1A9-275T > A/-2152C > T polymorphisms correlate with low MPA exposure and acute rejection in MMF/tacrolimus-treated kidney transplant patients. *Clin Pharmacol Ther*, **86**(**3**), 319–327.

34 Kuypers, D.R., de Jonge, H., Naesens, M., *et al.* (2008) Current target ranges of mycophenolic acid exposure and drug-related adverse events: a 5-year, open-label, prospective, clinical follow-up study in renal allograft recipients. *Clin Ther*, **30**(4), 673–683.

35 Sanchez-Fructuoso, A.I., Maestro, M.L., Calvo, N., *et al.* (2009) The prevalence of uridine diphosphate-glucuronosyltransferase 1A9 (UGT1A9) gene promoter region single-nucleotide polymorphisms T-275A and C-2152T and its influence on mycophenolic acid pharmacokinetics in stable renal transplant patients. *Transplant Proc*, **41**(6), 2313–2316.

36 Baldelli, S., Merlini, S., Perico, N., *et al.* (2007) C-440T/T-331C polymorphisms in the UGT1A9 gene affect the pharmacokinetics of mycophenolic acid in kidney transplantation. *Pharmacogenomics*, **8**(9), 1127–1141.

37 Johnson, L.A., Oetting, W.S., Basum S., *et al.* (2008) Pharmacogenetic effect of the UGT polymorphisms on mycophenolate is modified by calcineurin inhibitors. *Eur J Clin Pharmacol*, **64**(11), 1047–1056.

38 Huang, Y.H., Galijatovic, A., Nguyen, N., *et al.* (2002) Identification and functional characterization of UDP-glucuronosyltransferases UGT1A8*1, UGT1A8*2 and UGT1A8*3. *Pharmacogenetics*, **12**(4), 287–297.

39 Kagaya, H., Inoue, K., Miura, M., *et al.* (2007) Influence of UGT1A8 and UGT2B7 genetic polymorphisms on mycophenolic acid pharmacokinetics in Japanese renal transplant recipients. *Eur J Clin Pharmacol*, **63**(3), 279–288.

40 Zucker, K., Tsaroucha, A., Olson, L., *et al.* (1999) Evidence that tacrolimus augments the bioavailability of mycophenolate mofetil through the inhibition of mycophenolic acid glucuronidation. *Ther Drug Monit*, **21**(1), 35–43.

41 Woillard, J.B., Rerolle, J.P., Picard, N., *et al.* (2010) Risk of diarrhoea in a long-term cohort of renal transplant patients given mycophenolate mofetil: the significant role of the UGT1A8 2 variant allele. *Br J Clin Pharmacol*, **69**(6), 675–683.

42 Sawyer, M.B., Innocenti, F., Das, S., *et al.* (2003) A pharmacogenetic study of uridine diphosphate-glucuronosyltransferase 2B7 in patients receiving morphine. *Clin Pharmacol Ther*, **73**(6), 566–574.

43 Holthe, M., Klepstad, P., Zahlsen, K., *et al.* (2002) Morphine glucuronide-to-morphine plasma ratios are unaffected by the UGT2B7 H268Y and UGT1A1*28 polymorphisms in cancer patients on chronic morphine therapy. *Eur J Clin Pharmacol*, **58**(5), 353–356.

44 Coffman, B.L., King, C.D., Rios, G.R., *et al.* (1998) The glucuronidation of opioids, other xenobiotics, and androgens by human UGT2B7Y(268) and UGT2B7H (268). *Drug Metab Dispos*, **26**(1), 73–77.

45 Court, M.H., Krishnaswamy, S., Hao, Q., *et al.* (2003) Evaluation of 3′-azido-3′-deoxythymidine, morphine, and codeine as probe substrates for UDP-glucuronosyltransferase 2B7 (UGT2B7) in human liver microsomes: specificity and influence of the UGT2B7*2 polymorphism. *Drug Metab Dispos*, **31**(9), 1125–1133.

46 Duguay, Y., Baar, C., Skorpen, F., *et al.* (2004) A novel functional polymorphism in the uridine diphosphate-glucuronosyltransferase 2B7 promoter with significant impact on promoter activity. *Clin Pharmacol Ther*, **75**(3), 223–233.

47 Djebli, N., Picard, N., Rerolle, J.P., *et al.* (2007) Influence of the UGT2B7 promoter region and exon 2 polymorphisms and comedications on Acyl-MPAG production in vitro and in adult renal transplant patients. *Pharmacogenet Genomics*, **17**(5), 321–330.

48 Zhang, W.X., Chen, B., Jin, Z., *et al.* (2008) Influence of uridine diphosphate (UDP)-glucuronosyltransferases and ABCC2 genetic polymorphisms on the pharmacokinetics of mycophenolic acid and its metabolites in Chinese renal transplant recipients. *Xenobiotica*, **38**(11), 1422–1436.

49 van Agteren, M., Armstrong, V.W., van Schaik, R.H., *et al.* (2008) AcylMPAG plasma concentrations and mycophenolic acid-related side effects in patients undergoing renal transplantation are not related to the UGT2B7-840G > A gene polymorphism. *Ther Drug Monit*, **30**(4), 439–444.

50 Yang, J.W., Lee, P.H., Hutchinson, I.V., *et al.* (2009) Genetic polymorphisms of MRP2 and UGT2B7 and gastrointestinal symptoms in renal transplant recipients taking mycophenolic acid. *Ther Drug Monit*, **31**(5), 542–548.

51 Paulusma, C.C., Kool, M., Bosma, P.J., *et al.* (1997) A mutation in the human canalicular multispecific organic anion transporter gene causes the Dubin-Johnson syndrome. *Hepatology*, **25**(6), 1539–1542.

52 Haenisch, S., Zimmermann, U., Dazert, E., *et al.* (2007) Influence of polymorphisms of ABCB1 and ABCC2 on mRNA and protein expression in normal and cancerous kidney cortex. *Pharmacogenomics J*, **7**(1), 56–65.

53 Meyer zu Schwabedissen, H.E., Jedlitschky, G., *et al.* (2005) Variable expression of MRP2 (ABCC2) in human placenta: influence of gestational age and

cellular differentiation. *Drug Metab Dispos*, **33**(7), 896–904.

54 Hirouchi, M., Suzuki, H., Itoda, M., *et al.* (2004) Characterization of the cellular localization, expression level, and function of SNP variants of MRP2/ABCC2. *Pharm Res*, **21**(5), 742–748.

55 Miura, M., Satoh, S., Inoue, K., *et al.* (2007) Influence of SLCO1B1, 1B3, 2B1 and ABCC2 genetic polymorphisms on mycophenolic acid pharmacokinetics in Japanese renal transplant recipients. *Eur J Clin Pharmacol*, **63**(12), 1161–1169.

56 Naesens, M., Kuypers, D.R., Verbeke, K., *et al.* (2006) Multidrug resistance protein 2 genetic polymorphisms influence mycophenolic acid exposure in renal allograft recipients. *Transplantation*, **82**(8), 1074–1084.

57 Miura, M., Kagaya, H., Satoh, S., *et al.* (2008) Influence of drug transporters and UGT polymorphisms on pharmacokinetics of phenolic glucuronide metabolite of mycophenolic acid in Japanese renal transplant recipients. *Ther Drug Monit*, **30**(5), 559–564.

58 Niemi, M. (2007) Role of OATP transporters in the disposition of drugs. *Pharmacogenomics*, **8**(7), 787–802.

59 Letschert, K., Keppler, D., Konig, J. (2004) Mutations in the SLCO1B3 gene affecting the substrate specificity of the hepatocellular uptake transporter OATP1B3 (OATP8). *Pharmacogenetics*, **14**(7), 441–452.

60 Hamada, A., Sissung, T., Price, D.K., *et al.* (2008) Effect of SLCO1B3 haplotype on testosterone transport and clinical outcome in caucasian patients with androgen-independent prostatic cancer. *Clin Cancer Res*, **14**(11), 3312–3318.

61 Allison, A.C., Eugui, E.M. (2000) Mycophenolate mofetil and its mechanisms of action. *Immunopharmacology*, **47**(2–3), 85–118.

62 Zimmermann, A.G., Spychala, J., Mitchell, B.S. (1995) Characterization of the human inosine-5′-monophosphate dehydrogenase type II gene. *J Biol Chem*, **270**(12), 6808–6814.

63 Gensburger, O., Van Schaik, R.H., Picard, N., *et al.* (2010) Polymorphisms in type I and II inosine monophosphate dehydrogenase genes and association with clinical outcome in patients on mycophenolate mofetil. *Pharmacogenet Genomics*, **20**(9), 537–543.

64 Wu, T-Y., Peng, Y., Pelleymounter, L., *et al.* (2010) Pharmacogenetics of the mycophenolic acid targets inosine monophosphate dehydrogenase IMPDH1 and IMPDH2: gene sequence variation and functional genomics. *Br J Pharmacol.* DOI: 10.111/j.1476–5331.

65 Wang, J., Zeevi, A., Webber, S., *et al.* (2007) A novel variant L263F in human inosine 5′-monophosphate dehydrogenase 2 is associated with diminished enzyme activity. *Pharmacogenet Genomics*, **17**(4), 283–290.

66 Garat, A., Cauffiez, C., Hamdan-Khalil, R., *et al.* (2009) IMPDH2 genetic polymorphism: a promoter single-nucleotide polymorphism disrupts a cyclic adenosine monophosphate responsive element. *Genet Test Mol Biomarkers*, **13**(6), 841–847.

67 Sombogaard, F., van Schaik, R.H., Mathot, R.A., *et al.* (2009) Interpatient variability in IMPDH activity in MMF-treated renal transplant patients is correlated with IMPDH type II 3757T > C polymorphism. *Pharmacogenet Genomics*, **19**(8), 626–634.

68 Winnicki, W., Weigel, G., Sunder-Plassmann, G., *et al.* (2010) An inosine 5′-monophosphate dehydrogenase 2 single-nucleotide polymorphism impairs the effect of mycophenolic acid. *Pharmacogenomics J*, **10**(1), 70–76.

69 Grinyo, J., Vanrenterghem, Y., Nashan, B., *et al.* (2008) Association of four DNA polymorphisms with acute rejection after kidney transplantation. *Transpl Int*, **21**(9), 879–891.

70 Wang, J., Yang, J.W., Zeevi, A., *et al.* (2008) IMPDH1 gene polymorphisms and association with acute rejection in renal transplant patients. *Clin Pharmacol Ther*, **83**(5), 711–717.

71 Kagaya, H., Miura, M., Saito, M., *et al.* (2010) Correlation of IMPDH1 gene polymorphisms with subclinical acute rejection and mycophenolic acid exposure parameters on day 28 after renal transplantation. *Basic Clin Pharmacol Toxicol*, **107**(2), 631–636.

72 Kelly, P., Kahan, B.D. (2002) Review: metabolism of immunosuppressant drugs. *Curr Drug Metab*, **3**(3), 275–287.

73 Azarpira, N., Aghdaie, M.H., Behzad-Behbahanie, A., *et al.* (2006) Association between cyclosporine concentration and genetic polymorphisms of CYP3A5 and MDR1 during the early stage after renal transplantation. *Exp Clin Transplant*, **4**(1), 416–419.

74 Kronbach, T., Fischer, V., Meyer, U.A. (1988) Cyclosporine metabolism in human liver: identification of a cytochrome P-450III gene family as the major cyclosporine-metabolizing enzyme explains interactions of cyclosporine with other drugs. *Clin Pharmacol Ther*, **43**(6), 630–635.

75 Dai, Y., Iwanaga, K., Lin, Y.S., *et al.* (2004) In vitro metabolism of cyclosporine A by human kidney CYP3A5. *Biochem Pharmacol*, **68**(9), 1889–1902.

76 Benet, L.Z., Cummins, C.L., Wu, C.Y. (2003) Transporter-enzyme interactions: implications for predicting drug-drug interactions from in vitro data. *Curr Drug Metab*, **4**(**5**), 393–398.

77 Kato, R., Nishide, M., Kozu, C., *et al.* (2010) Is cyclosporine A transport inhibited by pravastatin via multidrug resistant protein 2? *Eur J Clin Pharmacol*, **66**(**2**), 153–158.

78 Shitara, Y., Itoh, T., Sato, H., *et al.* (2003) Inhibition of transporter-mediated hepatic uptake as a mechanism for drug–drug interaction between cerivastatin and cyclosporin A. *J Pharmacol Exp Ther*, **304**(**2**), 610–616.

79 Venkataramanan, R., Swaminathan, A., Prasad, T., *et al.* (1995) Clinical pharmacokinetics of tacrolimus. *Clin Pharmacokinet*, **29**(**6**), 404–430.

80 Moller, A., Iwasaki, K., Kawamura, A., *et al.* (1999) The disposition of 14C-labeled tacrolimus after intravenous and oral administration in healthy human subjects. *Drug Metab Dispos*, **27**(**6**), 633–636.

81 Dai, Y., Hebert, M.F., Isoherranen, N., *et al.* (2006) Effect of CYP3A5 polymorphism on tacrolimus metabolic clearance in vitro. *Drug Metab Dispos*, **34**(**5**), 836–847.

82 Iwasaki, K., Shiraga, T., Nagase, K., *et al.* (1993) Isolation, identification, and biological activities of oxidative metabolites of FK506, a potent immunosuppressive macrolide lactone. *Drug Metab Dispos*, **21**(**6**), 971–977.

83 Wu, C.Y., Benet, L.Z. (2003) Disposition of tacrolimus in isolated perfused rat liver: influence of troleandomycin, cyclosporine, and gg918. *Drug Metab Dispos*, **31**(**11**), 1292–1295.

84 Jeong, H., Chiou, W.L. (2006) Role of P-glycoprotein in the hepatic metabolism of tacrolimus. *Xenobiotica*, **36**(**1**), 1–13.

85 Lemahieu, W.P., Hermann, M., Asberg, A., *et al.* (2005) Combined therapy with atorvastatin and calcineurin inhibitors: no interactions with tacrolimus. *Am J Transplant*, **5**(**9**), 2236–2243.

86 Amirimani, B., Ning, B., Deitz, A.C., *et al.* (2003) Increased transcriptional activity of the CYP3A4*1B promoter variant. *Environ Mol Mutagen*, **42**(**4**), 299–305.

87 Spurdle, A.B., Goodwin, B., Hodgson, E., *et al.* (2002) The CYP3A4*1B polymorphism has no functional significance and is not associated with risk of breast or ovarian cancer. *Pharmacogenetics*, **12**(**5**), 355–366.

88 He, P., Court, M.H., Greenblatt, D.J., *et al.* (2005) Genotype–phenotype associations of cytochrome P450 3A4 and 3A5 polymorphism with midazolam clearance in vivo. *Clin Pharmacol Ther*, **77**(**5**), 373–387.

89 Kuehl, P., Zhang, J., Lin, Y., *et al.* (2001) Sequence diversity in CYP3A promoters and characterization of the genetic basis of polymorphic CYP3A5 expression. *Nat Genet*, **27**(**4**), 383–391.

90 Warrington, J.S., Shaw, L.M. (2005) Pharmacogenetic differences and drug–drug interactions in immunosuppressive therapy. *Expert Opin Drug Metab Toxicol*, **1**(**3**),487–503.

91 Roy, J.N., Lajoie, J., Zijenah, L.S., *et al.* (2005) CYP3A5 genetic polymorphisms in different ethnic populations. *Drug Metab Dispos*, **33**(**7**), 884–887.

92 Hesselink, D.A., van Schaik, R.H., van der Heiden, I.P., *et al.* (2003) Genetic polymorphisms of the CYP3A4, CYP3A5, and MDR-1 genes and pharmacokinetics of the calcineurin inhibitors cyclosporine and tacrolimus. *Clin Pharmacol Ther*, **74**(**3**), 245–254.

93 von Ahsen, N., Richter, M., Grupp, C., *et al.* (2001) No influence of the MDR-1 C3435T polymorphism or a CYP3A4 promoter polymorphism (CYP3A4-V allele) on dose-adjusted cyclosporin A trough concentrations or rejection incidence in stable renal transplant recipients. *Clin Chem*, **47**(**6**), 1048–1052.

94 Fanta, S., Niemi, M., Jonsson, S., *et al.* (2008) Pharmacogenetics of cyclosporine in children suggests an age-dependent influence of ABCB1 polymorphisms. *Pharmacogenet Genomics*, **18**(**2**), 77–90.

95 Min, D.I., Ellingrod, V.L. (2003) Association of the CYP3A4*1B 5'-flanking region polymorphism with cyclosporine pharmacokinetics in healthy subjects. *Ther Drug Monit*, **25**(**3**), 305–309.

96 Hesselink, D.A., van Gelder, T., van Schaik, R.H., *et al.* (2004) Population pharmacokinetics of cyclosporine in kidney and heart transplant recipients and the influence of ethnicity and genetic polymorphisms in the MDR-1, CYP3A4, and CYP3A5 genes. *Clin Pharmacol Ther*, **76**(**6**), 545–556.

97 Min, D.I., Ellingrod, V.L., Marsh, S., *et al.* (2004) CYP3A5 polymorphism and the ethnic differences in cyclosporine pharmacokinetics in healthy subjects. *Ther Drug Monit*, **26**(**5**), 524–528.

98 Haufroid, V., Mourad, M., Van Kerckhove, V., *et al.* (2004) The effect of CYP3A5 and MDR1 (ABCB1) polymorphisms on cyclosporine and tacrolimus dose requirements and trough blood levels in stable renal transplant patients. *Pharmacogenetics*, **14**(**3**), 147–154.

99 Chen, B., Zhang, W., Fang, J., *et al.* (2009) Influence of the MDR1 haplotype and CYP3A5 genotypes on

cyclosporine blood level in Chinese renal transplant recipients. *Xenobiotica*, **39**(**12**), 931–938.

100 Chu, X.M., Hao, H.P., Wang, G.J., *et al.* (2006) Influence of CYP3A5 genetic polymorphism on cyclosporine A metabolism and elimination in Chinese renal transplant recipients. *Acta Pharmacol Sin*, **27**(**11**), 1504–1508.

101 Eng, H.S., Mohamed, Z., Calne, R., *et al.* (2006) The influence of CYP3A gene polymorphisms on cyclosporine dose requirement in renal allograft recipients. *Kidney Int*, **69**(**10**), 1858–1864.

102 Hu, Y.F., Qiu, W., Liu, Z.Q., *et al.* (2006) Effects of genetic polymorphisms of CYP3A4, CYP3A5 and MDR1 on cyclosporine pharmacokinetics after renal transplantation. *Clin Exp Pharmacol Physiol*, **33**(**11**), 1093–1098.

103 Qiu, X.Y., Jiao, Z., Zhang, M., *et al.* (2008) Association of MDR1, CYP3A4*18B, and CYP3A5*3 polymorphisms with cyclosporine pharmacokinetics in Chinese renal transplant recipients. *Eur J Clin Pharmacol*, **64**(**11**),1069–1084.

104 Singh, R., Srivastava, A., Kapoor, R., *et al.* (2009) Impact of CYP3A5 and CYP3A4 gene polymorphisms on dose requirement of calcineurin inhibitors, cyclosporine and tacrolimus, in renal allograft recipients of North India. *Naunyn Schmiedebergs Arch Pharmacol*, **380**(**2**),169–177.

105 Anglicheau, D., Thervet, E., Etienne, I., *et al.* (2004) CYP3A5 and MDR1 genetic polymorphisms and cyclosporine pharmacokinetics after renal transplantation. *Clin Pharmacol Ther*, **75**(**5**), 422–433.

106 Kreutz, R., Zurcher, H., Kain, S., *et al.* (2004) The effect of variable CYP3A5 expression on cyclosporine dosing, blood pressure and long-term graft survival in renal transplant patients. *Pharmacogenetics*, **14**(**10**), 665–671.

107 Loh, P.T., Lou, H.X., Zhao, Y., *et al.* (2008) Significant impact of gene polymorphisms on tacrolimus but not cyclosporine dosing in Asian renal transplant recipients. *Transplant Proc*, **40**(**5**), 1690–1695.

108 Wang, Y., Wang, C., Li, J., *et al.* (2009) Effect of genetic polymorphisms of CYP3A5 and MDR1 on cyclosporine concentration during the early stage after renal transplantation in Chinese patients co-treated with diltiazem. *Eur J Clin Pharmacol*, **65**(**3**), 239–247.

109 Yates, C.R., Zhang, W., Song, P., *et al.* (2003) The effect of CYP3A5 and MDR1 polymorphic expression on cyclosporine oral disposition in renal transplant patients. *J Clin Pharmacol*, **43**(**6**), 555–564.

110 Zhao, Y., Song, M., Guan, D., *et al.* (2005) Genetic polymorphisms of CYP3A5 genes and concentration of the cyclosporine and tacrolimus. *Transplant Proc*, **37**(**1**),178–181.

111 Tang, H.L., Ma, L.L., Xie, H.G., *et al.* (2010) Effects of the CYP3A5*3 variant on cyclosporine exposure and acute rejection rate in renal transplant patients: a meta-analysis. *Pharmacogenet Genomics*, **20**(**9**), 525–531.

112 Zhu, H.J., Yuan, S.H., Fang, Y., *et al.* (2011) The effect of CYP3A5 polymorphism on dose-adjusted cyclosporine concentration in renal transplant recipients: a meta-analysis. *Pharmacogenomics J*, **11**,237–246.

113 Mourad, M., Mourad, G., Wallemacq, P., *et al.* (2005) Sirolimus and tacrolimus trough concentrations and dose requirements after kidney transplantation in relation to CYP3A5 and MDR1 polymorphisms and steroids. *Transplantation*, **80**(**7**), 977–984.

114 Renders, L., Frisman, M., Ufer, M., *et al.* (2007) CYP3A5 genotype markedly influences the pharmacokinetics of tacrolimus and sirolimus in kidney transplant recipients. *Clin Pharmacol Ther*, **81**(**2**), 228–234.

115 Kniepeiss, D., Renner, W., Trummer, O., *et al.* (2011) The role of CYP3A5 genotypes in dose requirements of tacrolimus and everolimus after heart transplantation. *Clin Transplant*, **25**,146–150.

116 Hesselink, D.A., van Schaik, R.H., van Agteren, M., *et al.* (2008) CYP3A5 genotype is not associated with a higher risk of acute rejection in tacrolimus-treated renal transplant recipients. *Pharmacogenet Genomics*, **18**(**4**), 339–348.

117 Zheng, H., Zeevi, A., Schuetz, E., *et al.* (2004) Tacrolimus dosing in adult lung transplant patients is related to cytochrome P4503A5 gene polymorphism. *J Clin Pharmacol*, **44**(**2**), 135–140.

118 Macphee, I.A., Fredericks, S., Mohamed, M., *et al.* (2005) Tacrolimus pharmacogenetics: the CYP3A5*1 allele predicts low dose-normalized tacrolimus blood concentrations in whites and South Asians. *Transplantation*, **79**(**4**), 499–502.

119 Tsuchiya, N., Satoh, S., Tada, H., *et al.* (2004) Influence of CYP3A5 and MDR1 (ABCB1) polymorphisms on the pharmacokinetics of tacrolimus in renal transplant recipients. *Transplantation*, **78**(**8**), 1182–1187.

120 Goto, M., Masuda, S., Kiuchi, T., *et al.* (2004) CYP3A5*1-carrying graft liver reduces the concentration/oral dose ratio of tacrolimus in recipients of living-donor liver transplantation. *Pharmacogenetics*, **14**(**7**), 471–478.

121 Wallemacq, P., Armstrong, V.W., Brunet, M., *et al.* (2009) Opportunities to optimize tacrolimus therapy in solid organ transplantation: report of the European consensus conference. *Ther Drug Monit*, **31**(2), 139–152.

122 Thervet, E., Loriot, M.A., Barbier, S., *et al.* (2010) Optimization of initial tacrolimus dose using pharmacogenetic testing. *Clin Pharmacol Ther*, **87**(6), 721–726.

123 Kimchi-Sarfaty, C., Oh, J.M., Kim, I.W., *et al.* (2007) A "silent" polymorphism in the MDR1 gene changes substrate specificity. *Science*, **315**(**5811**), 525–528.

124 Staatz, C.E., Goodman, L.K., Tett, S.E. (2010) Effect of CYP3A and ABCB1 single nucleotide polymorphisms on the pharmacokinetics and pharmacodynamics of calcineurin inhibitors: Part II. *Clin Pharmacokinet*, **49**(4),207–221.

125 Foote, C.J., Greer, W., Kiberd, B.A., *et al.* (2006) MDR1 C3435T polymorphisms correlate with cyclosporine levels in de novo renal recipients. *Transplant Proc*, **38**(9),2847–2849.

126 Bonhomme-Faivre, L., Devocelle, A., Saliba, F., *et al.* (2004) MDR-1 C3435T polymorphism influences cyclosporine a dose requirement in liver-transplant recipients. *Transplantation*, **78**(1), 21–25.

127 Jiang, Z.P., Wang, Y.R., Xu, P., *et al.* (2008) Meta-analysis of the effect of MDR1 C3435T polymorphism on cyclosporine pharmacokinetics. *Basic Clin Pharmacol Toxicol*, **103**(5), 433–444.

128 Anglicheau, D., Verstuyft, C., Laurent-Puig, P., *et al.* (2003) Association of the multidrug resistance-1 gene single-nucleotide polymorphisms with the tacrolimus dose requirements in renal transplant recipients. *J Am Soc Nephrol*, **14**(7), 1889–1896.

129 Fredericks, S., Moreton, M., Reboux, S., *et al.* (2006) Multidrug resistance gene-1 (MDR-1) haplotypes have a minor influence on tacrolimus dose requirements. *Transplantation*, **82**(5), 705–708.

130 Crettol, S., Venetz, J.P., Fontana, M., *et al.* (2008) Influence of ABCB1 genetic polymorphisms on cyclosporine intracellular concentration in transplant recipients. *Pharmacogenet Genomics*, **18**(4), 307–315.

131 Bandur, S., Petrasek, J., Hribova, P., *et al.* (2008) Haplotypic structure of ABCB1/MDR1 gene modifies the risk of the acute allograft rejection in renal transplant recipients. *Transplantation*, **86**(9), 1206–1213.

132 Masuda, S., Goto, M., Fukatsu, S., *et al.* (2006) Intestinal MDR1/ABCB1 level at surgery as a risk factor of acute cellular rejection in living-donor liver transplant patients. *Clin Pharmacol Ther*, **79**(1), 90–102.

133 Elens, L., Capron, A., Kerckhove, V.V., *et al.* (2007) 1199G > A and 2677G > T/A polymorphisms of ABCB1 independently affect tacrolimus concentration in hepatic tissue after liver transplantation. *Pharmacogenet Genomics*, **17**(10), 873–883.

134 Hauser, I.A., Schaeffeler, E., Gauer, S., *et al.* (2005) ABCB1 genotype of the donor but not of the recipient is a major risk factor for cyclosporine-related nephrotoxicity after renal transplantation. *J Am Soc Nephrol*, **16**(5), 1501–1511.

135 Woillard, J.B., Rerolle, J.P., Picard, N., *et al.* (2010) Donor P-gp polymorphisms strongly influence renal function and graft loss in a cohort of renal transplant recipients on cyclosporine therapy in a long-term follow-up. *Clin Pharmacol Ther*, **88**(1), 95–100.

136 Naesens, M., Lerut, E., de Jonge, H., *et al.* (2009) Donor age and renal P-glycoprotein expression associate with chronic histological damage in renal allografts. *J Am Soc Nephrol*, **20**(11), 2468–2480.

137 Feng, B., Stemmer, P.M. (1999) Interactions of calcineurin A, calcineurin B, and Ca2+. *Biochemistry*, **38**(38),12481–12489.

138 Zhu, D., Cardenas, M.E., Heitman, J. (1996) Calcineurin mutants render T lymphocytes resistant to cyclosporin A. *Mol Pharmacol*, **50**(3), 506–511.

139 Moscoso-Solorzano, G.T., Ortega, F., Rodriguez, I., *et al.* (2008) A search for cyclophilin-A gene variants in cyclosporine A-treated renal transplanted patients. *Clin Transplant*, **22**(6), 722–729.

140 Lampen, A., Zhang, Y., Hackbarth, I., *et al.* (1998) Metabolism and transport of the macrolide immunosuppressant sirolimus in the small intestine. *J Pharmacol Exp Ther*, **285**(3), 1104–1112.

141 Sattler, M., Guengerich, F.P., Yun, C.H., *et al.* (1992) Cytochrome P-450 3A enzymes are responsible for biotransformation of FK506 and rapamycin in man and rat. *Drug Metab Dispos*, **20**(5), 753–761.

142 Gallant-Haidner, H.L., Trepanier, D.J., Freitag, D.G., *et al.* (2000) Pharmacokinetics and metabolism of sirolimus. *Ther Drug Monit*, **22**(1), 31–35.

143 Picard, N., Djebli, N., Sauvage, F.L., *et al.* (2007) Metabolism of sirolimus in the presence or absence of cyclosporine by genotyped human liver microsomes and recombinant cytochromes P450 3A4 and 3A5. *Drug Metab Dispos*, **35**(3), 350–355.

144 Jacobsen, W., Serkova, N., Hausen, B., *et al.* (2001) Comparison of the in vitro metabolism of the macrolide immunosuppressants sirolimus and RAD. *Transplant Proc*, **33**(1–2), 514–515.

145 Crowe, A., Lemaire, M. (1998) In vitro and in situ absorption of SDZ-RAD using a human intestinal cell line (Caco-2) and a single pass perfusion model in rats: comparison with rapamycin. *Pharm Res*, **15**(11), 1666–1672.

146 Oswald, S., Nassif, A., Modess, C., *et al.* (2010) Pharmacokinetic and pharmacodynamic interactions between the immunosuppressant sirolimus and the lipid-lowering drug ezetimibe in healthy volunteers. *Clin Pharmacol Ther*, **87**(6), 663–667.

147 Anglicheau, D., Pallet, N., Rabant, M., *et al.* (2006) Role of P-glycoprotein in cyclosporine cytotoxicity in the cyclosporine-sirolimus interaction. *Kidney Int*, **70**(6),1019–1025.

148 Anglicheau, D., Le Corre, D., Lechaton, S., *et al.* (2005) Consequences of genetic polymorphisms for sirolimus requirements after renal transplant in patients on primary sirolimus therapy. *Am J Transplant*, **5**(3), 595–603.

149 Le Meur, Y., Djebli, N., Szelag, J.C., *et al.* (2006) CYP3A5*3 influences sirolimus oral clearance in de novo and stable renal transplant recipients. *Clin Pharmacol Ther*, **80**(1), 51–60.

150 Miao, L.Y., Huang, C.R., Hou, J.Q., *et al.* (2008) Association study of ABCB1 and CYP3A5 gene polymorphisms with sirolimus trough concentration and dose requirements in Chinese renal transplant recipients. *Biopharm Drug Dispos*, **29**(1), 1–5.

151 Picard, N., Rouguieg-Malki, K., Kamar, N., *et al.* (2011) CYP3A5 genotype does not influence everolimus in vitro metabolism and clinical pharmacokinetics in renal transplant recipients. *Transplantation*, **91**(6), 652–656.

152 Ameyaw, M.M., Regateiro, F., Li, T., *et al.* (2001) MDR1 pharmacogenetics: frequency of the C3435T mutation in exon 26 is significantly influenced by ethnicity. *Pharmacogenetics*, **11**(3), 217–221.

153 Johne, A., Kopke, K., Gerloff, T., *et al.* (2002) Modulation of steady-state kinetics of digoxin by haplotypes of the P-glycoprotein MDR1 gene. *Clin Pharmacol Ther*, **72**(5), 584–594.

154 Huang, S., Bjornsti, M.A., Houghton, P.J. (2003) Rapamycins: mechanism of action and cellular resistance. *Cancer Biol Ther*, **2**(3), 222–232.

155 Paoluzzi, L., Singh, A.S., Price, D.K., *et al.* (2004) Influence of genetic variants in UGT1A1 and UGT1A9 on the in vivo glucuronidation of SN-38. *J Clin Pharmacol*, **44**(8), 854–860.

CHAPTER 7

Pharmacogenomics of Cardiovascular Drugs

Linnea M. Baudhuin, PhD

Department of Laboratory Medicine and Pathology, Mayo Clinic, Rochester, Minnesota

Introduction

Cardiovascular disorders encompass a large variety of abnormalities and are important causes of both morbidity and mortality. There are numerous categories of cardiovascular-related drugs, including antihypertensives, lipid-lowering therapies, and anticoagulants. Current research has been attempting to address how genetic variations lead to variable response to these medications, and some of this research has translated into clinical practice. However, controversy with regard to the effect of PGx testing on clinical outcomes compared to more traditional therapeutic monitoring measurements exists for some applications. Additionally, there is uncertainty of how to apply pharmacogenetic information to clinical practice, in terms of dosing, alternative therapies, and other patient management issues. Below, we will discuss pharmacogenetic aspects of antiplatelet agents, beta blockers, and statins.

Antiplatelet agents

Acute coronary syndromes (ACS) represent a spectrum of thrombotic disorders including ST-elevation myocardial infarction (STEMI), non-ST-elevation myocardial infarction (NSTEMI), and unstable angina. ACS and other vascular diseases contribute significantly to worldwide morbidity and mortality.

For many years, aspirin was the only antiplatelet drug available for the management of ACS. But in recent years, numerous therapeutic advances have been made, allowing for more treatment options of ACS and other vascular diseases. Multiple clinical trials have demonstrated that antiplatelet drugs reduce thrombotic risk in patients with a history of previous vascular events or known risk factors for cardiovascular disease (1–4). More specifically, the major role of these drugs in clinical practice is to prevent thrombosis in atherosclerotic arteries of the heart (acute coronary syndrome), brain (ischemic stroke), limbs (peripheral arterial disease), veins (venous thromboembolism), and heart chambers (atrial fibrillation and heart failure).

Atherothrombosis is caused by injury to a vessel wall, due to either shear stress related to abnormal blood flow or rupture of an atherosclerotic plaque, which triggers an inflammatory response and platelet aggregation and thrombus formation. Atherothrombosis is the main pathological process associated with ACS, unstable angina, peripheral arterial disease (PAD), and certain types of ischemic stroke. Platelets, which are freely circulating cells, play a key role in this pathological process. Platelets are normally inactive, but become activated after vessel wall injury leads to exposure of subendothelial collagen, which attracts platelets in the presence of the von Willebrand factor (5). Once platelets are activated, they undergo morphological changes and release granule contents and generate lipid

Pharmacogenomics in Clinical Therapeutics, First Edition. Edited by Loralie J. Langman and Amitava Dasgupta.
© 2012 John Wiley & Sons, Ltd. Published 2012 by John Wiley & Sons, Ltd.

mediators, including adenosine diphosphate (ADP), adenosine triphosphate (ATP), and thromboxane A_2, which trigger a positive feedback mechanism leading to further platelet stimulation and aggregation. ADP-induced platelet aggregation is mediated by activation of nucleotide receptors on the platelet surface, including the P2Y1 and the P2Y12 receptors. Platelets aggregate together via fibrinogen, the von Willebrand factor, and transmembrane glycoprotein receptors, especially glycoproteins IIb and IIIa.

Antiplatelet drugs inhibit different aspects of platelet activity, including adhesion, activation, aggregation, and secretion, by targeting specific platelet surface proteins such as collagen receptor glycoproteins Ia/IIa (GP Ia/IIa), the fibrinogen glycoprotein receptors (GP IIb/IIIa), and the ADP-dependent receptors. There are three major families of antiplatelet agents with proven clinical efficacy: cyclo-oxygenase-1 (COX-1) inhibitors (e.g., aspirin), ADP receptor antagonists (e.g., clopidogrel, prasugrel), and GP IIb/IIIa antagonists (e.g., abciximab). Of these three families, the first two families have received the most attention recently in regard to "resistance" to these drugs, which may be more accurately described as low response or nonresponse. Decreased response to aspirin and clopidogrel has been identified as a risk factor for cardiovascular events. Although there is vast literature on this topic, there is great uncertainty regarding the clinical definition and measurement of antiplatelet resistance, as well as its causes and consequences.

Aspirin

Acetylsalicylic acid (ASA or aspirin) is recommended as a first-line antiplatelet drug and is the most commonly used antiplatelet agent worldwide. Aspirin is derived from the white willow tree, *Saliz alba*, and has been in use as a pharmacologic agent since the mid-1800s (6). The hemorrhagic properties of ASA were first documented in the 1940s. Compared to other antiplatelet agents, aspirin is a relatively weak antagonist of platelet action. However, aspirin's popularity is probably due to its widespread availability, low cost, lack of major adverse effects, and familiarity to both physicians and patients.

ASA is effective in reducing risk and mortality of cardiovascular events in patients at high risk for a serious vascular event. In recent years, it has been observed that there is a range of individual response to aspirin therapy. Reports have observed that 5% to 45% of patients who take therapeutic doses of aspirin do not achieve adequate antithrombotic protection, which is largely attributed to decreased bioavailability of aspirin, drug interferences (especially with other nonsteroidal anti-inflammatory drugs), and lack of compliance (7–12). This observation has been termed *aspirin resistance*, and it has been associated with increased risk of adverse events, including all-cause mortality, myocardial infarction, and cardiovascular death (8, 13). The concept of aspirin resistance is controversial, and the study of aspirin resistance is hindered by the lack of a standardized assay to determine clinical failure to aspirin treatment (12, 14, 15).

Upon absorption, aspirin (2-acetyloxybenzoic acid) is rapidly deacetylated to salicylic acid (2-hydroxybenzoic acid) by nonspecific esterases in the liver and stomach. In the liver, where the majority of aspirin conversion to salicylic acid occurs, salicylic acid is further metabolized to salicyluric acid (2-[(2-hydroxybenzoyl)amino]acetic acid) by the medium-chain fatty acid:CoA ligase ACSMB2. Other minor metabolic products of salicylic acid are also produced by UDP-glucuronosyl transferase 1A6 (UGT1A6) and other UGTs, as well as cytochrome P450 2C9 (CYP2C9).

ASA has a rapid onset of action, which occurs approximately 30 minutes after the first dose. It irreversibly inhibits cyclooxygenase-1 (COX-1) by acetylating the serine 529 site, and modifies the enzymatic activity of cyclooxygenase-2 (COX-2) by acetylating the serine 516 site. This results in decreased production of the potent platelet activator, thromboxane A_2 (TxA_2), and prevents platelet aggregation (16). The effect of aspirin on COX-1 activity is approximately 50- to 100-fold greater than its effect on COX-2 (17). Because anucleate platelets do not have the ability to make new COX-1 enzyme, the effect of aspirin persists for the life of the platelet. After discontinuation of therapy, new nonacetylated platelets are able to restore platelet aggregation capabilities.

As the primary target of aspirin, COX1 makes a logical enzyme for PGx investigation. Polymorphisms in the COX1 gene, *PTGS1*, have been associated with variable response of platelet aggregation to aspirin (18–20). The *PTGS1* −842A > G polymorphism was associated with nonresponders, but three other polymorphisms in the gene (R8W, 644C > T, and 714C > A) had no association (21). Another *PTGS1* variant, 50C > T, correlated with higher levels of 11-dehydroTxB$_2$ (a degradation product of TxA$_2$) and the *PTGS2* (encoding COX-2) -765G > C polymorphism showed slightly increased sensitivity to ASA (18). However, there is some discordance in the literature, and others have not found a convincing association of *PTGS1* variants and aspirin response (22).

Glycoprotein receptor polymorphisms have also been associated with variation in aspirin response. The GP IIIa P1$^{A1/A2}$ allele has been extensively studied, and carriers of the P1^{A2} allele were found to have increased platelet activity at baseline, which was predictive of resistance to drug effect (23–25). Macchi *et al.* showed that GP IIIa P1$^{A1/A1}$ homozygotes were less sensitive to inhibition by low-dose aspirin (26). Cooke *et al.* showed greater aspirin-induced inhibition of platelets with P1$^{A1/A2}$ compared to P1$^{A1/A1}$ (27). It was later described that ASA inhibition varies in an agonist-dependent matter and is associated with the GP IIIa P1$^{A1/A2}$ genotype (28). In contrast to these studies, others have not found any association with aspirin response and GP IIIa P1$^{A1/A2}$ genotype (18, 29). While studies investigating the relationship between the Pl$^{A1/A2}$ allele and aspirin resistance are somewhat conflicting, it should be noted that the association is complicated by the presence of cardiovascular disease, which may have not been taken into account in some PGx studies (15). Conversely, most studies have shown that polymorphisms in the genes encoding GP Ia/IIa and GP Ib were not associated with response to aspirin (18, 26, 30).

Plasma lipoprotein(a) [Lp(a)] has been associated with increased cardiovascular risk, especially atherogenesis and the promotion of thrombosis. The protein component of Lp(a), apolipoprotein(a) [apo (a)], is highly homologous to plasminogen and has mechanistically implicated a role for Lp(a) in hemostasis, thrombosis, and platelet function (31–33). The p.I4399M variant (rs3798220) in the *LPA* gene, which encodes apo(a), has been shown to be associated with elevated plasma Lp(a) and increased cardiovascular risk (32, 34, 35). This variant has a minor allele frequency of approximately 2% in Caucasians. A study investigating this allele in 25,131 Caucasian individuals reported that carriers of the variant allele who were taking aspirin (compared to placebo) had a decreased risk for major cardiovascular events (age-adjusted HR 0.44, 95% CI: 0.20–0.94, p = 0.033) (34).

Gastrointestinal complications, especially bleeding, can occur on aspirin therapy and may be associated with genetic variants. One study reported an association with the *CYP2C9* *2 polymorphism and development of acute gastrointestinal bleeding on NSAIDs (nonsteroidal anti-inflammatory drugs), including aspirin (36). Other studies have also demonstrated an association between CYP2C9 variants and gastrointestinal bleeding while on NSAIDs, including one study that reported an odds ratio of 1.73 for carriers of CYP2C9 variant alleles and gastrointestinal bleeding while on aspirin (37–39).

While it is commonly acknowledged that aspirin resistance, hypersensitivity, insensitivity, and adverse reactions occur on a relatively frequent basis, limited studies have been performed to robustly verify a genetic association. Studies with sufficient power are needed to determine whether genetic markers can play a role in determining clinical effects of aspirin.

Clopidogrel

Clopidogrel is in the thienopyridine class of antiplatelet drugs and is an effective and commonly used anticoagulant. Compared to aspirin, clopidogrel reduces the risk of serious vascular events among high-risk patients by about 10% (40). Clopidogrel is used to reduce atherosclerotic events (myocardial infarction, stroke, and vascular death) in patients with atherosclerosis documented by recent stroke, recent myocardial infarction, or established peripheral arterial disease. Clopidogrel is generally given as an alternative to aspirin in patients who require long-term secondary prevention or are at a very high risk of a vascular event and cannot tolerate aspirin or have found it ineffective. Clopidogrel is also often prescribed in combination with aspirin as a dual antiplatelet therapeutic regimen.

Clopidogrel has been widely prescribed for over a decade, but it wasn't until recently that its metabolism has been more fully understood. From a mechanistic standpoint, understanding the metabolism of clopidogrel is important since only 2% of ingested clopidogrel becomes bound to platelets (41). Therefore, small changes in metabolism could lead to large changes in how clopidogrel inhibits the action of platelets. This is important on many levels especially considering the risk of complications while on clopidogrel, including thrombotic and bleeding events, the "one-size-fits-all" dosing mentality and the lack of a measureable endpoint for titrating the drug, and the unavailability of alternative therapies until recently.

Clopidogrel metabolism

Clopidogrel is a $P2Y_{12}$ receptor-blocking agent that that can inhibit approximately 50% of ADP-induced platelet aggregation. It is given as a prodrug and is absorbed in the intestine and undergoes oxidation in the liver to 2-oxoclopidogrel by numerous cytochrome P450 (CYP) enzymes (predominantly CYP2C19, CYP1A2, and CYP2B6) (42) (Figure 7.1). Following oxidation, 2-oxoclopidogrel is converted to its active thiol metabolite (R-130964) by CYP2B6,

CYP2C9, CYP2C19, and CYP3A4. Only 15% of the prodrug becomes converted to its active thiol metabolite, with the rest (85%) being converted to an inactive metabolite by esterases, primarily human carboxylesterase 1 (CES1). The active metabolite inhibits adenosine diphosphate (ADP)-induced platelet aggregation by blocking the platelet ADP receptor resulting in decreased platelet aggregation. The effect of clopidogrel, whose half-life is only 8 hours, on platelets is irreversible and lasts approximately 7–10 days. Platelet inhibition by clopidogrel begins approximately 2 hours after the first dose and achieves a steady state value of 55–57% by day 7 (43). Approximately 4–30% of patients are refractory to clopidogrel at therapeutic doses, and variability in clopidogrel response is well established (44–46). Variation in platelet function in response to clopidogrel has been associated with numerous factors, including co-drugs (e.g., lipophilic statins, calcium channel blockers, proton pump inhibitors, and St. John's wort), smoking, and genetics.

On March 12, 2010, the FDA approved a new boxed warning label for clopidogrel to include information to warn about reduced effectiveness in

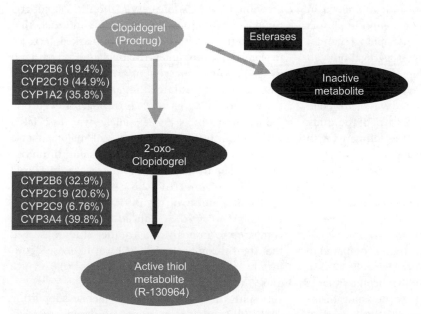

Figure 7.1 Clopidogrel pharmacokinetic metabolism. Clopidogrel is converted in the liver to an intermediate metabolite (2-oxo-clopidogrel) and active metabolite by several CYP enzymes. Esterases convert 85% of ingested clopidogrel to an inactive metabolite. Only 2% of ingested clopidogrel binds to platelets in its active thiol form.

patients who do not effectively convert clopidogrel to its active form; inform health care professionals that genetic tests (specifically for CYP2C19) are available; and advise health care professionals to consider using alternative medications or clopidogrel dosing strategies in patients who do not effectively convert clopidogrel to its active form (47). The FDA approved this boxed warning mainly because of concerns regarding cytochrome P450 (CYP)-dependent activation of clopidogrel and a decreased antiplatelet effect in CYP2C19-deficient patients taking clopidogrel.

CYP2C19

CYP2C19 is involved in oxidation of about 45% of clopidogrel to 2-oxo-clopidogrel and approximately 20% of the generation of 2-oxo-clopidogrel into the active thiol metabolite (48). A genomewide association study identified CYP2C19 as being associated with the pharmacodynamic response to clopidogrel (49). CYP2C19 poor metabolizers have a significantly lower response to clopidogrel, which is correlated to a decreased formation of the active metabolite (50, 51). Mega *et al.* demonstrated that healthy individuals receiving treatment with clopidogrel who carried at least one loss-of-function alleles in *CYP2C19* had a 32.4% relative reduction in plasma levels of the active metabolite of clopidogrel and a decreased ability to inhibit platelet aggregation with the usual induction dose of clopidogrel (52). Additionally, a relative 53% increased risk of death from cardiovascular causes, MI, or stroke was observed in carriers from the TRITON-TIMI 38 arm of the study who were treated with clopidogrel as compared with noncarriers. A threefold increase in risk of stent thrombosis was also observed in carriers versus noncarriers. Numerous studies have additionally demonstrated that patients with deficient CYP2C19 activity have higher rates of cardiovascular events after acute coronary syndromes (ACS) and percutaneous coronary interventions (PCIs) compared to individuals with normal CYP2C19 activity (49, 52–57).

CYP2C19 contains at least 25 polymorphic variants with varying frequency of these polymorphisms among ethnic groups. The *CYP2C19*2, variant encodes a loss of function allele in exon 5. Approximately 50% of Chinese, 34% of African Americans,

35% of Caucasians, and 19% of Mexican Americans carry one copy of the *CYP2C19*2 variant (58, 59). Other genetic polymorphisms in *CYP2C19*, such as *3, *4, *5, and *8, may also be associated with clopidogrel resistance, but occur at a much lower frequency in individuals of Caucasian, African American, and Hispanic descent. Overall, *CYP2C19* polymorphisms that result in inadequate platelet inhibition are found in approximately 30% of the North American population, but may be found at a higher frequency in specific populations (e.g., African Americans and some Asian and Oceanic populations).

*CYP2C19*2 has been the most widely implicated genetic variant associated with clopidogrel resistance. A genomewide association study (GWAS) of healthy Amish individuals receiving clopidogrel over a 7-day period identified a cluster of 13 SNPs spanning 1.5 megabases on chromosome 10q24, a region that spans the *CYP2C18-CYP2C19-CYP2C9-CYP2C8* gene cluster (49). Genotyping of the *CYP2C19*2 polymorphism as follow-up to the genome-wide association analyses demonstrated that this variant accounted for most of the association signal identified via GWAS and overall, accounted for 12% of the variation in clopidogrel response. Numerous studies have confirmed that the *2 variant is associated with a marked decrease in platelet responsiveness to clopidogrel as well as an increased rate of subsequent cardiovascular events. One study demonstrated that among patients treated with clopidogrel for PCI, carriage of even one reduced-function *CYP2C19* allele was associated with significantly increased risk of major adverse cardiovascular events (especially stent thrombosis) (60). The risk of stent thrombosis was increased in carriers of one (HR, 2.67; 95% CI 1.69–4.22; p < 0.0001) and two (HR, 3.97; 95% CI 1.75–9.02, p < 0.0001) *CYP2C19* reduced-function alleles as compared to noncarriers. Another study observed that stent thrombosis after PCI was likewise significantly associated with the presence of *CYP2C19* *2 and *3 (61).

Despite the large body of evidence supporting *CYP2C19*2 and its association with clopidogrel resistance and cardiovascular events, at least one study was not able to identify an association with

CYP2C19*2 or *3 and effect of clopidogrel in patients with ACS or atrial fibrillation (62). However, this study is limited by the analysis of only the *2, *3, and *17 variants in CYP2C19, and not taking into account additional variants in this and other genes. Additionally, the patients in this study were conservatively managed with only approximately 15% undergoing PCI as compared to other studies that showed a positive correlation and had more invasive patient management (> 75% of participants undergoing PCI).

The *17 promoter polymorphism in CYP2C19 (c. −806C > T) is associated with increased transcription of CYP2C19. This variant has been only recently described and occurs at a frequency of 41–46% in Caucasians, 4% in Chinese, and 30–46% in Africans (63). CYP2C19*17 carrier status has been shown to be associated with an enhanced response to clopidogrel, reduced clinical event rates, and an increased risk of bleeding (62, 64, 65). These effects were shown to be correlated to platelet function as measured by aggregometry. Patients homozygous for the *17 allele had an approximate fourfold increase in the occurrence of bleeding events (64).

Limited studies have investigated the interactive impact of CYP2C19 variants, including loss of function polymorphisms such as *2 and the *17 gain of function polymorphisms. Sibbing et al. investigated the effect of the CYP2C19 *2 and *17 polymorphisms in 986 CAD patients who had undergone PCI and were being treated with clopidogrel (66). Platelet function testing was also assessed by means of multiple electrode platelet aggregometry. The highest ADP-induced platelet aggregation was observed in individuals who were CYP2C19*2 but not 17 carriers [309 AU*min (IQR 172–409 AU*min)]. The lowest ADP-induced platelet aggregation occurred among individuals who carried the 17, but not the 2 allele (207AU*min [IQR 132–332 AU*min)].

ABCB1

Clopidogrel intestinal efflux occurs via the ATP-binding cassette transporter encoded by the ABCB1 gene (also known as the multidrug resistant (MDR1) gene). Carriers of the ABCB1 c.3435C > T variant allele have been shown to have reduced absorption of clopidogrel and an increased risk for cardiovas-

cular events (death, nonfatal myocardial infarction, or stroke) (56, 67). Individuals undergoing elective PCI had a significantly reduced bioavailability of clopidogrel if they carry one or two copies of the c.3435C > T variant (68). The frequency of the ABCB1 3435T allele is 54–62% in Caucasians, 38–40% in Chinese, 48% in Japanese, 55% in Hispanics, and 11–21% in Africans.

While most studies have investigated variants in only one gene (usually CYP2C19) in relation to clopidogrel resistance, less is known about the impact of multiple variants in multiple genes. The presence of the ABCB1 c.3435C > T variant in combination with two CYP2C19 loss of function alleles had the highest risk of events compared to other genotypes observed (adjusted HR 5.31, 95% CI 2.13–13.20, p = 0.009) (56). Mega et al. assessed the combined effect of reduced function alleles in CYP2C19 and the ABCB1 c.3435C > T variant in 2932 patients with ACS undergoing PCI (67). They observed that in this population, 47% of the individuals who were either CYP2C19 reduced function allele carriers, ABCB1 TT homozygotes, or both had a significantly increased risk of cardiovascular death, myocardial infarction, or stroke. Individuals who had were both CYP2C19 reduced function allele carriers and ABCB1 TT homozygotes had the highest rate of events (13.6%), followed by ABCB1 TT homozygotes (12.6%) and CYP2C19 reduced function allele carriers (11.5%), respectively.

CYP3A4

CYP3A4 activity is inversely associated with clopidogrel activation and is subject to drug–drug interaction that affects CYP3A4 function (69, 70). Carriers of the CYP3A4 IVS10 + 12G > A variant allele were found to have reduced glycoprotein IIb/IIIa activation and a better response to clopidogrel compared to individuals homozygous for the wild-type G allele. The CYP3A4 IVS10 + 12G > A variant allele is found at a frequency of 10% in Caucasians, 20% in Asians, 43% in Hispanics, and 70% in Africans (71). Until recently, the current utility of CYP3A4 as a PGx marker was low since common genetic variants associated with altered CYP3A4 activity were not well defined. However, a polymorphism (rs35599367 C > T) in intron 6 of CYP3A4 has been identified that is associated with decreased expression and enzymatic activity (72). This SNP was observed at a minor allele frequency of 5.2% of Caucasians and may at least partially explain variability in response to drugs metabolized by CYP3A4.

Other CYPs

In addition to CYP2C19 and CYP3A4, other CYP enzymes are involved in clopidogrel metabolism and variants in their genes may be associated with variable drug response (Figure 7.1). Variants in *CYP2C9*, *CYP3A5*, *CYP1A2*, and *CYP2B6* have been investigated on a limited basis. In one study, neither a consistent reduction of the plasma levels of the active clopidogrel metabolite nor platelet aggregation was observed in carriers of reduced function alleles of *CYP2C9*, *CYP3A5*, or *CYP1A2* (52). On the other hand, carriers of a reduced function *CYP2B6* allele did have lower levels of the active clopidogrel metabolite as well as reduced platelet aggregation (52, 73).

P2RY12

Clopidogrel targets the ADP receptor $P2Y_{12}$, which in part mediates platelet aggregation (74). Genetic variants in the *P2RY12* gene, which encodes $P2Y_{12}$, are associated with a range of activity levels both at baseline and in response to clopidogrel that correlates with the observed phenotype (75). The *P2RY12* gene has at least five common polymorphisms, four of which are in linkage disequilibrium and are the basis for the H2 haplotype designation and its controversial association with clopidogrel response (74, 76). Some authors have found the H2 haplotype to be less responsive to clopidogrel than the H1 haplotype (77–79). The *P2RY12* 744T > C polymorphism, which is part of the H2 haplotype, alone did not show a significant difference in its frequency in clopidogrel- or aspirin-sensitive or -insensitive patients (29, 80). Another *P2RY12* polymorphism, 32C > T, which is not in linkage disequilibrium with the other common polymorphisms, did not show a statistically significant difference in clopidogrel response (76). *P2RY12* c.18C > T variant carriers were found to have a fourfold increase in ischemic stroke and carotid revascularization compared to homozygous wild-type C individuals (79). Another

single nucleotide polymorphism (SNP), *P2Y12* c.36G > T, is 1 of 4 SNPs that comprise the H1/H2 haplotypes. The four variations (139C > T, 744T > C, 801_802insA, c.36G > T) are in complete linkage disequilibrium, with c.36G > T as the tagging SNP. The H1 haplotype is tagged by the wild-type G allele at nucleotide 36, whereas the minor H2 haplotype is tagged by the variant T allele at nucleotide 36. The H2 haplotype has been found to be associated with enhanced platelet reactivity, peripheral artery disease, coronary artery disease (particularly in nonsmokers) and with poor response to clopidogrel.

Platelet surface glycoproteins

Polymorphisms in genes encoding platelet surface glycoproteins have also been shown to contribute to refractory responses to clopidogrel. Polymorphisms in *ITGA2B* and *ITGB3*, which encode the alpha and beta subunits of the receptor complex GP IIb/IIIa, respectively, have been suggested as contributing to the variability of clopidogrel response. Heterozygotes for the *ITGB3* Leu33Pro polymorphism (a.k.a. $Pl^{A1/A2}$) were found to have higher platelet activation at 4 and 24 hours after loading dose of clopidogrel both by GP IIb/IIIa activation and P-selectin expression (81). However, similar studies investigating this polymorphism showed conflicting outcomes (28, 29).

Variability in clopidogrel response has also been linked to polymorphisms in *ITGA2*, encoding for GP Ia. The 807C > T variant, which is associated with increased GP Ia/IIa expression, has been reported as being linked to increased platelet activity and subsequently lower response to clopidogrel at 4 and 24 hours (82). The active metabolite of clopidogrel reduces collagen-induced platelet aggregation more effectively in individuals who are homozygous for the wild-type C allele at nucleotide 759, compared with carriers of the variant T allele. The c.759C > T variant allele is associated with increased glycoprotein Ia density, which results in an increase in collagen-induced platelet aggregation and an increase in thrombotic risk (83). Another study demonstrated that the 807T/873A allele of *ITGA2* was associated with higher platelet reactivity in MI patients undergoing PCI on dual antiplatelet treatment (84). Noncarriers of the variant 807T allele demonstrated reduced collagen-induced platelet aggregation in response to the active metabolite of clopidogrel.

Alternative dosing regimens in clopidogrel poor responders

Whether or not genetically defined poor responders to clopidogrel would benefit from high doses of the drug requires investigation. The GRAVITAS (Gauging Responsiveness with A Verifynow assay – Impact on Thrombosis And Safety) study is being undertaken to address this issue, and will examine approximately 2,800 patients and identify those with high residual platelet reactivity on clopidogrel therapy 12 to 24 hours post PCI (85). These patients will be randomized to clopidogrel therapy at the standard dose of 75 mg/day or the high-dose protocol (an additional loading dose followed by 150 mg/day maintenance dose). The primary endpoint of the study is time to first occurrence of event (cardiovascular death, nonfatal MI, or stent thrombosis). A pilot study of 41 patients (20 of whom were carriers of a CYP2C19 LOF allele) showed that increasing clopidogrel to a maintenance dose of 150 mg/day resulted in a significant reduction in platelet reactivity as determined by VerifyNow P2Y12 (86). This effect was independent of *CYP2C19* genotype; however, larger studies should be performed to confirm the observations from this pilot study. Another study investigated the effect of clopidogrel loading dose adjustment in 411 patients with ACS undergoing PCI (87). At least one copy of the CYP2C19 *2 allele was identified in 35.3% (n = 134) of the patients, and 103 of these individuals had high on-treatment platelet reactivity (HTPR) as determined by the vasodilator-stimulated phosphoprotein (VASP) index. Using the VASP index as a guide, patients with HTPR were given one 600 mg loading dose of clopidogrel, followed by up to three additional 600 mg loading doses. Dose adjustment enable the individuals with HTPR to achieve a VASP index <50% indicating the absence of HTPR (88).

Other studies have looked at the effect of adding another drug to the regimen of patients whom are poor responders to clopidogrel. One of these drugs is cilostazol, which has been approved for use in patients with peripheral vascular disease and clau-

dication. Cilostazol inhibits adenosine reuptake and nitric oxide PGI_2 production by endothelial cells (89). Jeong *et al.* investigated 60 patients with high posttreatment platelet reactivity (HPPR) undergoing coronary stenting (90). The patients were randomized to receive high maintenance dose clopidogrel (150 mg/day) with or without adjunctive cilostazol. They observed that cilostazol increased platelet inhibition to a greater degree than high-dose clopidogrel. Another study by the same authors found a similar effect in patients undergoing primary PCI for ST-segment elevation MI (91).

Other thienopyridines, including prasugrel and ticagrelor, have also been investigated as alternative therapies in clopidogrel poor responders. These thienopyridines are discussed in further detail below.

Dual antiplatelet therapy and proton pump inhibitors (PPIs)

Because of their different mechanisms of action, dual antiplatelet therapy with clopidogrel and aspirin has been recommended in some patients, including those with CAD, atherosclerotic ischemic stroke, and atrial fibrillation. Dual antiplatelet therapy has been demonstrated to be effective in reducing recurrent cardiac events after acute coronary syndromes (ACS) and in reducing stent thrombosis after percutaneous coronary intervention (PCI) (92, 93). Other studies have shown that dual antiplatelet therapy in patients with ST-segment elevation MI led to decreased odds of the composite death, recurrent MI or ischemia, as well as all-cause mortality (94, 95). However, an increased risk for gastrointestinal bleeding has been observed in patients taking dual antiplatelet therapy, especially in high-risk patients (94, 96). Therefore, proton pump inhibitors (PPIs) are often prescribed in these patients to help reduce the risk of gastrointestinal bleeding.

A decreased efficacy of clopidogrel when combined with PPIs has been reported, and an FDA announcement in November 2009 warned that patients should avoid using omeprazole and clopidogrel together (97, 98). Many PPIs, including omeprazole, esomeprazole, lansoprazole, and rabeprazole are both substrates and inhibitors of CYP2C19 (99). Pantoprazole, another PPI, is a

CYP2C19 substrate, but not a CYP2C19 inhibitor (100). Omeprazole is currently the most potent PPI on the market and it has been shown to reduce the inhibitory effect of clopidogrel on platelet aggregation (101–103). Results of four randomized crossover studies in healthy volunteers demonstrated that when clopidogrel and omeprazole were coadministered, exposure of the active metabolite of clopidogrel was consistently decreased by 40–47% (103). By comparison, coadministration of clopidogrel and pantoprazole resulted in a decrease of active metabolite of only 14%. Because of the observed differences between omeprazole and pantoprazole coadministration with clopidogrel, it could be argued that the effects of the PPI-clopidogrel interaction lie at the level of CYP2C19, rather than due to a more nonspecific PPI effect on clopidogrel caused by increased gastric pH.

Other antiplatelet agents
Ticlopidine
The thienopyridine, ticlopidine, is a first-generation ADP receptor antagonist that has been almost entirely replaced by clopidogrel. In 1991, ticlopidine became the first thienopyridine approved for the prevention of thrombosis after PCI (104). While ticlopidine has been shown to be efficacious, its use has been diminished because of concerns over serious side effects including neutropenia (1.0–2.4%) and thrombotic thrombocytopenic purpura (1:3000) (93). Ticlopidine also requires dosing twice daily and costs more. When compared with clopidogrel in the CLASSICS stenting trial, clopidogrel was more effective and had fewer major adverse cardiovascular events PCI (105). Thus, pharmacogenetic studies involving ticlopidine are limited. Von Beckerath et al. showed that in the setting of coronary artery stenting, GP Ia 807C > T polymorphism carriers were not at increased risk for thrombotic events in the first 30 days post intervention during therapy with aspirin and ticlopidine (106).

Prasugrel
Prasugrel, a potent antiplatelet agent, was approved by the FDA in July 2009 for the reduction of thrombotic cardiovascular events in patients with ACS managed with PCI. Prasugrel has been demonstrated to inhibit platelets to a greater and more consistent extent than clopidogrel, even when administered at high doses (107). Fewer recurrent atherothrombotic events, but more major bleeding events (especially coronary artery bypass surgery [CABG]-related bleeding) have been observed in patients with ACS being treated with prasugrel, as compared to clopidogrel (108).

Prasugrel is a third-generation thienopyridine and is chemically distinct from clopidogrel. Prasugrel, like clopidogrel, is administered as a prodrug that must be metabolized to its active form, mainly by CYP3A4/5 and CYP2B6 (and, to a lesser extent, CYP2C9 and CYP2C19) (109). Unlike clopidogrel, prasugrel is not inactivated by esterases, so the bioavailability of prasugrel is much higher than clopidogrel. Similar to clopidogrel, prasugrel also irreversibly blocks the P2Y$_{12}$ receptor in a mechanism similar to clopidogrel. Prasugrel is rapidly absorbed and metabolized, with a 30-minute median time for achieving active metabolite maximal blood concentration and a 3.7-hour mean elimination half-life of the active metabolite (110, 111).

In contrast to clopidogrel, a pharmacogenetic-dependent response to prasugrel has not been demonstrated. Healthy individuals with at least one reduced function allele in CYP2C19, CYP2C9, CYP2B6, CYP3A5, and CYP1A2 did not have a significant decrease in the plasma concentration of the prasugrel active metabolite or platelet inhibition compared to noncarriers (73). Similar results have been observed in patients with stable coronary disease (112). In TRITON-TIMI 38 patients taking prasugrel, one or two copies of ABCB1 c.3435C > T variant was not associated with cardiovascular outcome (67). There was also no observed association between healthy individuals, the presence of ABCB1 c.3435C > T, and pharmacodynamic or pharmacokinetic response to prasugrel in this study.

Since a pharmacogenetic-associated response to prasugrel has not been demonstrated, and because of the high variability in response to clopidogrel, some have supported the use of prasugrel instead of clopidogrel for ACS patients undergoing PCI. One study examined the effect of switching ACS patients from maintenance clopidogrel to prasugrel and observed a significant reduction in platelet function after one week (113). There were no significant bleeding concerns observed among patients switched from prasugrel to clopidogrel. However, the safety assessment aspect of the study was cited as being underpowered since the study included only 139 patients.

Since bleeding while on prasugrel is still likely a concern, it has been proposed by some to prescribe CYP2C19 reduced-metabolizers prasugrel as an alternative to clopidogrel. Sorich *et al.* genotyped ACS patients undergoing PCI (a subset of patients from TRITON-TIMI 38) and categorized them as CYP2C19 reduced metabolizers (carrying one or two copies of a CYP2C19 reduced function allele) or extensive metabolizers (114). They observed that individuals who were CYP2C19 reduced metabolizers were statistically significantly less likely to have CV or nonfatal MI on prasugrel compared to clopidogrel.

Ticagrelor

Ticagrelor is a nonthienopyridine and the first direct-acting reversibly binding oral $P2Y_{12}$ receptor antagonist. Unlike clopidogrel and prasugrel, ticagrelor is not given as a prodrug and thus does not undergo metabolic activation. Ticagrelor additionally does not undergo metabolism via the cytochrome P450 enzymes. An indirect meta-analysis of ticagrelor and prasugrel showed that they were both more efficacious than clopidogrel for ACS, with ticagrelor and prasugrel showing similar efficacy (115). Other studies have additionally demonstrated that ticagrelor is faster acting and more efficacious than clopidogrel (116–118). Additionally, platelet recovery following the last drug dose was faster for ticagrelor compared to clopidogrel, and PPI interactions were not observed with ticagrelor (117, 118). Ticagrelor was not as efficacious as prasugrel in preventing stent thrombosis, although unlike prasugrel, ticagrelor was not associated with a higher bleeding rate, and it was safer than clopidogrel in patients undergoing CABG (115, 119). On the other hand, ticagrelor was associated with more frequent non-CABG-related bleeding and side effects such as dyspnea, hypotension, nausea, and ventricular pauses compared to clopidogrel. An advantage to ticagrelor is its reversible inhibition, potentially allowing for more rapid surgical inter-

vention following discontinuation of therapy, as compared to clopidogrel.

Because ticagrelor is eliminated extensively via hepatic mechanisms, an investigation was undertaken to determine the effect of mild hepatic impairment on the pharmacokinetics, pharmacodynamics, and safety of the drug (120). Results of the study showed that exposure of ticagrelor and its active metabolite was modestly increased in the hepatic compromised group, but this did not have an effect on pharmacodynamics or tolerability.

Limited studies have been done to investigate an association between genetic polymorphisms and response to ticagrelor. Polymorphisms in *P2RY12*, *P2RY1*, and *ITGB3* were not demonstrated to influence ADP-induced platelet aggregation by ticagrelor (121). Wallentin *et al.* studied the effect of polymorphisms in *CY2C19* (*2–*8 and *17) and *ABCB1* (c.3435C > T) in the patient group from the PLATO trial of ticagrelor versus clopidogrel for treatment of ACS (122). They reported that ticagrelor was more efficacious than clopidogrel for ACS treatment and that its effect was not dependent on *CYP2C19* or *ABCB1* genotype. Another study demonstrated that ticagrelor effect on platelet reactivity was independent of *CYP2C19* genotype (*2–*8 and *17) or metabolizer status (123).

Platelet-function testing

Reduced response to antiplatelet agents has been widely demonstrated as a predictor of cardiovascular events. However, routine measurement of platelet reactivity has not been widely adopted for several reasons including a lack of reliable tests and consensus cutoff values for measuring reduced platelet responses, and limited outcomes data demonstrating support for altering therapy based on platelet function measurements.

Laboratory tests for platelet function associated with aspirin and clopidogrel response include optical light-transmittance aggregometry (LTA), thromboelastography (TEG), vasodilator-stimulated phosphoprotein (VASP), a platelet function analyzer system (PFA 100), and point-of-care assays VerifyNow and Plateletworks. The current gold standard is LTA, which has been used in studies demonstrating a link between poorer prognosis in patients with CAD who are treated with a combination of aspirin and clopidogrel (124–127). LTA is an ex vivo measurement of agonist-induced platelet aggregation, utilizing multiple agonists including ADP, thrombin, epinephrine, collagen, and arachidonic acid. The assay is based on the measurement of optical aggregation curves in platelet-rich plasma to measure dynamic clumping of platelets. While this test is considered the current gold standard, it has many pre-analytical and analytical variables and factors, and is affected by such factors as age, gender, race, diet, hematocrit, sample collection and processing, and operator variability. While LTA is one of the few assays that has predicted outcome in patients on aspirin, it is difficult to standardize, is labor intensive, has poor reproducibility, and has a longer turnaround time compared to other methods. Additionally, LTA is not specific for $P2Y_{12}$ receptor activation.

Other more user-friendly methods, such as the cartridge-based PFA 100, Plateletworks, and VerifyNow, have been proposed as alternatives to LTA for assessing platelet function as it relates to aspirin and clopidogrel resistance. The PFA-100 (Dade Behring, Deerfield, IL) utilizes collagen/ADP- or collagen/epinephrine-coated membranes and measures shear-induced platelet aggregation. In vitro bleeding time results from the PFA-100 can be obtained in 5 minutes, making it useful from the point of care testing (POCT) perspective, and the method is very sensitive to hemostatic disorders such as von Willebrand disease and platelet dysfunction (128). However, the PFA-100 has not been proven to be useful or specific for measuring the effects of aspirin or clopidogrel (129).

The VerifyNow assay (VerifyNow ASA and VerifyNow $P2Y_{12}$, Accumetrics, San Diego, CA) is a turbidimetric optical detection assay that measures aggregation of platelets to fibrinogen-coated beads in whole blood. The platelet induced aggregation of fibrinogen-coated microparticles is measured as an increase in light transmittance. Results can be achieved in fewer than 10 minutes and are expressed in arbitrary units (ARUs). Similar to the PFA-100, the VerifyNow system is advantageous from a POCT perspective. Additionally it may be better standardized than some of the other available methods. However, there are limited outcome studies with the VerifyNow ASA system and it has poor

concordance with other methods such as LTA. The VerifyNow $P2Y_{12}$ assay has better concordance with LTA and is more specific for ADP-induced $P2Y_{12}$ activation than LTA (130, 131). However, the VerifyNow $P2Y_{12}$ assay displays a wide variability in percent inhibition response to clopidogrel and is affected by many factors including platelet count and glycoprotein IIb/IIa inhibitors.

Plateletworks (Helena Laboratories, Beaumont, TX) measures platelet inhibition based on single platelet counting before and after exposure to ADP. This point of care method is easy to operate and can yield results in less than 5 minutes. However, the analysis needs to be performed within 10 minutes of blood draw in order to prevent overestimation of the degree of platelet inhibition and it does not compare well with LTA in terms of discrimination between different degrees of platelet inhibition in different patients (132).

Whole blood thromboelastography (TEG, Haemoscope Corporation, Niles, IL) is based on whole blood coagulation in a cup. TEG measures platelet expression of both activated GP IIb/IIa receptor and P-selectin following ADP stimulation in addition to ADP-induced platelet-fibrin clot strength. Similar to VerifyNow, multiple platelet agonists can be used to isolate the ADP effect on platelet aggregation. TEG is another relatively rapid assay with results in 20–30 minutes, and it has the advantage of providing information on clotting factors and fibrinogen. However, the disadvantages of TEG are that it requires fresh whole blood, is labor intensive, and has a high coefficient of variation.

Vasodilator-stimulated phosphoprotein (VASP) is a flow cytometric based assay which is a specific intracellular marker of residual $P2Y_{12}$ receptor reactivity in patients treated with $P2Y_{12}$ blockers. Because the phosphorylation of VASP is mediated by the $P2Y_{12}$ receptor, the VASP assay specifically measures $P2Y_{12}$ receptor activity. The drawbacks to the VASP system are that the instrument is more expensive and sophisticated compared to other platforms, and the assay is not sensitive to mild abnormalities of the receptor (133).

While there are different benefits to the various types of antiplatelet tests available, all of the testing platforms described have issues including, but not limited to, insufficient sensitivity (or oversensitivity) and specificity, inconsistent results, and lack of standardization. One study investigated the long-term effects of concomitant clopidogrel and aspirin therapy on platelet inhibition in 26 patients treated with elective PCI (134). They compared LTA, VerifyNow, and TEG, and observed a moderate correlation between LTA and VerifyNow, but poor correlation between TEG and the other methods. Most of the typical responders had concordant results between the different assays, whereas low responders often displayed discordant results. Breet *et al.* compared VerifyNow P2Y12, Plateletworks, and the PFA-100 (along with another method, IMPACT-R) in 1069 patients taking clopidogrel undergoing stent implantation in The Popular Study (Do Platelet Function Assays Predict Clinical Outcomes in Clopidogrel-Pretreated Patients Undergoing Elective PCI). They observed that only LTA, VerifyNow, and Plateletworks were significantly associated with the primary endpoint (all-cause death, MI, stent thrombosis, and ischemic stroke) (129). However, the area under the ROC curve for all of these methods was poor, ranging from 0.61 to 0.63 for the three methods. Thus the ability of any of these tests to properly classify those who will or will not have poor outcomes while taking clopidogrel is low. Another study investigated platelet function inhibition via four different methods (LTA, whole-blood aggregometry, PFA-100, and VerifyNow $P2Y_{12}$ in 116 stable CAD patients taking clopidogrel prior to diagnostic angiography (135). Correlation between the methods was poor and the authors concluded that platelet function testing for evaluating clopidogrel efficacy was not appropriate in routine clinical practice.

Anticoagulants

The other side of antithrombotic therapy involves altering hemostatic factors in the plasma. The vitamin K antagonist warfarin is one of the oldest and most studied anti-thrombotic drugs. In spite of it being one of the most prescribed drugs in the United States, clinical management of warfarin is often challenging and its administration frequently results in ADEs (136). Other anticoagulant drugs include hep-arin, low-molecular-weight heparin, and fondaparinux. Despite some promising findings regarding the PGx of unfractionated and low molecular weight heparin and interleukin-1 receptor genotype (137). PGx studies in predicting individual therapeutic response to parenteral anticoagulants are limited. The current state of knowledge regarding warfarin PGx is more advanced and is discussed in another chapter.

Beta blockers

Beta blocker drugs are used mainly to treat hypertension, cardiac arrhythmias, heart failure, and ischemic heart disease. There are multiple different beta blockers, but in the field of pharmacogenetics, the majority of the work related to beta blockers is focused on the three major beta blockers used to treat heart failure (HF): metoprolol, carvedilol, and bisoprolol. Consensus management guidelines recommend these beta blockers as essential drugs for patients with systolic HF who do not have contraindications to beta-blocker therapy (138).

In the cardiac myocyte, the beta-1-adrenergic receptor (B-1AR) stimulates adenylyl cyclase activity and intracellular cyclic-AMP through G-protein (G_s) signaling to mediate increased myocardial contractility and cardiomyopathic effects. The cardiomyopathic actions predominate in heart failure and the administration of beta blockers improves pathologic left ventricular remodeling and clinical outcomes. While clinical trials of beta-blocker therapy have shown significant overall survival benefits, approximately 25% of patients discontinue therapy due to drug intolerance (139). Substantial interindividual variability in response to therapy and outcome has been identified and is not readily explained on the basis of differences in baseline clinical characteristics. The basis of this variability may be related to polymorphisms in genes encoding for proteins involved in the pharmacokinetic and pharmacodynamic disposition of beta blockers.

Alpha- and beta-adrenergic receptors

The beta-1- and beta-2-adrenergic receptors are expressed at a ratio of 70:30 in the human heart. The B1-AR is the major beta-AR downregulated in heart failure and it is the main target of beta-blocker therapy and is encoded for by the *ADRB1* gene. Two common single nucleotide polymorphisms occur in the *ADRB1* gene at nucleotides 145 (A > G) and 1165 (G > C), resulting in serine (S) and arginine (R) to glycine (G) amino acid substitutions at codons 49 and 389, respectively. The S49G polymorphism occurs in the extracellular amino terminus, while the R389G polymorphism is located in a highly conserved intracellular G-protein coupling region of the carboxy terminus. The polymorphisms are found at allele frequencies of 9–21%, 15–34%, and 0% for Gly49 and 28–32%, 41–53%, and 15–25% for Gly389 in Caucasian, African, and Asian subjects, respectively (140). Both polymorphisms have been found to be functionally significant, and multiple studies have demonstrated their association, both alone and in haplotype, with blood pressure and blood pressure response to beta blockers, although some of these studies are controversial or inconclusive (reviewed in 141).

Liggett *et al.* examined the *ADRB1* Gly389Arg polymorphism and beta blockers in heart failure patients (142). In that study, genotyping of *ADRB1* was undertaken as a DNA substudy in 1,040 patients from the randomized, placebo-controlled Beta-Blocker Evaluation of Survival Trial (BEST) study, a trial of the beta blocker bucindolol in the treatment of NYHA Class III/IV heart failure. In vitro experiments revealed that the wild-type Arg389 allele exhibited higher basal and isoproterenol-stimulated adenylyl cyclase activity compared to the Gly389 variant (143). The results of that study suggested that the chronic heart failure patients with the *ADRB1* Gly389 variant did not respond well to treatment with bucindolol. This polymorphism was shown to significantly impact agonist-mediated contractility in failing and nonfailing myocardium and the response to antagonist and partial agonists in the failing heart. Arg389 homozygotes treated with bucindolol (vs. placebo) had an age-, sex-, and race-adjusted 38% reduction in mortality (p = 0.03) and 34% reduction in mortality or hospitalization (p = 0.004). In contrast, Gly389 carriers had no clinical response at all.

The findings with bucindolol do not necessarily apply to all beta blockers; in fact, Liggett *et al.* did not describe genotype-dependent differences in carvedilol-based contractility studies (142). However, other studies have demonstrated genotype-dependent effects of Arg389Gly in patients treated with carvedilol (144–146). Furthermore, a study by Rochais *et al.* demonstrated that carvedilol, compared to metoprolol and bisoprolol, showed marked inverse agonism on the Arg389 variant (147).

Studies examining the association with Arg389-Gly and left ventricular ejection fraction (LVEF), a surrogate marker whose improvement is correlated with survival in HF, have been inconclusive. Some studies with carvedilol and metoprolol have demonstrated a strong association between LVEF and Arg389Gly, with the greatest improvement in LVEF associated with homozygosity for Arg389Gly (142, 144, 148). Other studies have not been able to demonstrate an association with Arg389Gly and LVEF in HF patients taking carvedilol, bucindolol, or bisoprolol (142, 149, 150).

The *ADRB1* Ser49Gly polymorphism has also been studied in HF patients, although not as extensively as Arg389Gly. The variant Gly49 allele has been shown to be associated with significantly greater reduction in left ventricular end-diastolic diameter and lower risk of death or cardiac transplant in HF patients treated with beta blockers (151, 152). On the other hand, Ser49Gly was not found to be associated with LVEF in HF patients taking beta blockers (150).

The *ADRB2* gene, encoding for the beta-2 adrenergic receptor, has two common polymorphisms, Arg16Gly and Gln27Glu, both located in the extracellular amino terminus of the receptor. The variant alleles for Arg16Gly and Gln27Glu are found in 26–33% and 46–53% of Caucasians, 39–53% and 8–14% of Asians, and 48–54% and 8–18% of Africans, respectively. Both of the polymorphisms have been shown to be correlated to variable susceptibility and resistance to receptor downregulation after stimulation by agonist (153). In terms of an association with *ADRB2* polymorphisms and LVEF in HF patients taking beta blockers, studies have shown variable results. Metra *et al.* observed that in HF patients taking carvedilol, Gln27Glu but not Arg16-Gly (or *ADRB1* Arg389Gly) was associated with LVEF response (149). The strongest association was found in homozygotes for Gln27Glu. On the other hand, another study demonstrated the Gln27 homozygotes (compared to Glu27 carriers) actually had the most significant LVEF improvement in HF patients taking carvedilol (154), whereas another study found no association at all (150).

The alpha2C-adrenergic receptor (encoded for by *ADRA2C*) is an autoreceptor involved in regulating presynaptic norepinephrine release. An in-frame deletion polymorphism of four amino acids (p. 322–325) in *ADRA2C* has been shown to be associated with reduced auto-inhibitory function of the receptor (155). In the BEST trial substudy of response to bucindolol in HF patients with *ADRA2C* variants, it was observed that individuals with the deletion polymorphism exhibited a much greater response to bucindolol in terms of norepinephrine reduction (156). Individuals who did not carry the deletion polymorphism had a 30% reduction in mortality (HR 0.70, 95% CI, 0.51 to 0.96, p = 0.025) compared to carriers.

Cytochrome P450

Most beta blockers, including carvedilol, metoprolol, and bisoprolol, are either partially or extensively metabolized by the CYP2D6 enzyme (157–162). There are numerous genetic variants in the CYP2D6 gene which can lead to a poor (homozygous for nonfunctional alleles), intermediate (heterozygous for a nonfunctional allele or homozygous for partial function alleles), or ultra-rapid (three or more copies of the gene) metabolizer phenotypes. In the Caucasian population, approximately 5–10% of individuals are CYP2D6 poor metabolizers, 35% are intermediate metabolizers, and about 7% are ultra-rapid metabolizers (163).

Variants in *CYP2D6* have been found to be associated with various aspects of carvedilol and metoprolol metabolism (146, 164–171). Previous studies have demonstrated that plasma concentrations of metoprolol are higher in CYP2D6 poor metabolizers than nonpoor metabolizers (171, 172). *CYP2D6* genotypic differences in metoprolol-related heart rate reduction, diastolic blood pressure, mean arterial pressure, and adverse effects have also been observed (170, 172, 173). On the other hand, other studies have not demonstrated an association

between *CYP2D6* genotype and metoprolol adverse events or efficacy (174, 175). Although the studies are more limited than those involving metoprolol, variants in *CYP2D6* have also been associated with the pharmacokinetics of carvedilol (159, 167, 169). In addition to CYP2D6, CYP3A4 and CYP2C19 are also involved in carvedilol metabolism. CYP2D6 is only a minor metabolizer of bisoprolol, with CYP3A4 playing the major role in bisoprolol metabolism (162). Studies investigating the role of *CYP3A4* or *CYP2C19* variants in bisoprolol or carvedilol have not yet been published.

UDP-glucuronosyltransferase

UDP-glucuronosyltransferase (UGT) is an enzyme involved in phase II metabolism of many endogenous and exogenous compounds, including carvedilol. Approximately 35–40% of Caucasians carry that *28 (TA7) allele in the *UGT1A1* promoter, which is associated with decreased production of the enzyme (176). Carvedilol is mainly metabolized by the UGT1A1, UGT2B4, and UGT2B7 subtypes (177). The *UGT1A1* G71R, *UGT2B7* A71S, and *UGT2B7* H268Y polymorphisms have been shown to affect the pharmacokinetics and disposition of carvedilol in Japanese (159, 178). Other studies regarding UGT polymorphisms and carvedilol are limited.

Statins

Hydroxymethylglutaryl (HMG)-CoA reductase inhibitors (statins) are widely used for the treatment of hyperlipidemia and are effective at lowering LDL cholesterol because of their strong inhibition of the rate-limiting enzyme (HGM-CoA reductase) in cholesterol biosynthesis. Statins have been shown to reduce the incidence of coronary heart disease and are among the most widely prescribed medications worldwide.

Statin intolerance

Skeletal muscle side effects associated with statins may affect 10–20% of statin users. In fact, over 40% of patients with an indication for statin therapy are not treated, many of them because of concerns about statin-related side effects (179). Statin associated myopathic side effects include myalgia (with and without elevated creatine kinase [CK] levels), muscle weakness, muscle cramps, myositis, and rhabdomyolysis (180). Rhabdomyolysis, while rare (approximately 1.5 patients per 10 million prescriptions), is of clinical concern because of the risk for death as a result of cardiac arrhythmia, renal failure, and disseminated intravascular coagulation (181). The risk of statin myopathy generally increases with statin dose, although plasma drug levels do not entirely predict risk for statin myopathy (182).

While the underlying causes of statin-related myotoxicity are not known, several hypotheses have been formulated, including those related to the biochemical pathway of cholesterol synthesis inhibition. For example, levels of serum isoprenoids, such as ubiquinone (coenzyme Q10), and small GTP-binding proteins, such as Ras, Rac, and Rho, are decreased following statin treatment (183). The decreased levels of isoprenoids, which are necessary for posttranscriptional lipid modification of proteins, may lead to mitochondrial abnormalities which have been associated with statin therapy and myocyte apoptosis (184–186).

Another mechanism of statin-induced myopathy is myocyte coenzyme Q10 (CoQ10) deficiency resulting in defects in the mitochondrial oxidative phosphorylation pathway. CoQ10 is a product of the mevalonate pathway. Statins inhibit production of mevalonate, thereby leading to subsequent reduction of CoQ10. While statins have been shown to

reduce serum CoQ10 levels, intramuscular CoQ10 levels do not always correspondingly decrease with statin treatment (187–190). On the other hand, variants in the CoQ10 gene were correlated to statin intolerance in one study (191).

Although statins are structurally similar, they display different pharmacokinetic properties (Figure 7.2). Most statins (e.g., atorvastatin, fluvastatin, pravastatin, rosuvastatin, and pitavastatin) are administered as active hydroxy acids, although some (e.g., simvastatin and lovastatin) are given in the inactive δ-lactone prodrug form, whereupon they are converted to their respective hydroxy acids (SVA and LVA). The lactone forms are more strongly associated with skeletal muscle myopathy (192, 193). Lipophilic statins are readily distributed into peripheral tissues and undergo extensive metabolism by CYP3A4, CYP3A5, CYP2C8, and CYP2C9. Simvastatin, lovastatin, and atorvastatin are metabolized mainly through CYP3A4, while fluvastatin is metabolized primarily through CYP2C9 (194). One study demonstrated that patients who were taking atorvastatin and were homozygous for the CYP3A5*3 allele had higher serum CK levels compared to heterozygotes (195).

Statins are transported into hepatocytes by P-glycoprotein (MDR1) and the hepatic drug organic anion transporter 1B1 (OATP1B1 a.k.a. OATP2 a.k.a. OATPC), encoded for by the SLCO1B1 gene (Figure 7.2). Pravastatin, atorvastatin, rosuvastatin, simvastatin, and lovastatin are all transported into

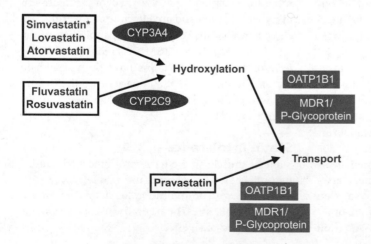

Figure 7.2 Statin pharmacokinetic metabolism. Statins in red are hydrophobic statins; statins in blue are hydrophilic statins. *Note*: Simvastatin and atorvastatin are administered in their inactive lactone form and converted to their active acid form. Most statins are metabolized by cytochrome P450 enzymes, although pravastatin does not undergo phase 1 metabolism though CYPs. All statins undergo phase 2 metabolism via OATP1B1 (encoded for by *SLCO1B1*) and MDR1/P-Glycoprotein (encoded for by *ABCB1*).

hepatocytes via this mechanism. The *5 allele (c.521T > C, p.Val174Ala) of *SLCO1B1* interferes with localization of the transporter to the plasma membrane, resulting in increased systemic statin concentrations. This allele is observed in 8–16% of Caucasians, 12–16% of Chinese, 10% of Japanese, and 1–2% of Africans. Another common polymorphism in *SLCO1B1* occurs at c.388A > G (rs2306283, p.Asn130Asp) and has been associated with increased transport activity of OATP1B1 and decreased plasma concentrations of pravastatin (196, 197).

In patients taking pravastatin, those with *SLCO1B1* variants (c.338A > G, c.521T > C, and c.1118G > A) had higher plasma pravastatin concentrations (AUC 130% higher compared to individuals without the variants) (198). Decreased liver transport of pravastatin, atorvastatin, and cerivastatin were associated with the *SLCO1B1**5 and *15 alleles (199). The *SLCO1B1* *15 variant was correlated with a higher incidence of pravastatin- or atorvastatin-related myopathy (200).

A genome-wide association study (SEARCH or Study of the Effectiveness of Additional Reductions in Cholesterol and Homocysteine Collaborative Group Study) identified the *SLCO1B1**5 polymorphism as a major cause of severe statin-induced myopathy (CK > 10X upper limit of normal [ULN] in symptomatic and > 3X in asymptomatic individuals) in patients taking simvastatin (80 mg/day) (201). Myopathy odds ratios were 4.5 for one *5 allele and 16.9 for two *5 alleles. The estimated 5-year cumulative risk or definite or incipient myopathy was predicted to be 0.6, 3, and 18% for none, one, or two *5 alleles, respectively.

Another study, the Statin Response Examined by Genetic HAP Markers (or STRENGTH) study which investigated variants in *CYP2D6*, *CYP2C8*, *CYP2C9*, *CYP3A4*, and *SLCO1B1* in 509 individuals randomized to atorvastatin (10 mg), simvastatin (20 mg), or pravastatin (10 mg) for 8 weeks followed by an additional 8 weeks of treatment with 80, 80, or 40 mg. Associations between genotype with discontinuation of statin treatment for any side effect, myalgia, or CK > 3X ULN demonstrated that the *SLCO1B1**5 variant was associated with mild statin-induced side effects, especially in individuals taking simvastatin (202). They observed that individuals with the *SLCO1B1**5 allele had a twofold relative risk of mild statin-induced side effects, and they concluded that individuals who carry this allele may want to opt for pravastatin, rather than simvastatin, as their first statin choice.

Several drugs, when administered concomitantly with statins, increase risk of statin-associated myopathy. One class of drugs that has received more widespread attention because of this phenomenon is the fibrates, which are also used for the treatment of dyslipidemia. Coadministration of the fibrate drug gemfibrozil with statin drugs is not recommended because of the increased risk of myopathy. On the other hand, coadministration of statins with fenofibrate, another fibrate drug, does not appear to be associated with increased risk of myopathy (203). A common pathway for clearance of active hydroxy statins is by glucuronidation at the dihydroxy heptanoic or heptenoic acid side chains by UDP-glucuronosyl transferases (UGTs), especially UGT1A1 and UGT1A3 (204). Interestingly, gemfibrozil is also metabolized via UGT1A1 and UGT1A3 and has been shown to inhibit statin glucuronidation, while fenofibrate does not have any known pharmacokinetic interaction with statins (203). Thus, inhibition of statin glucuronidation by gemfibrozil may potentially lead to myopathic side effects. Additionally, it may be speculated that because of common pathway of metabolism of gemfibrozil and statins through UGT1A, polymorphisms in *UGT1A1* and/or *UGT1A3* may affect statin intolerance.

Statin efficacy

Statin-induced reductions of LDL cholesterol (LDL-C) vary among individuals, and mechanisms of this variatbility are poorly understood. LDL cholesterol has been shown to be decreased by a given statin from less than 5% to greater than 60%, even when adherence to the medication regimen is taken into account (205). Thus, despite the widespread use of statins, many individuals taking statins fail to meet lipid-lowering goals. Interindividual variability in statin efficacy may be influenced by multiple factors, including age, gender, ethnicity, smoking status, and genetic differences. Genetic variations contributing to variable LDL-C lowering among statin users have been attributed to genes encoding regulators of cholesterol metabolism including *HMGCR*, *LDLR*, *PCSK9*, *APOE*, and *ABCB1*. Other genes involved in metabolism of statins, such as *CYP3A4*, and with unknown mechanistic relationship to statin pharmacology (e.g., *KIF6*) have also been implicated.

KIF6

The *KIF6* gene-encoding kinesin-like protein 6 was originally described as a marker for coronary heart disease (CHD) in the CARE (Cholesterol and Recurrent Events) and WOSCOPS (West of Scotland Coronary Prevention Study) trials (206). Several other studies, by the same group, additionally confirmed its correlation with CHD in other trials, with an up to 55% increased risk of CHD in untreated populations (207–209). KIF6 has also been shown to be associated with noncardioembolic stroke but not angiographically defined CAD (210, 211). The specific pathophysiological role of KIF6 is unknown. Kinesins are a family of dimeric motor proteins involved in the intracellular transport of organelles, protein complexes, and mRNAs. The Trp719Arg polymorphism in KIF6 is common, occurring in approximately 60% of Caucasians.

In the Pravastatin or Atorvastatin Evaluation and Infection Therapy, Thrombolysis in MI (PROVE IT - TIMI 22) trial, it was shown that carriers of the 719Arg allele received significant risk reduction (i. e., had fewer deaths or major CV events) from high dose atorvastatin (80 mg), compared to standard dose pravastatin (40 mg), and they also received significantly greater benefit than noncarriers (p = 0.018) over 30 months of study follow-up (207). The number need to treat with atorvastatin for two years to prevent one event was 10 for *KIF6* Arg carriers compared to 125 for noncarriers. Interestingly, *KIF6* Arg carriers and noncarriers did not have different on-treatment lipid or C-reactive protein (CRP) levels, suggesting that the difference in outcome was independent of LDL or CRP lowering by the statin drugs. Subsequent studies, by the same group, have additionally suggested that the Trp719Arg polymorphism may be predictive of response to statin therapy (212, 213).

Ongoing clinical trials are slated to assess the benefit of KIF6 Trp719Arg testing in the patient population. A prospective cohort study (AKRO-BATS, or Additional KIF6 Risk Offers Better Adherence to Statins) sponsored by Medco Health Solutions, in collaboration with Celera Corp., will investigate whether KIF6 testing will improve patient adherence to statin therapy. This clinical trial (NCT01068834) is scheduled to be completed in June 2011. Another ongoing study based at Brigham and Women's Hospital (Boston, MA) is investigating whether genetic factors can help identify individuals whom would benefit most from statin therapy. This clinical trial (1RC1HL099634-01) is scheduled to be completed in August 2011.

CYP3A4

CYP3A4 is involved in metabolism of several statins (e.g., atorvastatin, lovastatin, simvastatin, Figure 7.2) and has been shown to have 10- to 100-fold interindividual variation in activity (214–216). Inhibition of CYP3A4 activity dramatically increases the plasma concentrations of lovastatin and simvastatin (217, 218). Missense variants in *CYP3A4* are rare and have only accounted for a small percentage of variability in CYP3A4 activity. Recently, an intronic variant in CYP3A4 was identified as a functional SNP. This SNP (rs35599367 C > T) is located in intron 6 at c.522-190 and is present in 5–10% of the Caucasian population and approximately 4% of the African American and Chinese populations. The intron 6 SNP correlated with total mRNA level and enzyme activity and response to statin drugs (72). In 235 patients who were taking a CYP3A4-metabolized statin (atorvastatin, simvastatin, or lovastatin), carriers of the variant allele required significantly lower doses of statin drug than noncarriers (0.2–0.6-fold; p = 0.019). Investigations are necessary to further elucidate the role of this SNP (and other genetic variants in *CYP3A4*) in statin efficacy.

LDLR

The LDL receptor is involved in LDL clearance from the bloodstream and it is encoded by the *LDLR* gene. Mutations in *LDLR* are causative for familial hypercholesterolemia (FH), a common, autosomal dominant disorder of elevated LDL-C and premature coronary artery disease. Some of these mutations have also been associated with statin efficacy (219). *LDLR* is highly polymorphic and common sequence variants have been associated with response to statin treatment (220–224). Other studies have not demonstrated an association between *LDLR* variants and statin response (225–229). Most of the studies conducted were small in nature and thus larger studies that include additional genes or variants may be needed to clarify the role of *LDLR* in statin response.

HMGCR

The *HMGCR* gene encodes 3-hydroxy-3-methylglutaryl-coenzyme A reductase, the enzyme that catalyzes the rate limiting step in cholesterol biosynthesis. As the enzyme that is the target for statin drug inhibition, it is plausible that genetic variants in *HMGCR* may be associated with response to statins. Genetic variability in *HMGCR* has been associated with decreased lipid lowering by statins (230–234). Alternative splicing of HMGCR occurs due to a polymorphism in intron 13 (rs3846662) that leads to exon 13 skipping (*HMGCR13*[-]) (235). This allele has been shown to explain 6–15% of variability in statin response (231). The variant G allele for rs3846662 (c.1722 + 45A > G) occurs at a frequency of 38–46% in Caucasians, 53–60% in Japanese and Chinese, 52% in Hispanics, and 83–93% of African Americans. It has been observed that African Americans have, on average, a diminished response to statins compared to Caucasians, and this may be attributed, at least in part, to the high frequency of the rs3846662 G allele in the African American population (205).

Conclusion

Management of patient treatment with cardiovascular drugs using pharmacogenetics is an evolving area full of promise. Some of these areas are currently in use, in clinical practice, such as clopidogrel pharmacogenetics, and other areas require further investigation to determine their clinical utility (e.g., beta blockers and other antihypertensives). It is likely that the complexity of some of the gene–drug, gene–environment, and drug–environment interactions will require integration of clinical and lab test results and information in order to be optimally useful. The development of databases and guides for clinicians and patients will help to make pharmacogenetic testing more accessible and its results more meaningful and actionable.

References

1 CAPRIE Steering Committee (1996) A randomised, blinded, trial of clopidogrel versus aspirin in patients at risk of ischaemic events (CAPRIE). *Lancet*, **348**, 1329–1339.

2 Diener, H-C, Bogousslavsky, J, Brass, LM, Cimminiello, C, *et al.* (2004) Management of atherothrombosis with clopidogrel in high-risk patients with recent transient ischaemic attack or ischaemic stroke (MATCH): study design and baseline data. *Cerebrovascular Diseases*, **17**, 253–261.

3 Fox, KAA, Mehta, SR, Peters, R, Zhao, F, *et al.* (2004) Benefits and risks of the combination of clopidogrel and aspirin in patients undergoing surgical revascularization for non-ST-elevation acute coronary syndrome: the Clopidogrel in Unstable angina to prevent Recurrent ischemic Events (CURE) Trial. *Circulation*, **110**, 1202–1208.

4 Savi, P, Herbert, J-M (2005) Clopidogrel and ticlopidine: P2Y12 adenosine diphosphate-receptor antagonists for the prevention of atherothrombosis. *Seminars in Thrombosis & Hemostasis*, **31**, 174–183.

5 Turitto, VT, Weiss, HJ, Zimmerman, TS, Sussman, II (1985) Factor VIII/von Willebrand factor in subendothelium mediates platelet adhesion. *Blood*, **65**, 823–831.

6 Roth, GJ, Calverley, DC (1994) Aspirin, platelets, and thrombosis: theory and practice. *Blood*, **83**, 885–898.

7 Lev, EI, Patel, RT, Maresh, KJ, Guthikonda, S, *et al.* (2006) Aspirin and clopidogrel drug response in patients undergoing percutaneous coronary intervention: the role of dual drug resistance. *Journal of the American College of Cardiology*, **47**, 27–33.

8 Gum, PA, Kottke-Marchant, K, Welsh, PA, White, J, *et al.* (2003) A prospective, blinded determination of the natural history of aspirin resistance among stable patients with cardiovascular disease [erratum appears in *Journal of the American College of Cardiology*. 2006 Nov 7;48(9):1918]. *Journal of the American College of Cardiology*, **41**, 961–965.

9 Gum, PA, Kottke-Marchant, K, Poggio, ED, Gurm, H, *et al.* (2001) Profile and prevalence of aspirin resistance in patients with cardiovascular disease. *American Journal of Cardiology*, **88**, 230–235.

10 Grotemeyer, KH (1991) Effects of acetylsalicylic acid in stroke patients. Evidence of nonresponders in a subpopulation of treated patients. *Thrombosis Research*, **63**, 587–593.

11 Buchanan, MR, Brister, SJ (1995) Individual variation in the effects of ASA on platelet function: implications for the use of ASA clinically. *Canadian Journal of Cardiology*, **11**, 221–227.

12 Wang, TH, Bhatt, DL, Topol, EJ (2006) Aspirin and clopidogrel resistance: an emerging clinical entity. *European Heart Journal*, **27**, 647–654.

13 Eikelboom, JW, Hirsh, J, Weitz, JI, Johnston, M, *et al.* (2002) Aspirin-resistant thromboxane biosynthesis and the risk of myocardial infarction, stroke, or cardiovascular death in patients at high risk for cardiovascular events. *Circulation*, **105**, 1650–1655.

14 Macchi, L, Sorel, N, Christiaens, L (2006) Aspirin resistance: definitions, mechanisms, prevalence, and clinical significance. *Current Pharmaceutical Design*, **12**, 251–258.

15 Goodman, T, Ferro, A, Sharma, P (2008) Pharmacogenetics of aspirin resistance: a comprehensive systematic review. *British Journal of Clinical Pharmacology*, **66**, 222–232.

16 Awtry, EH, Loscalzo, J (2000) Aspirin. *Circulation*, **101**, 1206–1218.

17 Billett, HH (2008) Antiplatelet agents and arterial thrombosis. *Cardiol Clin*, **26**, 189–201, vi.

18 Gonzalez-Conejero, R, Rivera, J, Corral, J, Acuna, C, *et al.* (2005) Biological assessment of aspirin efficacy on healthy individuals: heterogeneous response or aspirin failure? *Stroke*, **36**, 276–280.

19 Catella-Lawson, F, Reilly, MP, Kapoor, SC, Cucchiara, AJ, *et al.* (2001) Cyclooxygenase inhibitors and the antiplatelet effects of aspirin. *New England Journal of Medicine*, **345**, 1809–1817.

20 Maree, AO, Curtin, RJ, Chubb, A, Dolan, C, *et al.* (2005) Cyclooxygenase-1 haplotype modulates platelet response to aspirin. *Journal of Thrombosis and Haemostasis*, **3**, 2340–2345.

21 Lepantalo, A, Mikkelsson, J, Resendiz, JC, Viiri, L, *et al.* (2006) Polymorphisms of COX-1 and GPVI associate with the antiplatelet effect of aspirin in coronary artery disease patients. *Thrombosis and Haemostasis*, **95**, 253–259.

22 Hillarp, A, Palmqvist, B, Lethagen, S, Villoutreix, BO, *et al.* (2003) Mutations within the cyclooxygenase-1 gene in aspirin non-responders with recurrence of stroke. *Thrombosis Research*, **112**, 275–283.

23 Papp, E, Havasi, V, Bene, J, Komlosi, K, *et al.* (2005) Glycoprotein IIIA gene (PlA) polymorphism and aspirin resistance: is there any correlation? *Annals of Pharmacotherapy*, **39**, 1013–1018.

24 Undas, A, Brummel, A, Musial, J, Mann, KG, *et al.* (2001) Pl(A2) polymorphism of beta(3) integrins is associated with enhanced thrombin generation and impaired antithrombotic action of aspirin at the site of microvascular injury. *Circulation*, **104**, 2666–2672.

25 Szczeklik, A, Undas, A, Sanak, M, Frolow, M, *et al.* (2000) Relationship between bleeding time, aspirin and the PlA1/A2 polymorphism of platelet glycoprotein IIIa. *British Journal of Haematology*, **110**, 965–967.

26 Macchi, L, Christiaens, L, Brabant, S, Sorel, N, *et al.* (2003) Resistance in vitro to low-dose aspirin is associated with platelet PlA1 (GP IIIa) polymorphism but not with C807T(GP Ia/IIa) and C-5T Kozak (GP Ibalpha) polymorphisms. *Journal of the American College of Cardiology*, **42**, 1115–1119.

27 Cooke, GE, Bray, PF, Hamlington, JD, Pham, DM, *et al.* (1998) PlA2 polymorphism and efficacy of aspirin. *Lancet*, **351**, 1253.

28 Cooke, GE, Liu-Stratton, Y, Ferketich, AK, Moeschberger, ML, *et al.* (2006) Effect of platelet antigen polymorphism on platelet inhibition by aspirin, clopidogrel, or their combination. *Journal of the American College of Cardiology*, **47**, 541–546.

29 Lev, EI, Patel, RT, Guthikonda, S, Lopez, D, *et al.* (2007) Genetic polymorphisms of the platelet receptors P2Y (12), P2Y(1) and GP IIIa and response to aspirin and clopidogrel. *Thrombosis Research*, **119**, 355–360.

30 Cambria-Kiely, JA, Gandhi, PJ (2002) Aspirin resistance and genetic polymorphisms. *Journal of Thrombosis & Thrombolysis*, **14**, 51–58.

31 Hancock, MA, Boffa, MB, Marcovina, SM, Nesheim, ME, *et al.* (2003) Inhibition of plasminogen activation by lipoprotein(a): critical domains in apolipoprotein (a) and mechanism of inhibition on fibrin and degraded fibrin surfaces. *J Biol Chem*, **278**, 23260–23269.

32 Luke, MM, Kane, JP, Liu, DM, Rowland, CM, *et al.* (2007) A polymorphism in the protease-like domain of apolipoprotein(a) is associated with severe coronary artery disease. *Arterioscler Thromb Vasc Biol*, **27**, 2030–2036.

33 Hancock, MA, Spencer, CA, Koschinsky, ML (2004) Definition of the structural elements in plasminogen required for high-affinity binding to apolipoprotein

(a): a study utilizing surface plasmon resonance. *Biochemistry*, **43**, 12237–12248.

34 Chasman, DI, Shiffman, D, Zee, RY, Louie, JZ, *et al.* (2009) Polymorphism in the apolipoprotein(a) gene, plasma lipoprotein(a), cardiovascular disease, and low-dose aspirin therapy. *Atherosclerosis*, **203**, 371–376.

35 Shiffman, D, O'Meara, ES, Bare, LA, Rowland, CM, *et al.* (2008) Association of gene variants with incident myocardial infarction in the Cardiovascular Health Study. *Arterioscler Thromb Vasc Biol*, **28**, 173–179.

36 Martinez, C, Blanco, G, Ladero, JM, Garcia-Martin, E, *et al.* (2004) Genetic predisposition to acute gastrointestinal bleeding after NSAIDs use. *British Journal of Pharmacology*, **141**, 205–208.

37 Vonkeman, HE, van de Laar, MA, van der Palen, J, Brouwers, JR, *et al.* (2006) Allele variants of the cytochrome P450 2C9 genotype in white subjects from The Netherlands with serious gastroduodenal ulcers attributable to the use of NSAIDs. *Clin Ther*, **28**, 1670–1676.

38 Pilotto, A, Seripa, D, Franceschi, M, Scarcelli, C, *et al.* (2007) Genetic susceptibility to nonsteroidal anti-inflammatory drug-related gastroduodenal bleeding: role of cytochrome P450 2C9 polymorphisms. *Gastroenterology*, **133**, 465–471.

39 Blanco, G, Martinez, C, Ladero, JM, Garcia-Martin, E, *et al.* (2008) Interaction of CYP2C8 and CYP2C9 genotypes modifies the risk for nonsteroidal anti-inflammatory drugs-related acute gastrointestinal bleeding. *Pharmacogenetic Genomics*, **18**, 37–43.

40 Hankey, GJ, Eikelboom, JW (2003) Antiplatelet drugs. *Med J Aust* **178**: 568–74.

41 Steinhubl, SR. Genotyping, clopidogrel metabolism, and the search for the therapeutic window of thienopyridines. *Circulation*, **121**, 481–483.

42 Kazui, M, Nishiya, Y, Ishizuka, T, Hagihara, K, *et al.* (2010) Identification of the human cytochrome P450 enzymes involved in the two oxidative steps in the bioactivation of clopidogrel to its pharmacologically active metabolite. *Drug Metabolism and Disposal*, **38**, 92–99.

43 Denninger, MH, Necciari, J, Serre-Lacroix, E, Sissmann, J. (1999) Clopidogrel antiplatelet activity is independent of age and presence of atherosclerosis. *Semin Thromb Hemost*, **25**(**Suppl. 2**), 41–45.

44 Angiolillo, DJ, Fernandez-Ortiz, A, Bernardo, E, Alfonso, F, *et al.* (2007) Variability in individual responsiveness to clopidogrel: clinical implications, management, and future perspectives. *Journal of the American College of Cardiology*, **49**, 1505–1516.

45 Gurbel, PA, Bliden, KP, Hiatt, BLO'Connor, CM (2003) Clopidogrel for coronary stenting: response variability, drug resistance, and the effect of pretreatment platelet reactivity. *Circulation*, **107**, 2908–2913.

46 Michelson, AD, Linden, MD, Furman, MI, Li, Y, *et al.* (2007) Evidence that pre-existent variability in platelet response to ADP accounts for 'clopidogrel resistance'. *Journal of Thrombosis and Haemostasis*, **5**, 75–81.

47 U.S. Food and Drug Administration (2011) *FDA Drug Safety Communication: reduced effectiveness of Plavis (clopidogrel) in patients who are poor metabolizers of the drug* [WWW document]. URL http://www.fda.gov/drugs/drugsafety/PostmarketDrugSafetyInformationforPatientsandProviders/ucm203888.htm [accessed on 19 June 2011]

48 Holmes, DR, Jr., Dehmer, GJ, Kaul, S, Leifer, D, *et al.* (2010) ACCF/AHA clopidogrel clinical alert: approaches to the FDA "boxed warning": a report of the American College of Cardiology Foundation Task Force on clinical expert consensus documents and the American Heart Association endorsed by the Society for Cardiovascular Angiography and Interventions and the Society of Thoracic Surgeons. *Journal of the American College of Cardiology*, **56**, 321–341.

49 Shuldiner, AR, O'Connell, JR, Bliden, KP, Gandhi, A, *et al.* (2009) Association of cytochrome P450 2C19 genotype with the antiplatelet effect and clinical efficacy of clopidogrel therapy. *JAMA*, **302**, 849–857.

50 Umemura, K, Furuta, T, Kondo, K. (2008) The common gene variants of CTP2C19 affect pharmacokinetics and pharmacodynmics in an active metabolite of clopidogrel in healthy subjects. *Journal of Thrombosis and Haemostasis*, **6**, 1439–1441.

51 Hulot, JS, Bura, A, Villard, E, Azizi, M, *et al.* (2006) Cytochrome P450 2C19 loss-of-function polymorphism is a major determinant of clopidogrel responsiveness in healthy subjects. *Blood*, **108**, 2244–2247.

52 Mega, JL, Close, SL, Wiviott, SD, Shen, L, *et al.* (2009) Cytochrome p-450 polymorphisms and response to clopidogrel. *New England Journal of Medicine*, **360**, 354–362.

53 Collet, JP, Hulot, JS, Pena, A, Villard, E, *et al.* (2009) Cytochrome P450 2C19 polymorphism in young patients treated with clopidogrel after myocardial infarction: a cohort study. *Lancet*, **373**, 309–317.

54 Giusti, B, Gori, AM, Marcucci, R, Saracini, C, *et al.* (2009) Relation of cytochrome P450 2C19 loss-of-function polymorphism to occurrence of drug-eluting

coronary stent thrombosis. *American Journal of Cardiology*, **103**, 806–811.

55 Sibbing, D, Stegherr, J, Latz, W, Koch, W, *et al.* (2009) Cytochrome P450 2C19 loss-of-function polymorphism and stent thrombosis following percutaneous coronary intervention. *Eur Heart J*, **30**, 916–922.

56 Simon, T, Verstuyft, C, Mary-Krause, M, Quteineh, L, *et al.* (2009) Genetic determinants of response to clopidogrel and cardiovascular events. *New England Journal of Medicine*, **360**, 363–375.

57 Trenk, D, Hochholzer, W, Fromm, MF, Chialda, LE, *et al.* (2008) Cytochrome P450 2C19 681G>A polymorphism and high on-clopidogrel platelet reactivity associated with adverse 1-year clinical outcome of elective percutaneous coronary intervention with drug-eluting or bare-metal stents. *Journal of the American College of Cardiology*, **51**, 1925–1934.

58 Luo, HR, Poland, RE, Lin, KM, Wan, YJ (2006) Genetic polymorphism of cytochrome P450 2C19 in Mexican Americans: a cross-ethnic comparative study. *Clinical Pharmacology & Therapeutics*, **80**, 33–40.

59 Man, M, Farmen, M, Dumaual, C, Teng, CH, *et al.* (2010) Genetic variation in metabolizing enzyme and transporter genes: comprehensive assessment in 3 major East asian subpopulations with comparison to Caucasians and Africans. *J Clin Pharmacol*, **50**, 929–940.

60 Mega, JL, Simon, T, Collet, JP, Anderson, JL, *et al.* (2010) Reduced-function CYP2C19 genotype and risk of adverse clinical outcomes among patients treated with clopidogrel predominantly for PCI: a meta-analysis. *JAMA*, **304**, 1821–1830.

61 Harmsze, AM, van Werkum, JW, Ten Berg, JM, Zwart, B, *et al.* (2010) CYP2C19*2 and CYP2C9*3 alleles are associated with stent thrombosis: a case-control study. *Eur Heart J*, epub ahead of print.

62 Pare, G, Mehta, S, Yusuf, S, Anand, S, *et al.* (2010) Effects of CYP2C19 genotype on outcomes of clopidogrel treatment. *New England Journal of Medicine*, **363**, 1704–1714.

63 Sim, SC, Risinger, C, Dahl, ML, Aklillu, E, *et al.* (2006) A common novel CYP2C19 gene variant causes ultra-rapid drug metabolism relevant for the drug response to proton pump inhibitors and antidepressants. *Clinical Pharmacology & Therapeutics*, **79**, 103–113.

64 Sibbing, D, Koch, W, Gebhard, D, Schuster, T, *et al.* (2010) Cytochrome 2C19*17 allelic variant, platelet aggregation, bleeding events, and stent thrombosis in clopidogrel-treated patients with coronary stent placement. *Circulation*, **121**, 512–518.

65 Tiroch, KA, Sibbing, D, Koch, W, Roosen-Runge, T, *et al.* (2010) Protective effect of the CYP2C19 *17 polymorphism with increased activation of clopidogrel on cardiovascular events. *Am Heart J*, **160**, 506–512.

66 Sibbing, D, Gebhard, D, Koch, W, Braun, S, *et al.* (2010) Isolated and interactive impact of common CYP2C19 genetic variants on the antiplatelet effect of chronic clopidogrel therapy. *Journal of Thrombosis and Haemostasis*, **8**, 1685–1693.

67 Mega, JL, Close, SL, Wiviott, SD, Shen, L, *et al.* (2010) Genetic variants in ABCB1 and CYP2C19 and cardiovascular outcomes after treatment with clopidogrel and prasugrel in the TRITON-TIMI 38 trial: a pharmacogenetic analysis. *Lancet*, **376**, 1312–1319.

68 Taubert, D, von Beckerath, N, Grimberg, G, Lazar, A, *et al.* (2006) Impact of P-glycoprotein on clopidogrel absorption. *Clinical Pharmacology & Therapeutics*, **80**, 486–501.

69 Lau, WC, Gurbel, PA, Watkins, PB, Neer, CJ, *et al.* (2004) Contribution of hepatic cytochrome P450 3A4 metabolic activity to the phenomenon of clopidogrel resistance. *Circulation*, **109**, 166–171.

70 Lau, WC, Waskell, LA, Watkins, PB, Neer, CJ, *et al.* (2003) Atorvastatin reduces the ability of clopidogrel to inhibit platelet aggregation: a new drug–drug interaction. *Circulation*, **107**, 32–37.

71 Angiolillo, DJ, Fernandez-Ortiz, A, Bernardo, E, Ramirez, C, *et al.* (2006) Contribution of gene sequence variations of the hepatic cytochrome P450 3A4 enzyme to variability in individual responsiveness to clopidogrel. *Arteriosclerosis, Thrombosis & Vascular Biology*, **26**, 1895–1900.

72 Wang, D, Guo, Y, Wrighton, SA, Cooke, GE, *et al.* (2010) Intronic polymorphism in CYP3A4 affects hepatic expression and response to statin drugs. *Pharmacogenomics Journal*, epub ahead of print.

73 Mega, JL, Close, SL, Wiviott, SD, Shen, L, *et al.* (2009) Cytochrome P450 genetic polymorphisms and the response to prasugrel: relationship to pharmacokinetic, pharmacodynamic, and clinical outcomes. *Circulation*, **119**, 2553–2560.

74 Conley, PB, Delaney, SM (2003) Scientific and therapeutic insights into the role of the platelet P2Y12 receptor in thrombosis. *Current Opinion in Hematology*, **10**, 333–338.

75 Hollopeter, G, Jantzen, HM, Vincent, D, Li, G, *et al.* (2001) Identification of the platelet ADP receptor targeted by antithrombotic drugs. *Nature*, **409**, 202–207.

76 von Beckerath, N, von Beckerath, O, Koch, W, Eichinger, M, *et al.* (2005) P2Y12 gene H2 haplotype is not associated with increased adenosine diphosphate-induced platelet aggregation after initiation of clopidogrel therapy with a high loading dose. *Blood Coagulation & Fibrinolysis*, **16**, 199–204.

77 Fontana, P, Gaussem, P, Aiach, M, Fiessinger, J-N, *et al.* (2003) P2Y12 H2 haplotype is associated with peripheral arterial disease: a case-control study. *Circulation*, **108**, 2971–2973.

78 Bura, A, Bachelot-Loza, C, Ali, FD, Aiach, M, *et al.* (2006) Role of the P2Y12 gene polymorphism in platelet responsiveness to clopidogrel in healthy subjects. *Journal of Thrombosis and Haemostasis*, **4**, 2096–2097.

79 Fontana, P, Dupont, A, Gandrille, S, Bachelot-Loza, C, *et al.* (2003) Adenosine diphosphate-induced platelet aggregation is associated with P2Y12 gene sequence variations in healthy subjects. *Circulation*, **108**, 989–995.

80 Angiolillo, DJ, Fernandez-Ortiz, A, Bernardo, E, Ramirez, C, *et al.* (2005) Lack of association between the P2Y12 receptor gene polymorphism and platelet response to clopidogrel in patients with coronary artery disease. *Thrombosis Research*, **116**, 491–497.

81 Angiolillo, DJ, Fernandez-Ortiz, A, Bernardo, E, Alfonso, F, *et al.* (2004) PlA polymorphism and platelet reactivity following clopidogrel loading dose in patients undergoing coronary stent implantation. *Blood Coagulation & Fibrinolysis*, **15**, 89–93.

82 Angiolillo, DJ, Fernandez-Ortiz, A, Bernardo, E, Ramirez, C, *et al.* (2004) 807 C/T Polymorphism of the glycoprotein Ia gene and pharmacogenetic modulation of platelet response to dual antiplatelet treatment. *Blood Coagulation & Fibrinolysis*, **15**, 427–433.

83 Beitelshees, AL, McLeod, HL (2006) Clopidogrel pharmacogenetics: promising steps towards patient care? *Arterioscler Thromb Vasc Biol*, **26**, 1681–1683.

84 Giusti, B, Gori, AM, Marcucci, R, Sestini, I, *et al.* (2008) Role of glycoprotein Ia gene polymorphisms in determining platelet function in myocardial infarction patients undergoing percutaneous coronary intervention on dual antiplatelet treatment. *Atherosclerosis*, **196**, 341–348.

85 Price, MJ, Berger, PB, Angiolillo, DJ, Teirstein, PS, *et al.* (2009) Evaluation of individualized clopidogrel therapy after drug-eluting stent implantation in patients with high residual platelet reactivity: design and rationale of the GRAVITAS trial. *Am Heart J*, **157**, 818–824, 824 e1.

86 Barker, CM, Murray, SS, Teirstein, PS, Kandzari, DE, *et al.* (2010) Pilot study of the antiplatelet effect of increased clopidogrel maintenance dosing and its relationship to CYP2C19 genotype in patients with high on-treatment reactivity. *JACC Cardiovasc Interv*, **3**, 1001–1007.

87 Bonello, L, Armero, S, Ait Mokhtar, O, Mancini, J, *et al.* (2010) Clopidogrel loading dose adjustment according to platelet reactivity monitoring in patients carrying the 2C19 2* loss of function polymorphism. *Journal of the American College of Cardiology*, **56**, 1630–6.

88 Bonello, L, Tantry, US, Marcucci, R, Blindt, R, *et al.* (2010) Consensus and future directions on the definition of high on-treatment platelet reactivity to adenosine diphosphate. *Journal of the American College of Cardiology*, **56**, 919–933.

89 Gurbel, PA, Tantry, US. (2010) Combination antithrombotic therapies. *Circulation*, **121**, 569–583.

90 Jeong, YH, Lee, SW, Choi, BR, Kim, IS, *et al.* (2009) Randomized comparison of adjunctive cilostazol versus high maintenance dose clopidogrel in patients with high post-treatment platelet reactivity: results of the ACCEL-RESISTANCE (Adjunctive Cilostazol Versus High Maintenance Dose Clopidogrel in Patients With Clopidogrel Resistance) randomized study. *Journal of the American College of Cardiology*, **53**, 1101–1109.

91 Jeong, YH, Hwang, JY, Kim, IS, Park, Y, *et al.* (2010) Adding cilostazol to dual antiplatelet therapy achieves greater platelet inhibition than high maintenance dose clopidogrel in patients with acute myocardial infarction: Results of the adjunctive cilostazol versus high maintenance dose clopidogrel in patients with AMI (ACCEL-AMI) study. *Circ Cardiovasc Interv*, **3**, 17–26.

92 Yusuf, S, Zhao, F, Mehta, SR, Chrolavicius, S, *et al.* (2001) Effects of clopidogrel in addition to aspirin in patients with acute coronary syndromes without ST-segment elevation. *New England Journal of Medicine*, **345**, 494–502.

93 Steinhubl, SR, Berger, PB, Mann, JT, 3rd, Fry, ET, *et al.* (2002) Early and sustained dual oral antiplatelet therapy following percutaneous coronary intervention: a randomized controlled trial. *JAMA*, **288**, 2411–2420.

94 Bhatt, DL, Fox, KA, Hacke, W, Berger, PB, *et al.* (2006) Clopidogrel and aspirin versus aspirin alone for the prevention of atherothrombotic events. *New England Journal of Medicine*, **354**, 1706–1717.

95 Sabatine, MS, Cannon, CP, Gibson, CM, Lopez-Sendon, JL, *et al.* (2005) Addition of clopidogrel to aspirin

and fibrinolytic therapy for myocardial infarction with ST-segment elevation. *New England Journal of Medicine*, **352**, 1179–1789.

96 Aronow, HD, Steinhubl, SR, Brennan, DM, Berger, PB, *et al.* (2009) Bleeding risk associated with 1 year of dual antiplatelet therapy after percutaneous coronary intervention: Insights from the Clopidogrel for the Reduction of Events During Observation (CREDO) trial. *Am Heart J*, **157**, 369–374.

97 Ho, PM, Maddox, TM, Wang, L, Fihn, SD, *et al.* (2009) Risk of adverse outcomes associated with concomitant use of clopidogrel and proton pump inhibitors following acute coronary syndrome. *JAMA*, **301**, 937–944.

98 Juurlink, DN, Gomes, T, Ko, DT, Szmitko, P, *et al.* (2009) A population-based study of the drug interaction between proton pump inhibitors and clopidogrel. *Cmaj*, **180**, 713–718.

99 Li, XQ, Andersson, TB, Ahlstrom, M, Weidolf, L (2004) Comparison of inhibitory effects of the proton pump-inhibiting drugs omeprazole, esomeprazole, lansoprazole, pantoprazole, and rabeprazole on human cytochrome P450 activities. *Drug Metabolism and Disposal*, **32**, 821–827.

100 Blume, H, Donath, F, Warnke, A, Schug, BS. (2006) Pharmacokinetic drug interaction profiles of proton pump inhibitors. *Drug Safety*, **29**, 769–784.

101 Gilard, M, Arnaud, B, Cornily, JC, Le Gal, G, *et al.* (2008) Influence of omeprazole on the antiplatelet action of clopidogrel associated with aspirin: the randomized, double-blind OCLA (Omeprazole CLopidogrel Aspirin) study. *Journal of the American College of Cardiology*, **51**, 256–260.

102 Gilard, M, Arnaud, B, Le Gal, G, Abgrall, JF, *et al.* (2006) Influence of omeprazol on the antiplatelet action of clopidogrel associated to aspirin. *Journal of Thrombosis and Haemostasis*, **4**, 2508–2509.

103 Angiolillo, DJ, Gibson, CM, Cheng, S, Ollier, C, *et al.* (2010) Differential effects of omeprazole and pantoprazole on the pharmacodynamics and pharmacokinetics of clopidogrel in healthy subjects: randomized, placebo-controlled, crossover comparison studies. *Clinical Pharmacology & Therapeutics*, epub ahead of print.

104 Leon, MB, Baim, DS, Popma, JJ, Gordon, PC, *et al.* (1998) A clinical trial comparing three antithrombotic-drug regimens after coronary-artery stenting: Stent Anticoagulation Restenosis Study Investigators. *New England Journal of Medicine*, **339**, 1665–1671.

105 Bertrand, ME, Rupprecht, HJ, Urban, P, Gershlick, AH (2000) Double-blind study of the safety of clopidogrel with and without a loading dose in combination with aspirin compared with ticlopidine in combination with aspirin after coronary stenting: the clopidogrel aspirin stent international cooperative study (CLASSICS). *Circulation*, **102**, 624–629.

106 von Beckerath, N, Koch, W, Mehilli, J, Bottiger, C, *et al.* (2000) Glycoprotein Ia gene C807T polymorphism and risk for major adverse cardiac events within the first 30 days after coronary artery stenting. *Blood*, **95**, 3297–3301.

107 Wiviott, SD, Trenk, D, Frelinger, AL, O'Donoghue, M, *et al.* (2007) Prasugrel compared with high loading- and maintenance-dose clopidogrel in patients with planned percutaneous coronary intervention: the Prasugrel in Comparison to Clopidogrel for Inhibition of Platelet Activation and Aggregation-Thrombolysis in Myocardial Infarction 44 trial. *Circulation*, **116**, 2923–2932.

108 Wiviott, SD, Braunwald, E, McCabe, CH, Montalescot, G, *et al.* (2007) Prasugrel versus clopidogrel in patients with acute coronary syndromes. *New England Journal of Medicine*, **357**, 2001–2015.

109 Rehmel, JL, Eckstein, JA, Farid, NA, Heim, JB, *et al.* (2006) Interactions of two major metabolites of prasugrel, a thienopyridine antiplatelet agent, with the cytochromes P450. *Drug Metabolism and Disposal*, **34**, 600–6907.

110 Wallentin, L, Varenhorst, C, James, S, Erlinge, D, *et al.* (2008) Prasugrel achieves greater and faster P2Y12receptor-mediated platelet inhibition than clopidogrel due to more efficient generation of its active metabolite in aspirin-treated patients with coronary artery disease. *Eur Heart J*, **29**, 21–30.

111 Payne, CD, Li, YG, Small, DS, Ernest, CS, II, *et al.* (2007) Increased active metabolite formation explains the greater platelet inhibition with prasugrel compared to high-dose clopidogrel. *J Cardiovasc Pharmacol*, **50**, 555–562.

112 Varenhorst, C, James, S, Erlinge, D, Brandt, JT, *et al.* (2009) Genetic variation of CYP2C19 affects both pharmacokinetic and pharmacodynamic responses to clopidogrel but not prasugrel in aspirin-treated patients with coronary artery disease. *Eur Heart J*, **30**, 1744–1752.

113 Angiolillo, DJ, Saucedo, JF, Deraad, R, Frelinger, AL, *et al.* (2010) Increased platelet inhibition after switching from maintenance clopidogrel to prasugrel in patients with acute coronary syndromes: results of the SWAP (SWitching Anti Platelet) study. *Journal of the American College of Cardiology*, **56**, 1017–1023.

114 Sorich, MJ, Vitry, A, Ward, MB, Horowitz, J.D. *et al.* (2010) Prasugrel versus clopidogrel for Cytochrome P450 2C19 genotyped subgroups: integration of the TRITON-TIMI 38 trial data. *Journal of Thrombosis and Haemostasis*, **8**, 1678–84.

115 Biondi-Zoccai, G, Lotrionte, M, Agostoni, P, Abbate, A, *et al.* (2010) Adjusted indirect comparison meta-analysis of prasugrel versus ticagrelor for patients with acute coronary syndromes. *Int J Cardiol*, epub ahead of print.

116 Husted, S, Emanuelsson, H, Heptinstall, S, Sandset, PM, *et al.* (2006) Pharmacodynamics, pharmacokinetics, and safety of the oral reversible P2Y12 antagonist AZD6140 with aspirin in patients with atherosclerosis: a double-blind comparison to clopidogrel with aspirin. *Eur Heart J*, **27**, 1038–1047.

117 Gurbel, PA, Bliden, KP, Butler, K, Tantry, US, *et al.* (2009) Randomized double-blind assessment of the ONSET and OFFSET of the antiplatelet effects of ticagrelor versus clopidogrel in patients with stable coronary artery disease: the ONSET/OFFSET study. *Circulation*, **120**, 2577–2585.

118 Storey, RF, Angiolillo, DJ, Patil, SB, Desai, B, *et al.* (2010) Inhibitory Effects of Ticagrelor Compared With Clopidogrel on Platelet Function in Patients With Acute Coronary Syndromes The PLATO (PLATelet inhibition and patient Outcomes) PLATELET Substudy. *Journal of the American College of Cardiology*, **56**, 1456–1462.

119 Wallentin, L, Becker, RC, Budaj, A, Cannon, CP, *et al.* (2009) Ticagrelor versus clopidogrel in patients with acute coronary syndromes. *New England Journal of Medicine*, **361**, 1045–1057.

120 Butler, K, Teng, R (2010) Pharmacokinetics, pharmacodynamics, and safety of ticagrelor in volunteers with mild hepatic impairment. *J Clin Pharmacol*, epub ahead of print.

121 Storey, RF, Melissa Thornton, S, Lawrance, R, Husted, S, *et al.* (2009) Ticagrelor yields consistent dose-dependent inhibition of ADP-induced platelet aggregation in patients with atherosclerotic disease regardless of genotypic variations in P2RY12, P2RY1, and ITGB3. *Platelets*, **20**, 341–348.

122 Wallentin, L, James, S, Storey, RF, Armstrong, M, *et al.* (2010) Effect of CYP2C19 and ABCB1 single nucleotide polymorphisms on outcomes of treatment with ticagrelor versus clopidogrel for acute coronary syndromes: a genetic substudy of the PLATO trial. *Lancet*, **376**, 1320–1328.

123 Tantry, US, Bliden, KP, Wei, C, Storey, RF, *et al.* (2010) First Analysis of the Relation Between CYP2C19 Genotype and Pharmacodynamics in Patients Treated With Ticagrelor Versus Clopidogrel: The ONSET/OFFSET and RESPOND Genotype Studies. *Circ Cardiovasc Genet*, epub ahead of print.

124 Gurbel, PA, Bliden, KP, Guyer, K, Cho, PW, *et al.* (2005) Platelet reactivity in patients and recurrent events post-stenting: results of the PREPARE POST-STENTING Study. *Journal of the American College of Cardiology*, **46**, 1820–1826.

125 Geisler, T, Langer, H, Wydymus, M, Gohring, K, *et al.* (2006) Low response to clopidogrel is associated with cardiovascular outcome after coronary stent implantation. *Eur Heart J*, **27**, 2420–2425.

126 Cuisset, T, Frere, C, Quilici, J, Barbou, F, *et al.* (2006) High post-treatment platelet reactivity identified low-responders to dual antiplatelet therapy at increased risk of recurrent cardiovascular events after stenting for acute coronary syndrome. *Journal of Thrombosis and Haemostasis*, **4**, 542–549.

127 Matetzky, S, Shenkman, B, Guetta, V, Shechter, M, *et al.* (2004) Clopidogrel resistance is associated with increased risk of recurrent atherothrombotic events in patients with acute myocardial infarction. *Circulation*, **109**, 3171–3175.

128 Hayward, CP, Harrison, P, Cattaneo, M, Ortel, TL, *et al.* (2006) Platelet function analyzer (PFA)-100 closure time in the evaluation of platelet disorders and platelet function. *Journal of Thrombosis and Haemostasis*, **4**, 312–319.

129 Breet, NJ, van Werkum, JW, Bouman, HJ, Kelder, JC, *et al.* (2010) Comparison of platelet function tests in predicting clinical outcome in patients undergoing coronary stent implantation. *JAMA*, **303**, 754–762.

130 von Beckerath, N, Pogatsa-Murray, G, Wieczorek, A, Sibbing, D, *et al.* (2006) Correlation of a new point-of-care test with conventional optical aggregometry for the assessment of clopidogrel responsiveness. *Thrombosis and Haemostasis*, **95**, 910–911.

131 van Werkum, JW, van der Stelt, CA, Seesing, TH, Hackeng, CM, *et al.* (2006) A head-to-head comparison between the VerifyNow P2Y12 assay and light transmittance aggregometry for monitoring the individual platelet response to clopidogrel in patients undergoing elective percutaneous coronary intervention. *Journal of Thrombosis and Haemostasis*, **4**, 2516–2518.

132 van Werkum, JW, Kleibeuker, M, Postma, S, Bouman, HJ, *et al.* (2010) A comparison between the

Plateletworks-assay and light transmittance aggrego-metry for monitoring the inhibitory effects of clopido-grel. *Int J Cardiol*, **140**, 123–126.

133 Cattaneo, M. (2007) Resistance to antiplatelet drugs: molecular mechanisms and laboratory detection. *Journal of Thrombosis and Haemostasis*, **5** (**Suppl. 1**), 230–237.

134 Madsen, EH, Saw, J, Kristensen, SR, Schmidt, EB, *et al.* (2010) Long-term aspirin and clopidogrel response evaluated by light transmission aggregometry, Verify-Now, and thrombelastography in patients undergoing percutaneous coronary intervention. *Clin Chem*, **56**, 839–847.

135 Lordkipanidze, M, Pharand, C, Nguyen, TA, Scham-paert, E, *et al.* (2008) Comparison of four tests to assess inhibition of platelet function by clopidogrel in stable coronary artery disease patients. *Eur Heart J*, **29**, 2877–2785.

136 Budnitz, DS, Shehab, N, Kegler, SR, Richards, CL (2007) Medication use leading to emergency depart-ment visits for adverse drug events in older adults. *Annals of Internal Medicine*, **147**, 755–765.

137 Ray, KK, Francis, S, Crossman, DC (2005) A potential pharmacogenomic strategy for anticoagulant treat-ment in non-ST elevation acute coronary syndromes: the role of interleukin-1 receptor antagonist genotype. *Journal of Thrombosis and Haemostasis*, **3**, 287–291.

138 Hunt, SA, Abraham, WT, Chin, MH, Feldman, AM, *et al.* (2005) ACC/AHA 2005 guideline update for the diagnosis and management of chronic heart failure in the adult: a report of the American College of Cardi-ology/American Heart Association Task Force on Prac-tice Guidelines (Writing Committee to Update the 2001 Guidelines for the Evaluation and Management of Heart Failure): developed in collaboration with the American College of Chest Physicians and the Inter-national Society for Heart and Lung Transplantation: endorsed by the Heart Rhythm Society. *Circulation*, **112**, e154–3235.

139 Tandon, P, McAlister, FA, Tsuyuki, RT, Hervas-Malo, M, *et al.* (2004) The use of beta blockers in a tertiary care heart failure clinic: dosing, tolerance, and out-comes. *Archives of Internal Medicine*, **164**, 769–774.

140 Moore, JD, Mason, DA, Green, SA, Hsu, J, *et al.* (1999) Racial differences in the frequencies of cardiac beta (1)-adrenergic receptor polymorphisms: analysis of c145A>G and c1165G>C. *Hum Mutat*, **14**, 271.

141 Muszkat, M, Stein, CM (2005) Pharmacogenetics and response to beta-adrenergic receptor antagonists in heart failure. *Clinical Pharmacology & Therapeutics*, **77**, 123–126.

142 Liggett, SB, Mialet-Perez, J, Thaneemit-Chen, S, Weber, SA, *et al.* (2006) A polymorphism within a conserved beta(1)-adrenergic receptor motif alters cardiac function and beta-blocker response in human heart failure. *Proceedings of the National Academy of Sciences of the United States of America*, **103**, 11288–11293.

143 Mason, DA, Moore, JD, Green, SA, Liggett, SB (1999) A gain-of-function polymorphism in a G-protein cou-pling domain of the human beta1-adrenergic recep-tor. *J Biol Chem*, **274**, 12670–12674.

144 Chen, L, Meyers, D, Javorsky, G, Burstow, D, *et al.* (2007) Arg389Gly-beta1-adrenergic receptors deter-mine improvement in left ventricular systolic function in nonischemic cardiomyopathy patients with heart failure after chronic treatment with carvedilol. *Phar-macogenetic Genomics*, **17**, 941–949.

145 Molenaar, P, Chen, L, Semmler, AB, Parsonage, WA, *et al.* (2007) Human heart beta-adrenoceptors: beta1-adrenoceptor diversification through 'affinity states' and polymorphism. *Clin Exp Pharmacol Physiol*, **34**, 1020–1028.

146 Baudhuin, LM, Miller, WL, Train, L, Bryant, S, *et al.* (2010) Relation of ADRB1, CYP2D6, and UGT1A1 polymorphisms with dose of, and response to, carve-dilol or metoprolol therapy in patients with chronic heart failure. *American Journal of Cardiology*, **106**, 402–408.

147 Rochais, F, Vilardaga, JP, Nikolaev, VO, Bunemann, M, *et al.* (2007) Real-time optical recording of beta1-adrenergic receptor activation reveals supersensitivity of the Arg389 variant to carvedilol. *J Clin Invest*, **117**, 229–235.

148 Mialet Perez, J, Rathz, DA, Petrashevskaya, NN, Hahn, HS, *et al.* (2003) Beta 1-adrenergic receptor poly-morphisms confer differential function and predispo-sition to heart failure. *Nat Med*, **9**, 1300–1305.

149 Metra, M, Covolo, L, Pezzali, N, Zaca, V, *et al.* (2010) Role of beta-adrenergic receptor gene polymorphisms in the long-term effects of beta-blockade with carve-dilol in patients with chronic heart failure. *Cardiovasc Drugs Ther*, **24**, 49–60.

150 de Groote, P, Helbecque, N, Lamblin, N, Hermant, X, *et al.* (2005) Association between beta-1 and beta-2 adrenergic receptor gene polymorphisms and the response to beta-blockade in patients with stable congestive heart failure. *Pharmacogenetic Genomics*, **15**, 137–142.

151 Borjesson, M, Magnusson, Y, Hjalmarson, A, Andersson, B (2000) A novel polymorphism in the gene coding for the beta(1)-adrenergic receptor associated with survival in patients with heart failure. *Eur Heart J*, **21**, 1853–1858.

152 Terra, SG, Hamilton, KK, Pauly, DF, Lee, CR, *et al.* (2005) Beta1-adrenergic receptor polymorphisms and left ventricular remodeling changes in response to beta-blocker therapy. *Pharmacogenetic Genomics*, **15**, 227–234.

153 Green, SA, Turki, J, Innis, M, Liggett, SB (1994) Amino-terminal polymorphisms of the human beta 2-adrenergic receptor impart distinct agonist-promoted regulatory properties. *Biochemistry*, **33**, 9414–9419.

154 Kaye, DM, Smirk, B, Williams, C, Jennings, G, *et al.* (2003) Beta-adrenoceptor genotype influences the response to carvedilol in patients with congestive heart failure. *Pharmacogenetics*, **13**, 379–382.

155 Small, KM, Forbes, SL, Rahman, FF, Bridges, KM, *et al.* (2000) A four amino acid deletion polymorphism in the third intracellular loop of the human alpha 2C-adrenergic receptor confers impaired coupling to multiple effectors. *J Biol Chem*, **275**, 23059–23064.

156 Bristow, MR, Murphy, GA, Krause-Steinrauf, H, Anderson, JL, *et al.* (2010) An alpha2C-adrenergic receptor polymorphism alters the norepinephrine-lowering effects and therapeutic response of the beta-blocker bucindolol in chronic heart failure. *Circ Heart Fail*, **3**, 21–28.

157 Cice, G, Ferrara, L, D'Andrea, A, D'Isa, S, *et al.* (2003) Carvedilol increases two-year survival in dialysis patients with dilated cardiomyopathy: a prospective, placebo-controlled trial. *Journal of the American College of Cardiology*, **41**, 1438–1444.

158 Keating, GM, Jarvis, B. (2003) Carvedilol: a review of its use in chronic heart failure. *Drugs*, **63**, 1697–1741.

159 Takekuma, Y, Takenaka, T, Kiyokawa, M, Yamazaki, K, *et al.* (2006) Contribution of polymorphisms in UDP-glucuronosyltransferase and CYP2D6 to the individual variation in disposition of carvedilol. *J Pharm Pharm Sci*, **9**, 101–112.

160 Lennard, MS, Silas, JH, Freestone, S, Ramsay, LE, *et al.* (1982) Oxidation phenotype: a major determinant of metoprolol metabolism and response. *New England Journal of Medicine*, **307**, 1558–1560.

161 McGourty, JC, Silas, JH, Lennard, MS, Tucker, GT, *et al.* (1985) Metoprolol metabolism and debrisoquine oxidation polymorphism: population and family studies. *British Journal of Clinical Pharmacology*, **20**, 555–566.

162 Horikiri, Y, Suzuki, T, Mizobe, M (1998) Pharmacokinetics and metabolism of bisoprolol enantiomers in humans. *J Pharm Sci*, **87**, 289–294.

163 Bradford, LD (2002) CYP2D6 allele frequency in European Caucasians, Asians, Africans and their descendants. *Pharmacogenomics*, **3**, 229–243.

164 Jin, SK, Chung, HJ, Chung, MW, Kim, JI, *et al.* (2008) Influence of CYP2D6*10 on the pharmacokinetics of metoprolol in healthy Korean volunteers. *J Clin Pharm Ther*, **33**, 567–573.

165 Goryachkina, K, Burbello, A, Boldueva, S, Babak, S, *et al.* (2008) CYP2D6 is a major determinant of metoprolol disposition and effects in hospitalized Russian patients treated for acute myocardial infarction. *Eur J Clin Pharmacol*, **64**, 1163–1173.

166 Ismail, R, Teh, LK (2006) The relevance of CYP2D6 genetic polymorphism on chronic metoprolol therapy in cardiovascular patients. *J Clin Pharm Ther*, **31**, 99–109.

167 Honda, M, Nozawa, T, Igarashi, N, Inoue, H, *et al.* (2005) Effect of CYP2D6*10 on the pharmacokinetics of R- and S-carvedilol in healthy Japanese volunteers. *Biol Pharm Bull*, **28**, 1476–1479.

168 Nozawa, T, Taguchi, M, Tahara, K, Hashimoto, Y, *et al.* (2005) Influence of CYP2D6 genotype on metoprolol plasma concentration and beta-adrenergic inhibition during long-term treatment: a comparison with bisoprolol. *J Cardiovasc Pharmacol*, **46**, 713–720.

169 Zhou, HH, Wood, AJ (1995) Stereoselective disposition of carvedilol is determined by CYP2D6. *Clinical Pharmacology & Therapeutics*, **57**, 518–524.

170 Wuttke, H, Rau, T, Heide, R, Bergmann, K, *et al.* (2002) Increased frequency of cytochrome P450 2D6 poor metabolizers among patients with metoprolol-associated adverse effects. *Clinical Pharmacology & Therapeutics*, **72**, 429–437.

171 Huang, J, Chuang, SK, Cheng, CL, Lai, ML (1999) Pharmacokinetics of metoprolol enantiomers in Chinese subjects of major CYP2D6 genotypes. *Clinical Pharmacology & Therapeutics*, **65**, 402–407.

172 Rau, T, Wuttke, H, Michels, LM, Werner, U, *et al.* (2009) Impact of the CYP2D6 genotype on the clinical effects of metoprolol: a prospective longitudinal study. *Clinical Pharmacology & Therapeutics*, **85**, 269–272.

173 Rau, T, Heide, R, Bergmann, K, Wuttke, H, *et al.* (2002) Effect of the CYP2D6 genotype on metoprolol metabolism persists during long-term treatment. *Pharmacogenetics*, **12**, 465–472.

174 Fux, R, Morike, K, Prohmer, AM, Delabar, U, *et al.* (2005) Impact of CYP2D6 genotype on adverse effects during treatment with metoprolol: a prospective clinical study. *Clinical Pharmacology & Therapeutics*, **78**, 378–387.

175 Zineh, I, Beitelshees, AL, Gaedigk, A, Walker, JR, *et al.* (2004) Pharmacokinetics and CYP2D6 genotypes do not predict metoprolol adverse events or efficacy in hypertension. *Clinical Pharmacology & Therapeutics*, **76**, 536–544.

176 Monaghan, G, Ryan, M, Seddon, R, Hume, R, *et al.* (1996) Genetic variation in bilirubin UPD-glucuronosyltransferase gene promoter and Gilbert's syndrome. *Lancet*, **347**, 578–581.

177 Ohno, A, Saito, Y, Hanioka, N, Jinno, H, *et al.* (2004) Involvement of human hepatic UGT1A1, UGT2B4, and UGT2B7 in the glucuronidation of carvedilol. *Drug Metabolism and Disposal*, **32**, 235–239.

178 Takekuma, Y, Takenaka, T, Yamazaki, K, Ueno, K, *et al.* (2007) Stereoselective metabolism of racemic carvedilol by UGT1A1 and UGT2B7, and effects of mutation of these enzymes on glucuronidation activity. *Biol Pharm Bull*, **30**, 2146–2153.

179 Mitka, M (2003) Expanding statin use to help more at-risk patients is causing financial heartburn. *JAMA*, **290**, 2243–2245.

180 Joy, TR, Hegele, RA (2009) Narrative review: statin-related myopathy. *Ann Intern Med*, **150**, 858–868.

181 Staffa, JA, Chang, J, Green, L (2002) Cerivastatin and reports of fatal rhabdomyolysis. *New England Journal of Medicine*, **346**, 539–540.

182 Jacobson, TA (2006) Statin safety: lessons from new drug applications for marketed statins. *American Journal of Cardiology*, **97**, 44C–51C.

183 Thompson, PD, Clarkson, P, Karas, RH (2003) Statin-associated myopathy. *JAMA*, **289**, 1681–1690.

184 Schick, BA, Laaksonen, R, Frohlich, JJ, Paiva, H, *et al.* (2007) Decreased skeletal muscle mitochondrial DNA in patients treated with high-dose simvastatin. *Clinical Pharmacology & Therapeutics*, **81**, 650–653.

185 Gambelli, S, Dotti, MT, Malandrini, A, Mondelli, M, *et al.* (2004) Mitochondrial alterations in muscle biopsies of patients on statin therapy. *J Submicrosc Cytol Pathol*, **36**, 85–89.

186 Matzno, S, Yasuda, S, Juman, S, Yamamoto, Y, *et al.* (2005) Statin-induced apoptosis linked with membrane farnesylated Ras small G protein depletion, rather than geranylated Rho protein. *J Pharm Pharmacol*, **57**, 1475–1484.

187 Lamperti, C, Naini, AB, Lucchini, V, Prelle, A, *et al.* (2005) Muscle coenzyme Q10 level in statin-related myopathy. *Arch Neurol*, **62**, 1709–1712.

188 Laaksonen, R, Jokelainen, K, Sahi, T, Tikkanen, MJ, *et al.* (1995) Decreases in serum ubiquinone concentrations do not result in reduced levels in muscle tissue during short-term simvastatin treatment in humans. *Clinical Pharmacology & Therapeutics*, **57**, 62–66.

189 Laaksonen, R, Jokelainen, K, Laakso, J, Sahi, T, *et al.* (1996) The effect of simvastatin treatment on natural antioxidants in low-density lipoproteins and high-energy phosphates and ubiquinone in skeletal muscle. *American Journal of Cardiology*, **77**, 851–854.

190 Paiva, H, Thelen, KM, Van Coster, R, Smet, J, *et al.* (2005) High-dose statins and skeletal muscle metabolism in humans: a randomized, controlled trial. *Clinical Pharmacology & Therapeutics*, **78**, 60–68.

191 Oh, J, Ban, MR, Miskie, BA, Pollex, RL, *et al.* (2007) Genetic determinants of statin intolerance. *Lipids Health Dis*, **6**, 7.

192 Hermann, M, Bogsrud, MP, Molden, E, Asberg, A, *et al.* (2006) Exposure of atorvastatin is unchanged but lactone and acid metabolites are increased several-fold in patients with atorvastatin-induced myopathy. *Clinical Pharmacology & Therapeutics*, **79**, 532–539.

193 Skottheim, IB, Gedde-Dahl, A, Hejazifar, S, Hoel, K, *et al.* (2008) Statin induced myotoxicity: the lactone forms are more potent than the acid forms in human skeletal muscle cells in vitro. *Eur J Pharm Sci*, **33**, 317–325.

194 Neuvonen, PJ, Niemi, M, Backman, JT (2006) Drug interactions with lipid-lowering drugs: mechanisms and clinical relevance. *Clinical Pharmacology & Therapeutics*, **80**, 565–581.

195 Wilke, RA, Moore, JH, Burmester, JK (2005) Relative impact of CYP3A genotype and concomitant medication on the severity of atorvastatin-induced muscle damage. *Pharmacogenetic Genomics*, **15**, 415–421.

196 Pasanen, MK, Neuvonen, PJ, Niemi, M (2008) Global analysis of genetic variation in SLCO1B1. *Pharmacogenomics*, **9**, 19–33.

197 Mwinyi, J, Johne, A, Bauer, S, Roots, I, *et al.* (2004) Evidence for inverse effects of OATP-C (SLC21A6) 5 and 1b haplotypes on pravastatin kinetics. *Clinical Pharmacology & Therapeutics*, **75**, 415–421.

198 Niemi, M, Pasanen, MKNeuvonen, PJ (2006) SLCO1B1 polymorphism and sex affect the pharmacokinetics of pravastatin but not fluvastatin. *Clinical Pharmacology & Therapeutics*, **80**, 356–366.

199 Kameyama, Y, Yamashita, K, Kobayashi, K, Hoso-kawa, M, *et al.* (2005) Functional characterization of SLCO1B1 (OATP-C) variants, SLCO1B1*5, SLCO1B1*15 and SLCO1B1*15 + C1007G, by using transient expression systems of HeLa and HEK293 cells. *Pharmacogenetic Genomics*, **15**, 513–522.

200 Morimoto, K, Oishi, T, Ueda, S, Ueda, M, *et al.* (2004) A novel variant allele of OATP-C (SLCO1B1) found in a Japanese patient with pravastatin-induced myopathy. *Drug Metab Pharmacokinet*, **19**, 453–455.

201 Link, E, Parish, S, Armitage, J, Bowman, L, *et al.* (2008) SLCO1B1 variants and statin-induced myopathy: a genomewide study. *New England Journal of Medicine*, **359**, 789–799.

202 Voora, D, Shah, SH, Spasojevic, I, Ali, S. *et al.* (2009) The SLCO1B1*5 genetic variant is associated with statin-induced side effects. *Journal of the American College of Cardiology*, **54**, 1609–1616.

203 Jones, PH, Davidson, MH (2005) Reporting rate of rhabdomyolysis with fenofibrate + statin versus gemfibrozil + any statin. *American Journal of Cardiology*, **95**, 120–122.

204 Fujino, H, Saito, T, Tsunenari, Y, Kojima, J, *et al.* (2004) Metabolic properties of the acid and lactone forms of HMG-CoA reductase inhibitors. *Xenobiotica*, **34**, 961–971.

205 Simon, JA, Lin, F, Hulley, SB, Blanche, PJ *et al.* (2006) Phenotypic predictors of response to simvastatin therapy among African-Americans and Caucasians: the Cholesterol and Pharmacogenetics (CAP) Study. *American Journal of Cardiology*, **97**, 843–850.

206 Iakoubova, OA, Tong, CH, Rowland, CM, Kirchgess-ner, TG, *et al.* (2008) Association of the Trp719Arg polymorphism in kinesin-like protein 6 with myocar-dial infarction and coronary heart disease in 2 pro-spective trials: the CARE and WOSCOPS trials. *Journal of the American College of Cardiology*, **51**, 435–443.

207 Iakoubova, OA, Sabatine, MS, Rowland, CM, Tong, CH, *et al.* (2008) Polymorphism in KIF6 gene and benefit from statins after acute coronary syndromes: results from the PROVE IT-TIMI 22 study. *Journal of the American College of Cardiology*, **51**, 449–455.

208 Shiffman, D, Chasman, DI, Zee, RY, Iakoubova, OA, *et al.* (2008) A kinesin family member 6 variant is associated with coronary heart disease in the Women's Health Study. *Journal of the American College of Cardiology*, **51**, 444–448.

209 Bare, LA, Morrison, AC, Rowland, CM, Shiffman, D, *et al.* (2007) Five common gene variants identify elevated genetic risk for coronary heart disease. *Genet Med*, **9**, 682–689.

210 Luke, MM, Lalouschek, W, Rowland, CM, Catanese, JJ, *et al.* (2009) Polymorphisms associated with both noncardioembolic stroke and coronary heart disease: vienna stroke registry. *Cerebrovasc Dis*, **28**, 499–504.

211 Stewart, AF, Dandona, S, Chen, L, Assogba, O, *et al.* (2009) Kinesin family member 6 variant Trp719Arg does not associate with angiographically defined cor-onary artery disease in the Ottawa Heart Genomics Study. *Journal of the American College of Cardiology*, **53**, 1471–1472.

212 Shiffman, D, Sabatine, MS, Louie, JZ, Kirchgessner, TG, *et al.* (2010) Effect of pravastatin therapy on coronary events in carriers of the KIF6 719Arg allele from the cholesterol and recurrent events trial. *American Journal of Cardiology*, **105**, 1300–5.

213 Iakoubova, OA, Robertson, M, Tong, CH, Rowland, CM, *et al.* (2010) KIF6 Trp719Arg polymorphism and the effect of statin therapy in elderly patients: results from the PROSPER study. *Eur J Cardiovasc Prev Rehabil*, **17**, 455–461.

214 Shimada, T, Yamazaki, H, Mimura, M, Inui, Y, *et al.* (1994) Interindividual variations in human liver cyto-chrome P-450 enzymes involved in the oxidation of drugs, carcinogens and toxic chemicals: studies with liver microsomes of 30 Japanese and 30 Caucasians. *J Pharmacol Exp Ther*, **270**, 414–423.

215 Lamba, JK, Lin, YS, Schuetz, EG, Thummel, KE (2002) Genetic contribution to variable human CYP3A-mediated metabolism. *Adv Drug Deliv Rev*, **54**, 1271–1294.

216 Westlind, A, Lofberg, L, Tindberg, N, Andersson, TB, *et al.* (1999) Interindividual differences in hepatic expression of CYP3A4: relationship to genetic poly-morphism in the 5'-upstream regulatory region. *Bio-chem Biophys Res Commun*, **259**, 201–205.

217 Neuvonen, PJ, Kantola, T, Kivisto, KT (1998) Simva-statin but not pravastatin is very susceptible to inter-action with the CYP3A4 inhibitor itraconazole. *Clinical Pharmacology & Therapeutics*, **63**, 332–341.

218 Jalava, KM, Olkkola, KTNeuvonen, PJ (1997) Itraco-nazole greatly increases plasma concentrations and effects of felodipine. *Clinical Pharmacology & Therapeu-tics*, **61**, 410–415.

219 Choumerianou, DM, Dedoussis, GV (2005) Familial hypercholesterolemia and response to statin therapy according to LDLR genetic background. *Clin Chem Lab Med*, **43**, 793–801.

220 Leitersdorf, E, Eisenberg, S, Eliav, O, Friedlander, Y, *et al.* (1993) Genetic determinants of responsiveness to the HMG-CoA reductase inhibitor fluvastatin in patients with molecularly defined heterozygous familial hypercholesterolemia. *Circulation*, **87**, III35–III44.

221 Vohl, MC, Szots, F, Lelievre, M, Lupien, PJ, *et al.* (2002) Influence of LDL receptor gene mutation and apo E polymorphism on lipoprotein response to simvastatin treatment among adolescents with heterozygous familial hypercholesterolemia. *Atherosclerosis*, **160**, 361–368.

222 Couture, P, Brun, LD, Szots, F, Lelievre, M, *et al.* (1998) Association of specific LDL receptor gene mutations with differential plasma lipoprotein response to simvastatin in young French Canadians with heterozygous familial hypercholesterolemia. *Arterioscler Thromb Vasc Biol*, **18**, 1007–1012.

223 Chaves, FJ, Real, JT, Garcia-Garcia, AB, Civera, M, *et al.* (2001) Genetic diagnosis of familial hypercholesterolemia in a South European outbreed population: influence of low-density lipoprotein (LDL) receptor gene mutations on treatment response to simvastatin in total, LDL, and high-density lipoprotein cholesterol. *J Clin Endocrinol Metab*, **86**, 4926–4932.

224 Kajinami, K, Yagi, K, Higashikata, T, Inazu, A, *et al.* (1998) Low-density lipoprotein receptor genotype-dependent response to cholesterol lowering by combined pravastatin and cholestyramine in familial hypercholesterolemia. *American Journal of Cardiology*, **82**, 113–117.

225 Brorholt-Petersen, JU, Jensen, HK, Raungaard, B, Gregersen, N, *et al.* (2001) LDL-receptor gene mutations and the hypocholesterolemic response to statin therapy. *Clin Genet*, **59**, 397–405.

226 Sijbrands, EJ, Lombardi, MP, Westendorp, RG, Leuven, JA, *et al.* (1998) Similar response to simvastatin in patients heterozygous for familial hypercholesterolemia with mRNA negative and mRNA positive mutations. *Atherosclerosis*, **136**, 247–254.

227 Sun, XM, Patel, DD, Knight, BL, Soutar, AK (1998) Influence of genotype at the low density lipoprotein (LDL) receptor gene locus on the clinical phenotype and response to lipid-lowering drug therapy in heterozygous familial hypercholesterolaemia: the Familial Hypercholesterolaemia Regression Study Group. *Atherosclerosis*, **136**, 175–185.

228 Vuorio, AF, Ojala, JP, Sarna, S, Turtola, H. *et al.* (1995) Heterozygous familial hypercholesterolaemia: the influence of the mutation type of the low-density-lipoprotein receptor gene and PvuII polymorphism of the normal allele on serum lipid levels and response to lovastatin treatment. *Journal of Internal Medicine*, **237**, 43–48.

229 Leren, TP, Hjermann, I (1995) Is responsiveness to lovastatin in familial hypercholesterolaemia heterozygotes influenced by the specific mutation in the low-density lipoprotein receptor gene? *Eur J Clin Invest*, **25**, 967–973.

230 Chasman, DI, Posada, D, Subrahmanyan, L, Cook, NR, *et al.* (2004) Pharmacogenetic study of statin therapy and cholesterol reduction. *JAMA*, **291**, 2821–2827.

231 Krauss, RM, Mangravite, LM, Smith, JD, Medina, MW, *et al.* (2008) Variation in the 3-hydroxyl-3-methylglutaryl coenzyme a reductase gene is associated with racial differences in low-density lipoprotein cholesterol response to simvastatin treatment. *Circulation*, **117**, 1537–1544.

232 Thompson, JF, Man, M, Johnson, KJ, Wood, LS, *et al.* (2005) An association study of 43 SNPs in 16 candidate genes with atorvastatin response. *Pharmacogenomics Journal*, **5**, 352–358.

233 Donnelly, LA, Doney, AS, Dannfald, J, Whitley, AL, *et al.* (2008) A paucimorphic variant in the HMG-CoA reductase gene is associated with lipid-lowering response to statin treatment in diabetes: a GoDARTS study. *Pharmacogenetic Genomics*, **18**, 1021–1026.

234 Poduri, A, Khullar, M, Bahl, A, Sehrawat, BS, *et al.* (2010) Common variants of HMGCR, CETP, APOAI, ABCB1, CYP3A4, and CYP7A1 genes as predictors of lipid-lowering response to atorvastatin therapy. *DNA Cell Biology*, **29**, 629–637.

235 Burkhardt, R, Kenny, EE, Lowe, JK, Birkeland, A, *et al.* (2008) Common SNPs in HMGCR in micronesians and whites associated with LDL-cholesterol levels affect alternative splicing of exon13. *Arterioscler Thromb Vasc Biol*, **28**, 2078–2084.

CHAPTER 8

Pharmacogenomic Aspects of Antiretroviral Therapy

Natella Y. Rakhmanina, MD, PhD[1] and John N. van den Anker, MD, PhD[2]

[1]Division of Infectious Disease and Department of Pediatrics, The George Washington University School of Medicine, Washington, DC, and Children's National Medical Center, Washington, DC

[2]Division of Pediatric Clinical Pharmacology and Departments of Pediatrics, Pharmacology and Physiology, The George Washington University School of Medicine, Washington, DC, and Children's National Medical Center, Washington, DC

Introduction

More than 33 million people with multiple racial and ethnical backgrounds live with HIV infection in different regions of the world (1). The current management of HIV infection focuses on the long-term delivery of effective and safe antiretroviral therapy (ART) to affected individuals. Of the estimated 15 million people living with HIV infection in low- and middle-income countries who need treatment today, more than 30% (5.2 million) have access to combination ART comprised of a minimum of three antiretroviral (ARV) drugs (1). Currently available ARV drugs represent five classes of therapeutic agents with different metabolic pathways and mechanisms of action: nucleoside reverse transcriptase inhibitors (NRTIs), nonnucleoside reverse transcriptase inhibitors (NNRTIs), protease inhibitors (PIs), entry and fusion inhibitors, and integrase inhibitors.

Marked interindividual variability in pharmacokinetics (P) and pharmacodynamics (PD) of ARV drugs has been reported in populations of diverse ethnic and racial backgrounds. Variations in the genes involved in the metabolism and disposition of ARV drugs may affect efficacy and toxicity of ART. Several important relationships between genetic variants in drug-metabolizing cytochrome P450 (CYP450) enzymes and drug transporters on the

variability in plasma concentrations and the adverse events of ARV drugs have been established. This chapter reviews the available data on the influence of patient genetic variations on the PK/PD of ARV drugs. Tables 8.1 and 8.2 summarize the established associations between host genetic variants in drug-metabolizing enzymes and transporters, and the exposure and side effects of ART.

Nucleoside reverse transcriptase inhibitors

In order to inhibit HIV-1 reverse transcriptase NRTIs require the addition of three phosphate groups by cellular kinases, forming active intracellular triphosphate metabolites. NRTIs zidovudine (ZDV), and abacavir (ABC), are cleared through a mechanism involving uridine diphosphate (UDP)-glucuronosyltransferase (UGT), while lamivudine (3TC) and tenofovir (TFV) are excreted renally unchanged. While the significance of the genetic polymorphisms in cellular kinases in intracellular phosphorylation of NRTIs is unknown, the *UGT2B7*1C* polymorphism has been associated with faster ZDV clearance (CL) and glucuronidation in Ghanian tuberculosis/HIV co-infected patients (2).

Drug transporter polymorphisms have been reported to affect PK and PD of NRTIs. Multidrug

Table 8.1 Pharmacogenomic Associations with Pharmacokinetics of Antiretroviral Drugs

Gene Allele (SNP)	NRTIs	NNRTIs	PIs	Entry and Fusion Inhibitors	Integrase Inhibitors
Drug-Metabolizing Enzymes					
CYP3A4/5	N/A	Trend to higher EFV AUC[a,b]	Decreased plasma IDV levels Increased SQV metabolite ratio[b] Decreased ATV CL and plasma levels[b,c,d]	NAR	N/A
CYP3A4*1B(−392A > G)[a]					
CYP3A5*3 (6986A > G)[b]					
CYP3A5*6 (14690G > A)[c]					
CYP3A5*7 (G27131-32insT)[d]					
CYP2C19	N/A		Increased NFV AUC	NAR	N/A
CYP2C19*2 (681G > A)					
CYP2D6	N/A	Increased plasma EFV levels	Increased plasma NFV levels	N/A	N/A
CYP2D6*3, *4, *6 (2549A > del, 1846G > A, 1707T > del)					
CYP2B6	N/A	Increased EFV and NVP plasma levels	NAR	N/A	N/A
CYP2B6*5, *6, *7, *9, *16: (516G > T, 983 T > C, 785A > G)					
CYP2B6*26: (499C > G, 516G > T, 785A > G)					
CYP2A6	N/A	Increased EFV and NVP plasma levels	NAR	N/A	NAR
CYP2A6*9B (1836G > T)					
CYP2A6*17 (1093G > A)					
UGT	Increased ZDV CL[a]	N/A	NAR	N/A	Higher plasma RAL levels[b]
UGT2B7*1c (735A > G)[a]					
UGT1A1*28 (A(TA)7TAA)[b]					
NR1/2	NAR	NAR	Decreased ATV plasma levels	NAR	NAR
Pregnane X receptor (63396C > T)					

Drug Transporters

MDR1					
MDR1 (3435T > C)	NAR	Increased EFV plasma levels Increased intracellular NFV levels	Increased/decreased NFV plasma levels and CL Increased ATV plasma levels	NAR	NAR
MRP2(ABCC2)					
MRP2 (-24C > T)[a]	Increased TFV CL	NAR	Increased IDV CL	NAR	NAR
MRP4(ABCC4)					
MRP4(ABCC4) MRP4 (4131T > G)[a] MRP4 (3724G > A)[b] MRP4 (3463A > G)[c]	Increased intracellular ZDV[a], 3TC[b] triphospates Decreased TFV CL and increased TFV AUC[c]	NAR	NAR	NAR	NAR
OAT					
SLCO1B1 (521T > C)	NAR	NAR	Increased LPV plasma levels	Increased MVC plasma levels	NAR

NAR: No association reported; and N/A: not applicable.

Table 8.2 Pharmacogenomic Associations with Toxicities of Antiretroviral Drugs

Gene Allele (SNP)	NRTIs	NNRTIs	PIs	Entry and Fusion Inhibitors	Integrase Inhibitors
CYP2B6 CYP2B6*6: (516G > T, 983T > C)	NAR	Increased EFV CNS toxicity	NAR	NAR	NAR
HLA-B HLA-B*5701[a] HLA-B*3505[b] HLA-B*4001[c]	Increased ABC hypersensitivity[a] Increased d4T lipoatrophy[c]	Increased NVP rash[b]	NAR	NAR	NAR
HLA-Cw HLA-B*14 HLA-Cw*8		Increased NVP hepatotoxicity			
HLA-DR HLA-DRB1*0101	NAR	Increased: NVP and EFV rash NVP hypersensitivity NVP hepatotoxicity	NAR	NAR	NAR
UGT1A UGT1A1*28 (A(TA)7TAA,-43-42insTA)[a] UGT1A1*6 (211G > A)[b] UGT1A1-TA7[c] UGT1A3[d] UGT1A7[e]	No data	N/A	Increased: ATV hyperbilirubinemia[a,b,c] IDV hyperbilirubinemia[d,e]	NAR	NAR
MDR1 MDR1 3435C > T[a] MDR1 2677G > T[b]	NAR	Decreased NVP hepatotoxicity[a] Increased HDL-cholesterol with EFV[a]	Increased ATV hyperbilirubinemia[a,b]	NAR	NAR
MRP2 MRP2 (1249G > A) CATC haplotype	Increased TFV nephrotoxicity	N/A	NAR	NAR	NAR
mtDNA MT-ND1 MT-ND1 (4216T > C, 4917A > G)	Increased NRTI neuropathy	N/A	NAR	NAR	NAR

CFTR		
CFTR (1717-1G > A)	Increased amylasemia	NAR	NAR	NAR
IVS8 5T	Increased d4T pancreatitis			
SPINK-1		
SPINK-1 (112C > T)	Increased amylasemia	NAR	NAR	NAR
	Increased d4T pancreatitis			

Non-drug specific

Gene / Variant	Association
TNF-α	
TNF-α (238G > A)	Earlier onset of lipoatrophy	NAR
APO	
APOC3 (-455C > T, -482C > T, 3238C > g)[a]	
ARbeta2[b]	Lipoatrophy[a], fat accumulation[b], dyslipidemia[a,c,d,e,f]
APOE ε2 & APOE ε3 haplotypes (2060T/2198T)[c]	
APOA1[d]	
APOA5 (-1131T > C)[e]	
CETP	
CETP (279A > G)	Dyslipidemia

NAR: No association reported; and N/A: not applicable.

resistance protein 4 (MRP4), a nucleoside efflux transporter loss-of-function polymorphism, has been associated with increased intracellular concentrations of ZDV and 3TC. Moreover, higher intracellular ZDV and 3TC concentrations have been correlated with improved CD4 + cell counts and a higher degree of virologic control (3, 4). Drug transporter polymorphisms affect another NRTI, TFV, whose secretion by renal tubular cells depends on uptake on the basolateral side by human ATP-binding cassette (ABC) transporters. Polymorphisms in drug transporters MRP2 and MRP4 have been shown to significantly influence TFV renal CL and the plasma area under the concentration versus time curve (AUC) (5). Since higher TFV exposure has been linked to TFV related renal proximal tubulopathy, MRP2 haplotypes have also been associated with TFV-induced nephrotoxicity (6). The CATC MRP2 haplotype was present in 40.9% of those with TFV tubulopathy versus only 13.7% of controls, while CGAC appeared to be a protective haplotype being observed in 20.2% of the control subjects and absent in patients with renal disease (P < 0.01) (6). Further studies confirmed that homozygosity for the C allele at position -24 of the MRP2 gene is strongly associated with TFV-associated tubulopathy. Screening for this polymorphism may help to identify patients at greater risk for developing TFV-associated tubulopathy, and suggest close monitoring of renal function in these patients (7).

Possible genetic predisposition has been suggested for didanosine (ddI) (±d4T) induced pancreatitis in HIV-infected patients. Limited data suggest that cystic fibrosis transmembrane conductance regulators (CFTR) mutations and serine protease inhibitor kazal-1 (SPINK-1) polymorphisms (both known genetic risk factors for the development of pancreatitis) may increase the susceptibility to ddI pancreatitis. Indeed, an association between CFTR and SPINK-1 mutations and higher amylase concentrations and clinical pancreatitis has been reported (8).

NRTIs-associated lipodystrophy, peripheral neuropathy, and lactic acidosis affect selected populations, suggesting that genetic factors may be involved (9). Tumor necrosis factor (TNF-α), which promotes adipocyte apoptosis, has been linked to the development of lipodystrophy in HIV-infected patients. Two studies have shown that a functional promoter polymorphism TNF-α (238G > A) has been associated with more frequent and more rapid onset of lipoatrophy in patients of ART (10, 11). These findings, however, were not confirmed in the further study evaluating the role of apoptosis and TNF polymorphisms in the development of ART-associated lipid disorders (12). In addition to TNF, major histocompatibility complex (MHC) has been linked to the development of the lipodystrophy in a recent study of Thai patients (13). The presence of HLA-B*4001 (OR 14.05; 95% CI, 2.57–76.59; P = 0.002) and a longer duration of stavudine (d4T) treatment were associated with d4T-induced lipoatrophy. HLA-B*4001 had a high specificity (95.8%) and positive predictive value (88.9%) for lipodystrophy and could potentially be considered as a screening tool for identifying the patients at risk for d4T-asscoated lipoatrophy (13). Genetic polymorphisms of genes involved in apoptosis and adipocyte metabolism have been shown to be significantly associated with ART associated lipodystrophy. Polymorphisms in apolipoproteins (APO) APOC3 and APOE have been associated with increased risk of developing lipoatrophy, and two genetic variants of adrenergic beta3 receptor (ARbeta3) were linked to fat accumulation in patients with ART (12, 14).

The inhibition of gamma polymerase by NRTIs leads to the depletion of mitochondrial DNA (mtDNA) and inhibition of the transcription of proteins encoded by mtDNA, leading to the depletion of the electronic transport system enzymes involved in oxidative phosphorylation. Underlying human variations of mtDNA have been associated with different predisposition to ART-related neuropathy. In particular, increased susceptibility to NRTIs induced peripheral neuropathy has been associated with a European mitochondrial DNA (mtDNA) haplogroup among non-Hispanic white persons (15). In further studies the same group of investigators established that African mtDNA subhaplogroup L1c was an independent predictor of peripheral neuropathy in non-Hispanic black persons (16).

Among all ART toxicity related host polymorphisms, hypersensitivity to abacavir (ABC) has become the best example of the successful application of pharmacogenomic screening into clinical practice. Hypersensitivity to ABC, observed in ~5–8% of patients, develops within 6 weeks of initiation of therapy and leads to a serious systemic reaction including rash, fever, and gastrointestinal, constitutional, and respiratory symptoms associated with high mortality (17, 18). Non-Caucasian race has been associated with a lower risk of ABC hypersensitivity, and familial predisposition has been reported (18). A series of studies has established a strong association between carriage of HLA-B*5701 and hypersensitivity to ABC (19–21). Most importantly, this association has been proven to predict the risk of ABC toxicity. The predictive positive value and negative value of the HLA-B*5701 allele were greater in Caucasians (>70% and >90%, respectively) and decreased for other populations, suggesting that screening for this allele reduces (but does not completely eliminate) the incidence of the hypersensitivity reaction and allows one to avoid overdiagnosis of this condition (22–24). In the U.S. study, however, the 100% sensitivity of HLA-B*5701 as a marker for ABC hypersensitivity has been reported both in white and black patients, suggesting similar implications of the association between HLA-B*5701 positivity and risk of ABC induced hypersensitivity in both races (25). In a large randomized, double-blind prospective study conducted in 19 countries, prospective screening for HLA-B*5701 eliminated (0% compared with 2.7% in the control group) immunologically confirmed (skin patch testing) hypersensitivity reactions to ABC and significantly (>twofold) reduced the rate of clinically suspected reactions (26). Open screening studies and successful implementation of this genetic screening into clinical practice globally have supported the usefulness of the HLA-B*5701 test in predicting ABC hypersensitivity reactions in populations of diverse racial background (23). The fact that 45% of those carrying HLA-B*5701 allele can tolerate ABC without developing hypersensitivity reaction is unclear and deserves further investigation (22). Moreover, this unique model of successful application of pharmacogenetic screening as a widely used clinical tool was shown cost-effective only in a setting where an ABC-based regimen was as effective and cheaper than an ART regimen without ABC (27).

Nonnucleoside reverse transcriptase inhibitors

First-generation NNRTIs efavirenz (EFV) and nevirapine (NVP) are extensively metabolized primarily by hepatic CYP2B6 with partial involvement of CYP3A4, and with a lesser involvement of CYP2D6, CYP2C19, and CYP2A6 (28–32). In vitro studies have shown that CYP2B6 genetic polymorphisms markedly influence the metabolism of EFV and NVP (29–31, 33). The CYP2B6*6 allele harboring two SNPs (516G > T and 785A > G) was significantly associated with a pronounced decrease in CYP2B6 expression and a low rate of 8-hydroxylation of EFV. In fact, the data from in vitro studies suggested that 8-hydroxylation of EFV is a specific marker of CYP2B6 activity and can be used as a phenotyping probe to evaluate expression of CYP2B6 in humans, and the choice of this probe has been supported by the FDA guidelines on genomic studies (30, 31).

CYP2B6 polymorphisms have been associated with altered PK of EFV and NVP in HIV-infected humans (33–37). The CYP2B6 G to T polymorphism at position 516 has been strongly associated with elevated EFV plasma concentrations and an increase in neurotoxicity (29, 38), while up to 20% of subjects with wild-type genotype have been reported to have subtherapeutic EFV concentrations (39). The CYP2B6 516G > T polymorphism has also been associated with a prolonged elimination serum half-life and an increased risk of developing drug resistance after discontinuation of an EFV-based regimen (40). Recently the CYP2B6 983T > C and CYP2A6 (CYP2A6*9B and CYP2A6*17) genotypes have also been reported to affect EFV and NVP plasma concentrations (41–44). Individuals with a poor metabolizer genotype had a likelihood ratio of 35 (95% CI, 11–110) of very high EFV plasma levels (42). CYP2B6 516G > T has been shown to significantly influence NVP and EFV plasma trough concentrations in HIV-infected patients in Africa and Asia (45–48). Non-Caucasian ethnicity and CYP2B6 polymorphism have been both associated with elevated plasma trough NVP concentrations in ethnically diverse patients (49). In Chinese patients, however, the association between CYP2B6 516G > T polymorphism was only significant for EFV, and not for NVP (50). It is also important to recognize that polymorphisms in accessory metabolic pathways, for example CYP2A6 for EFV, can lead to extremely high EFV and NVP concentrations in patients who are already CYP2B6 slow metabolizers, or can compensate for the deficiency in the main drug-metabolizing enzyme (51). Indeed, the CYP2D6*3, *4, and *6, representing the most frequent inactivating mutations in Caucasians leading to a poor metabolizer phenotype, have been shown to affect the plasma concentrations of EFV (52). The polymorphisms in CYP3A4 and CYP3A5 have been associated with a trend to higher EFV AUC (37, 52, 53).

The effect of CYP2B6 polymorphisms on the PK and clinical response of EFV and NVP has been also evaluated in HIV-infected children (54–56). CYP2B6 516G > T polymorphisms were shown to significantly change the clearance of EFV in children, but there was no significant association between CYP2B6 516G > T polymorphism and virologic and immunologic responses (55). Another study on the effects of CYP2B6 polymorphisms on the PK/PD of NVP in children suggested that the CYP2B6 516G > T polymorphism may affect the immunological response to NVP based ART through differences in NVP exposure as a result of altered metabolism of the drug (54).

CYP2B6 poor metabolizer genotypes can identify individuals at risk of high EFV and NVP plasma concentrations. High EFV plasma concentrations and successful genotype-based EFV dose reduction were further demonstrated in individuals with the haplotypes CYP2B6*6/*6 (516G > T and 785A > G) and *6/*26 (499C > G, 516G > T, and 785A > G) (57). CYP2B6 genotype-based dose reduction has been proposed in several population PK models (58, 59). Reducing the dose of EFV for patients who are already receiving, or about to start EFV, on the basis of CYP2B6 screening has been shown as a viable strategy to maintain virologic suppression and minimize risk of CNS toxicity by maintaining therapeutic EFV plasma concentrations in adults (57). In children, successful EFV dose reduction in adolescent patients with extremely high EFV exposure due to the CYP2B6 516G > T polymorphism has been described as well (60, 61). No studies on NVP dose reduction have been published to date.

Of great importance is the high prevalence of CYP2B6 polymorphisms in patients of African descent who currently represent the majority of the HIV-infected population worldwide (36, 37, 40, 41, 62–65). The 516T allelic frequency is significantly higher in Sub-Saharan Africans (45.5%) and African Americans (46.7%) as compared to Hispanic (27.3%), European (21.4%), and Asian (17.4%) populations, indicating the need for prospective clinical dose optimization studies to evaluate the utility of genotype-driven dose adjustments in diverse populations (34, 63, 66). Simulations indicate that an a priori 35% EFV dose reduction in homozygous CYP2B6*6 patients would maintain drug exposure within the therapeutic range in African patients (63). While low EFV exposure has been reported to be associated with virologic failure (67), no studies have evaluated the long-term consequences of high EFV exposure to date, and no cost analysis of EFV dose adjustment has been conducted. We believe that selective genotyping of populations with high prevalence of CYP2B6 polymorphism deserves strong consideration and future studies need to be conducted.

The relationship between drug transporter polymorphism and EFV plasma concentrations has been reported for MDR1. In the study by Fellay *et al.*, median EFV plasma concentrations differed significantly between patients with MDR1 3435TT, CT, and CC genotypes being at 30th, 50th, and 75th percentiles, respectively (52). Interestingly, the same polymorphism has also been associated with more robust immunological recovery and lesser degree of virologic failure for EFV-based ART (52). This finding, however, was not confirmed in a subsequent study (68). Equally, this and other studies questioned the role of MDR1 in EFV disposition (37, 68, 69). MDR1 3435C > T polymorphism was shown, however, to be associated with an increase in high-density lipoprotein cholesterol in patients treated with EFV-based ART (70).

NVP- and EFV-induced hypersensitivity is similar to ABC hypersensitivity as it also develops within first 6 weeks of therapy in susceptible individuals. For NVP the development of rash and significant (frequently fulminant) hepatitis, more prominent in presence of high CD4+ cell counts, is consistent with T-cell dependent immune response to NVP antigens and participation of HLA class II alleles (71, 72). HLA-DRB1*0101 has been significantly associated with NVP- and EFV-induced hypersensitivity (fever, rash, and hepatitis) (73, 74). HLA B*3505 was linked to isolated NVP rash in a Thai population with no HLA DRB1*0101 (75), highlighting the importance of differences in polymorphism distributions by race. Additional HLA alleles have also been associated with NVP-induced hepatotoxicity in Sardinian (HLA-C*w/HLA-B*14) and Japanese (HLA-Cw*8) populations (76, 77). The polymorphism multidrug resistance transporter (encoding P-glycoprotein) MDR1 C3435T, shown to predict immune recovery after initiation of NVP based-ART, has also been associated with NVP-induced hepatotoxicity (52, 78–80).

Second-generation NNRTIs etravirine (ETV) is a substrate of the CYP450 enzyme system including CYP3A4, CYP2C9, and CYP2C19 and drug transporter P-glycoprotein. Its spectrum of side effects is very close to that of the first-generation NNRTIs. While it is possible that polymorphisms in CYP enzymes and MDR1 may affect the PK and toxicity of ETV, no data have been published to date on this subject.

Protease inhibitors

Protease inhibitors (Pis) are all metabolized to a major extent by the CYP450 enzymes, mainly CYP3A4, and are not only substrates but also potent inhibitors and inducers of CYP enzymes; some are inhibitors of UGT enzymes. All PIs are substrates of P-gp drug transport and many have also been found to be transported by the organic anion transporter (OAT) family. All these factors create ground for a potentially significant association between the polymorphisms of CYP450 enzymes and drug transporters with the PK and PD of the PIs.

While multiple studies investigated the relationship between CYP3A4 and CYP3A5 polymorphisms and the PK of the PIs, the majority did not find any significant association with the plasma concentrations of PIs. The CYP3A*5 (6986A > G) polymorphisms were associated with the metabolic ratio of saquinavir (SQV) to its urinary hydroxymetabolites (81, 82), and CYP3A4 1B*/1B* genotype was associated with 25% reduced peak plasma IDV concentrations, 70% reduced overall bioavailability, and a significant correlation between both indinavir (IDV) AUC and C_{trough} and short-term change in viral load (83). The wild-type ABCB1 CGC haplotype was associated with a slower CL of another PI atazanavir (ATV) (84).

Nelfinavir (NFV) is extensively metabolized by CYP2C19 with partial involvement of CYP3A and CYP2D6. The CYP2C19*2 (681G > A) polymorphism (less frequent in Caucasian [2–3%] and African [4%] populations, and more frequent in Asians [10–25%]) has been significantly associated with higher NFV AUC and reduced risk of viral failure (37, 85). The rate of metabolism of NFV to its main metabolite M8 has been reported to be reduced by 50% in patients with *1/*2 or *2/*2 for CYP2C19 compared with those with *1/*1 genotype (86). In another study of the NFV and CYP2C19 in adults, mutation in CYP2C19 increased the systemic exposure to NFV and reduced the exposure to M8, but no significant differences were noted among heterozygous (*1/*2) and homozygous (*2/*2) mutants (87). In children, CYP2C19 681G > A has been found to be strongly associated with M8/NFV ratios ranging from 0.45 in the GG genotype to 0.02 in the AA genotype (P < 0.001), and at week 24, 46% of the GG group versus 63% of the AA group had a viral load <400 copies/mL (p = 0.01) (88). A possible trend to higher NFV plasma concentrations has also been reported in association with CYP2D6 (CYP2D6*3, *4 and *6) polymorphisms (52).

Several transporter genes have been linked to the PK and toxicity of PIs. The MRP2-24C/T polymorphisms were shown to affect the PK of IDV by increasing oral clearance of IDV by 24% (4). The P-gp MDR1 3435C > T polymorphism has been shown to affect the plasma NFV concentrations and clearance in children with the CT genotype associated with a higher 8-hour postdose concentration (p = 0.02) and lower clearance (p = 0.04) compared to patients with the CC genotype (53). Ninety-one percent of children with the CT genotype reached undetectable plasma HIV–RNA viral load by week 8 compared to 59% of children with the CC genotype (p = 0.01), suggesting the role of P-gp in the PK and virologic response to NFV. These results, however, were questioned by other studies where the intracellular accumulation of NFV correlated with P-gp function, but not with P-gp expression, and in vitro results contradicting clinical findings about the significance of MDR1 polymorphism in the disposition of NFV (89, 90). Recently, studies have reported the significance of another drug transporter from the OAT family coded by the *SLCO* genes in the exposure to lopinavir (LPV) (91, 92). The trough plasma concentrations of LPV have been reported to be significantly increased in patients with the *SLCO1B1* 521T > C polymorphism (92). Reduced uptake of LPV by hepatocytes in carriers of *SLCO1B1* 521T > C genotype has been suggested to be responsible for this effect (91). In our study of pediatric patients, we have found that *SLCO1B1* 521T > C polymorphism was significantly associated with higher LPV AUC, but was not associated with virological outcome (unpublished data). In addition to the genetic variations, CYP450 enzymes and drug transporters can be modulated by activation of the nuclear receptor Pregnane X Receptor (PXR) (93). PXR has been shown to be responsible for the activation of CYP3A4, CYP2B6, and CYP2C9 transcription as well as for the efflux transporter MDR1 (94–96). The PXR 63396C > T polymorphism has been associated with an increase in diurnal ATV clearance and overall decrease in ATV plasma concentrations (97, 98).

ATV and IDV both are capable of producing clinically significant unconjugated hyperbilirubinemia related to inhibition of UGT by these PIs. Indeed, UGT1A1*28 and UGT1A1*6 genotypes has been associated with increased levels of bilirubin in the presence of IDV or ATV through a mechanism similar to the one seen in Gilbert's syndrome (99–102). In addition to UGT1A1, other UGT enzymes (UGT1A3 and UGT1A7) were reported to be associated with IDV-induced hyperbilirubinemia (100). Besides UGT metabolic mechanism, the drug transporters involved in moving the unconjugated bilirubin inside hepatocytes have been linked to the development of IDV- and ATV-induced hyperbilirubinemia. MDR1 3435CC genotype has been associated with increased ATV plasma concentrations. MDR1 3435 CC homozygotes had a threefold higher ATV plasma trough concentration (C_{trough}) (P = 0.001) than heterozygotes or homozygote TT, and the odds of hyperbilirubinemia increased 1.3-fold for every 100 ng/mL increase in ATV C_{trough} (P = 0.03) (103). In addition to MDR1 polymorphism, ATV plasma concentrations directly correlate with bilirubin levels, the risk of severe hyperbilirubinemia was further increased in the presence of the UGT1A1-TA7 allele (103). Genetic screening before the initiation of IDV (UGT1A1) and ATV (MDR1 3435T > C and UGT1A1-TA7) therapy could potentially help identify the patients at risk of greater plasma exposures and significant hyperbilirubinemia.

The use of PI-based regimens has been associated with a high degree of hyperlipidemia and lipoatrophy. The polymorphisms in APOC3 and APOE have been reported to be associated with a higher risk of developing severe hypertriglyceridemia, while lipoatrophy was related to the APOC3 and TNF polymorphisms (12). Further studies have confirmed the association of APOC3 and APOE with plasma triglycerides and offered data on other APO genotypes associations with abnormal lipids such as APOA1, APOA5, and cholesteryl esters transfer protein (CETP) (104–106). Future studies will allow identifying which genetic profile can be useful in identifying patients at risk for developing ART associated hyperlipidemia.

Integrase inhibitors

Raltegravir (RAL) is a novel integrase strand transfer inhibitor metabolized by glucuronidation via UGT1A1. Since UGT1A1*28/*28 is known to be associated with decreased activity of UGT1A1, it is reasonable to expect that this polymorphism might have an impact on the PK of RAL. The study by Wenning *et al.* has evaluated the RAL PK in a cohort of 30 subjects with known UGT1A1*28/*28 genotype and 27 control subjects with UGT1A1*1/*1 genotype (107). RAL plasma concentrations were slightly higher in the patients with UGT1A1 polymorphism, but this increase was not clinically significant. In another study of drug–drug interaction between RAL and ATV, the UGT1A1 polymorphism was not associated with RAL metabolite formation (108).

Entry and fusion inhibitors

Enfuvirtide (ENF) is the only ARV agent administered parenterally, and is not metabolized by CYP450 enzymes. As a peptide, ENF undergoes catabolism to its constituent amino acids with subsequent recycling of the amino acids in the body pool. No genetic polymorphisms in drug-metabolizing enzymes or transporters have been studied in relationship to the PK and PD of ENF. Maraviroc (MVC) is a novel chemokine receptor (CCR5) antagonist that interferes with viral entry process inside the human cell. This drug is unique in its principle of action because its ability to treat HIV depends on the genetic factors of the human host cell. Genetic variation in the CCR5 chemokine receptor genes have been studied extensively, but they have not been shown to affect the virological response to MVC-based regimen (109). MVC is metabolized by the CYP450 enzymes, primarily by CYP3A. No data on the significance of CYP3A polymorphisms on the metabolism of MVC is available to date. The drug transporter OAT has been linked to the disposition of MVC with *SLCO1B1* 521T > C polymorphism associated with elevated plasma MVC concentrations (98).

Conclusions

The association between host genetic factors and PK and PD of ART has been proven to be significant for some ARV agents. Genetic screening for the HLA-B*5701 has significantly reduced the incidence of ABC-associated hypersensitivity. Other significant associations such as CYP2B6 polymorphisms and PK and CNS toxicity of EFV may equally find their application in prescreening for the specific drug-induced toxicity or consideration of the reduced

dose of certain ARV drugs. Possible pharmacogenetic associations between ART and ARV induced metabolic complications, and cardiovascular, oncologic, and renal diseases are being investigated in multiple clinical projects globally. Most importantly, growing evidence of differences in ARV drugs tolerability and therapeutic efficacy in ethnically and racially diverse populations of the world prompts ongoing investigations about the role of the human genome in the response and toxicity of ART.

References

1 World Health Organization (2010) *Global report: UNAIDS report on the global AIDS epidemic 2010* [WWW document]. URL http://www.who.int/hiv/pub/global_report2010/en/index.html [accessed on 19 June 2011]

2 Kwara A, Lartey M, Boamah I, Rezk NL, Oliver-Commey J, Kenu E, *et al.* (2009) Interindividual variability in pharmacokinetics of generic nucleoside reverse transcriptase inhibitors in TB/HIV-coinfected Ghanaian patients: UGT2B7*1c is associated with faster zidovudine clearance and glucuronidation. *J Clin Pharmacol*, **49**(**9**), 1079–1090.

3 Fletcher CV, Kawle SP, Kakuda TN, Anderson PL, Weller D, Bushman LR, *et al.* (2000) Zidovudine triphosphate and lamivudine triphosphate concentration-response relationships in HIV-infected persons. *AIDS*, **14**(**14**), 2137–2144.

4 Anderson PL, Lamba J, Aquilante CL, Schuetz E, Fletcher CV (2006) Pharmacogenetic characteristics of indinavir, zidovudine, and lamivudine therapy in HIV-infected adults: a pilot study. *J Acquir Immune Defic Syndr*, **42**(**4**), 441–449.

5 Kiser JJ, Carten ML, Aquilante CL, Anderson PL, Wolfe P, King TM, *et al.* (2008) The effect of lopinavir/ritonavir on the renal clearance of tenofovir in HIV-infected patients. *Clin Pharmacol Ther*, **83**(**2**), 265–272.

6 Izzedine H, Hulot JS, Villard E, Goyenvalle C, Dominguez S, Ghosn J, *et al.* (2006) Association between ABCC2 gene haplotypes and tenofovir-induced proximal tubulopathy. *J Infect Dis*, **194**(**11**), 1481–1491.

7 Rodriguez-Novoa S, Labarga P, Soriano V, Egan D, Albalater M, Morello J, *et al.* (2009) Predictors of kidney tubular dysfunction in HIV-infected patients treated with tenofovir: a pharmacogenetic study. *Clin Infect Dis*, **48**(**11**), e108–e116.

8 Felley C, Morris MA, Wonkam A, Hirschel B, Flepp M, Wolf K, *et al.* (2004) The role of CFTR and SPINK-1 mutations in pancreatic disorders in HIV-positive patients: a case-control study. *AIDS*, **18**(**11**), 1521–1527.

9 Maagaard A, Kvale D. (2009) Mitochondrial toxicity in HIV-infected patients both off and on antiretroviral treatment: a continuum or distinct underlying mechanisms? *J Antimicrob Chemother*, **64**(**5**), 901–909.

10 Nolan D, Moore C, Castley A, Sayer D, Mamotte C, John M, *et al.* (2003) Tumour necrosis factor-alpha gene -238G/A promoter polymorphism associated with a more rapid onset of lipodystrophy. *AIDS*, **17**(**1**),121–123.

11 Maher B, Alfirevic A, Vilar FJ, Wilkins EG, Park BK, Pirmohamed M. (2002) TNF-alpha promoter region gene polymorphisms in HIV-positive patients with lipodystrophy. *AIDS*, **16**(**15**), 2013–2018.

12 Tarr PE, Taffe P, Bleiber G, Furrer H, Rotger M, Martinez R, *et al.* (2005) Modeling the influence of APOC3, APOE, and TNF polymorphisms on the risk of antiretroviral therapy-associated lipid disorders. *J Infect Dis*, **191**(**9**), 1419–1426.

13 Wangsomboonsiri W, Mahasirimongkol S, Chantarangsu S, Kiertiburanakul S, Charoenyingwattana A, Komindr S, *et al.* (2010) Association between HLA-B*4001 and lipodystrophy among HIV-infected patients from Thailand who received a stavudine-containing antiretroviral regimen. *Clin Infect Dis*, **50**(**4**),597–604.

14 Zanone Poma B, Riva A, Nasi M, Cicconi P, Broggini V, Lepri AC, *et al.* (2008) Genetic polymorphisms differently influencing the emergence of atrophy and fat accumulation in HIV-related lipodystrophy. *AIDS*, **22**(**14**),1769–1778.

15 Canter JA, Haas DW, Kallianpur AR, Ritchie MD, Robbins GK, Shafer RW, *et al.* (2008) The mitochondrial pharmacogenomics of haplogroup T: MTND2* LHON4917G and antiretroviral therapy-associated peripheral neuropathy. *Pharmacogenomics J*, **8**(**1**), 71–77.

16 Canter JA, Robbins GK, Selph D, Clifford DB, Kallianpur AR, Shafer R, *et al.* (2010) African mitochondrial DNA subhaplogroups and peripheral neuropathy during antiretroviral therapy. *J Infect Dis*, **201**(**11**), 1703–1707.

17 Cutrell AG, Hernandez JE, Fleming JW, Edwards MT, Moore MA, Brothers CH, *et al.* (2004) Updated clinical risk factor analysis of suspected hypersensitivity reactions to abacavir. *Ann Pharmacother*, **38**(**12**),2171–2172.

18 Hewitt RG (2002) Abacavir hypersensitivity reaction. *Clin Infect Dis*, **34**(**8**), 1137–42.

19 Hetherington S, Hughes AR, Mosteller M, Shortino D, Baker KL, Spreen W, *et al.* (2002) Genetic variations in HLA-B region and hypersensitivity reactions to abacavir. *Lancet*, **359**(**9312**), 1121–1122.

20 Mallal S, Nolan D, Witt C, Masel G, Martin AM, Moore C, *et al.* (2002) Association between presence of HLA-B*5701, HLA-DR7, and HLA-DQ3 and hypersensitivity to HIV-1 reverse-transcriptase inhibitor abacavir. *Lancet*, **359**(**9308**), 727–732.

21 Martin AM, Nolan D, Gaudieri S, Almeida CA, Nolan R, James I, *et al.* (2004) Predisposition to abacavir hypersensitivity conferred by HLA-B*5701 and a haplotypic Hsp70-Hom variant. *Proceedings of the National Academy of Sciences of the United States of America*, **101**(**12**),4180–4185.

22 Phillips EJ, Mallal SA (2009) HLA and drug-induced toxicity. *Curr Opin Mol Ther*, **11**(**3**), 231–242.

23 Hughes AR, Mosteller M, Bansal AT, Davies K, Haneline SA, Lai EH, *et al.* (2004) Association of genetic variations in HLA-B region with hypersensitivity to abacavir in some, but not all, populations. *Pharmacogenomics*, **5**(**2**), 203–311.

24 Rauch A, Nolan D, Thurnheer C, Fux CA, Cavassini M, Chave JP, *et al.* (2008) Refining abacavir hypersensitivity diagnoses using a structured clinical assessment and genetic testing in the Swiss HIV Cohort Study. *Antivir Ther*, **13**(**8**), 1019–1028.

25 Saag M, Balu R, Phillips E, Brachman P, Martorell C, Burman W, *et al.* (2008) High sensitivity of human leukocyte antigen-b*5701 as a marker for immunologically confirmed abacavir hypersensitivity in white and black patients. *Clin Infect Dis*, **46**(**7**), 1111–1118.

26 Mallal S, Phillips E, Carosi G, Molina JM, Workman C, Tomazic J, *et al.* (2008) HLA-B*5701 screening for hypersensitivity to abacavir. *N Engl J Med*, **358**(**6**), 568–579.

27 Schackman BR, Scott CA, Walensky RP, Losina E, Freedberg KA, Sax PE. (2008) The cost-effectiveness of HLA-B*5701 genetic screening to guide initial antiretroviral therapy for HIV. *AIDS*, **22**(**15**), 2025–2033.

28 Mutlib AE, Chen H, Nemeth GA, Markwalder JA, Seitz SP, Gan LS, *et al.* (1999) Identification and characterization of efavirenz metabolites by liquid chromatography/mass spectrometry and high field NMR: species differences in the metabolism of efavirenz. *Drug Metab Dispos*, **27**(**11**), 1319–1333.

29 Desta Z, Saussele T, Ward B, Blievernicht J, Li L, Klein K, *et al.* (2007) Impact of CYP2B6 polymorphism on hepatic efavirenz metabolism in vitro. *Pharmacogenomics*, **8**(**6**), 547–458.

30 Ward BA, Gorski JC, Jones DR, Hall SD, Flockhart DA, Desta Z. (2003) The cytochrome P450 2B6 (CYP2B6) is the main catalyst of efavirenz primary and secondary metabolism: implication for HIV/AIDS therapy and utility of efavirenz as a substrate marker of CYP2B6 catalytic activity. *J Pharmacol Exp Ther*, **306**(**1**), 287–300.

31 Bumpus NN, Kent UM, Hollenberg PF (2006) Metabolism of efavirenz and 8-hydroxyefavirenz by P450 2B6 leads to inactivation by two distinct mechanisms. *J Pharmacol Exp Ther*, **318**(**1**), 345–351.

32 Wen B, Chen Y, Fitch WL(20089) Metabolic activation of nevirapine in human liver microsomes: dehydrogenation and inactivation of cytochrome P450 3A4. *Drug Metab Dispos*, **37**(**7**), 1557–1562.

33 Rotger M, Colombo S, Furrer H, Bleiber G, Buclin T, Lee BL, *et al.* (2005) Influence of CYP2B6 polymorphism on plasma and intracellular concentrations and toxicity of efavirenz and nevirapine in HIV-infected patients. *Pharmacogenet Genomics*, **15**(**1**), 1–5.

34 Lang T, Klein K, Richter T, Zibat A, Kerb R, Eichelbaum M, *et al.* (2004) Multiple novel nonsynonymous CYP2B6 gene polymorphisms in Caucasians: demonstration of phenotypic null alleles. *J Pharmacol Exp Ther*, **311**(**1**), 34–43.

35 Tsuchiya K, Gatanaga H, Tachikawa N, Teruya K, Kikuchi Y, Yoshino M, *et al.* (2004) Homozygous CYP2B6 *6 (Q172H and K262R) correlates with high plasma efavirenz concentrations in HIV-1 patients treated with standard efavirenz-containing regimens. *Biochem Biophys Res Commun*, **319**(**4**), 1322–1326.

36 Klein K, Lang T, Saussele T, Barbosa-Sicard E, Schunck WH, Eichelbaum M, *et al.* (2005) Genetic variability of CYP2B6 in populations of African and Asian origin: allele frequencies, novel functional variants, and possible implications for anti-HIV therapy with efavirenz. *Pharmacogenet Genomics*, **15**(**12**), 861–873.

37 Haas DW, Smeaton LM, Shafer RW, Robbins GK, Morse GD, Labbe L, *et al.* (2005) Pharmacogenetics of long-term responses to antiretroviral regimens containing Efavirenz and/or Nelfinavir: an Adult Aids Clinical Trials Group Study. *J Infect Dis*, **192**(**11**), 1931–1942.

38 Haas DW, Ribaudo HJ, Kim RB, Tierney C, Wilkinson GR, Gulick RM, *et al.* (2004) Pharmacogenetics of

efavirenz and central nervous system side effects: an Adult AIDS Clinical Trials Group study. *AIDS*, **18**(**18**), 2391–2400.

39 Rodriguez-Novoa S, Barreiro P, Rendon A, Jimenez-Nacher I, Gonzalez-Lahoz J, Soriano V. (2005) Influence of 516G>T polymorphisms at the gene encoding the CYP450-2B6 isoenzyme on efavirenz plasma concentrations in HIV-infected subjects. *Clin Infect Dis*, **40**(**9**), 1358–1361.

40 Ribaudo HJ, Haas DW, Tierney C, Kim RB, Wilkinson GR, Gulick RM, *et al.* (2006) Pharmacogenetics of plasma efavirenz exposure after treatment discontinuation: an Adult AIDS Clinical Trials Group Study. *Clin Infect Dis*, **42**(**3**), 401–407.

41 Wyen C, Hendra H, Vogel M, Hoffmann C, Knechten H, Brockmeyer NH, *et al.* (2008) Impact of CYP2B6 983T>C polymorphism on non-nucleoside reverse transcriptase inhibitor plasma concentrations in HIV-infected patients. *J Antimicrob Chemother*, **61**(**4**), 914–918.

42 Rotger M, Tegude H, Colombo S, Cavassini M, Furrer H, Decosterd L, *et al.* (2007) Predictive value of known and novel alleles of CYP2B6 for efavirenz plasma concentrations in HIV-infected individuals. *Clin Pharmacol Ther*, **81**(**4**), 557–566.

43 Kwara A, Lartey M, Sagoe KW, Rzek NL, Court MH. (2009) CYP2B6 (c.516G -->T) and CYP2A6 (*9B and/or *17) polymorphisms are independent predictors of efavirenz plasma concentrations in HIV-infected patients. *Br J Clin Pharmacol*, **67**(**4**), 427–436.

44 Haas DW, Gebretsadik T, Mayo G, Menon UN, Acosta EP, Shintani A, *et al.* (2009) Associations between CYP2B6 polymorphisms and pharmacokinetics after a single dose of nevirapine or efavirenz in African americans. *J Infect Dis*, **199**(**6**), 872–880.

45 Penzak SR, Kabuye G, Mugyenyi P, Mbamanya F, Natarajan V, Alfaro RM, *et al.* (2007) Cytochrome P450 2B6 (CYP2B6) G516T influences nevirapine plasma concentrations in HIV-infected patients in Uganda. *HIV Med*, **8**(**2**), 86–91.

46 Ramachandran G, Ramesh K, Hemanth Kumar AK, Jagan I, Vasantha M, Padmapriyadarsini C, *et al.* (2009) Association of high T allele frequency of CYP2B6 G516T polymorphism among ethnic south Indian HIV-infected patients with elevated plasma efavirenz and nevirapine. *J Antimicrob Chemother*, **63**(**4**), 841–843.

47 Uttayamakul S, Likanonsakul S, Manosuthi W, Wichukchinda N, Kalambaheti T, Nakayama EE,

et al. (2010) Effects of CYP2B6 G516T polymorphisms on plasma efavirenz and nevirapine levels when co-administered with rifampicin in HIV/TB co-infected Thai adults. *AIDS Res Ther*, **7**, 8.

48 Chou M, Bertrand J, Segeral O, Verstuyft C, Borand L, Comets E, *et al.* (2010) Population pharmacokinetic-pharmacogenetic study of nevirapine in HIV-infected Cambodian patients. *Antimicrob Agents Chemother*, **54**(**10**), 4432–4439.

49 Mahungu T, Smith C, Turner F, Egan D, Youle M, Johnson M, *et al.* (2009) Cytochrome P450 2B6 516G-->T is associated with plasma concentrations of nevirapine at both 200 mg twice daily and 400 mg once daily in an ethnically diverse population. *HIV Med*, **10**(**5**), 310–317.

50 Chen J, Sun J, Ma Q, Yao Y, Wang Z, Zhang L, *et al.* (2010) CYP2B6 polymorphism and nonnucleoside reverse transcriptase inhibitor plasma concentrations in Chinese HIV-infected patients. *Ther Drug Monit*, **32**(**5**),573–578.

51 di Iulio J, Fayet A, Arab-Alameddine M, Rotger M, Lubomirov R, Cavassini M, *et al.* (2009) In vivo analysis of efavirenz metabolism in individuals with impaired CYP2A6 function. *Pharmacogenet Genomics*, **19**(**4**), 300–309.

52 Fellay J, Marzolini C, Meaden ER, Back DJ, Buclin T, Chave JP, *et al.* (2002) Response to antiretroviral treatment in HIV-1-infected individuals with allelic variants of the multidrug resistance transporter 1: a pharmacogenetics study. *Lancet*, **359**(**9300**), 30–36.

53 Saitoh A, Singh KK, Powell CA, Fenton T, Fletcher CV, Brundage R, *et al.* (2005) An MDR1-3435 variant is associated with higher plasma nelfinavir levels and more rapid virologic response in HIV-1 infected children. *AIDS*, **19**(**4**), 371–380.

54 Saitoh A, Sarles E, Capparelli E, Aweeka F, Kovacs A, Burchett SK, *et al.* (2007) CYP2B6 genetic variants are associated with nevirapine pharmacokinetics and clinical response in HIV-1-infected children. *AIDS*, **21**(**16**), 2191–2199.

55 Saitoh A, Fletcher CV, Brundage R, Alvero C, Fenton T, Hsia K, *et al.* (2007) Efavirenz pharmacokinetics in HIV-1-infected children are associated with CYP2B6-G516T polymorphism. *J Acquir Immune Defic Syndr*, **45**(**3**),280–285.

56 ter Heine R, Scherpbier HJ, Crommentuyn KM, Bekker V, Beijnen JH, Kuijpers TW, *et al.* (2008) A pharmacokinetic and pharmacogenetic study of efavirenz in children: dosing guidelines can result in subtherapeutic concentrations. *Antivir Ther*, **13**(**6**), 779–787.

57 Gatanaga H, Hayashida T, Tsuchiya K, Yoshino M, Kuwahara T, Tsukada H, *et al.* (2007) Successful efavirenz dose reduction in HIV type 1-infected individuals with cytochrome P450 2B6 *6 and *26. *Clin Infect Dis*, **45**(**9**), 1230–1237.

58 Cabrera SE, Santos D, Valverde MP, Dominguez-Gil A, Gonzalez F, Luna G, *et al.* (2009) Influence of the cytochrome P450 2B6 genotype on population pharmacokinetics of efavirenz in human immunodeficiency virus patients. *Antimicrob Agents Chemother*, **53**(**7**), 2791–2798.

59 Arab-Alameddine M, Di Iulio J, Buclin T, Rotger M, Lubomirov R, Cavassini M, *et al.* (2009) Pharmacogenetics-based population pharmacokinetic analysis of efavirenz in HIV-1-infected individuals. *Clin Pharmacol Ther*, **85**(**5**), 485–494.

60 Rakhmanina NY, van den Anker JN, Soldin SJ, van Schaik RH, Mordwinkin N, Neely MN (2010) Can therapeutic drug monitoring improve pharmacotherapy of HIV infection in adolescents? *Ther Drug Monit*, **32**(**3**), 273–281.

61 Neely M, Jelliffe R (2008) Practical therapeutic drug management in HIV-infected patients: use of population pharmacokinetic models supplemented by individualized Bayesian dose optimization. *J Clin Pharmacol*, **48**(**9**), 1081–1091.

62 Wang J, Sonnerborg A, Rane A, Josephson F, Lundgren S, Stahle L, *et al.* (2006) Identification of a novel specific CYP2B6 allele in Africans causing impaired metabolism of the HIV drug efavirenz. *Pharmacogenet Genomics*, **16**(**3**), 191–198.

63 Nyakutira C, Roshammar D, Chigutsa E, Chonzi P, Ashton M, Nhachi C, *et al.* (2008) High prevalence of the CYP2B6 516G-->T(*6) variant and effect on the population pharmacokinetics of efavirenz in HIV/AIDS outpatients in Zimbabwe. *Eur J Clin Pharmacol*, **64**(**4**), 357–365.

64 Gross R, Aplenc R, Tenhave T, Foulkes AS, Thakur R, Mosepele M, *et al.* (2008) Slow efavirenz metabolism genotype is common in Botswana. *J Acquir Immune Defic Syndr*, **49**(**3**), 336–337.

65 Leger P, Dillingham R, Beauharnais CA, Kashuba AD, Rezk NL, Fitzgerald DW, *et al.* (2009) CYP2B6 Variants and Plasma Efavirenz Concentrations during Antiretroviral Therapy in Port-au-Prince, *Haiti. J Infect Dis*, **200**(**6**), 955–964.

66 Mehlotra RK, Ziats MN, Bockarie MJ, Zimmerman PA. (2006) Prevalence of CYP2B6 alleles in malaria-endemic populations of West Africa and Papua New Guinea. *Eur J Clin Pharmacol*, **62**(**4**), 267–275.

67 Marzolini C, Telenti A, Decosterd LA, Greub G, Biollaz J, Buclin T. (2001) Efavirenz plasma levels can predict treatment failure and central nervous system side effects in HIV-1-infected patients. *AIDS*, **15**(**1**), 71–75.

68 Winzer R, Langmann P, Zilly M, Tollmann F, Schubert J, Klinker H, *et al.* (2003) No influence of the P-glycoprotein genotype (MDR1 C3435T) on plasma levels of lopinavir and efavirenz during antiretroviral treatment. *Eur J Med Res*, **8**(**12**), 531–534.

69 Motsinger AA, Ritchie MD, Shafer RW, Robbins GK, Morse GD, Labbe L, *et al.* (2006) Multilocus genetic interactions and response to efavirenz-containing regimens: an adult AIDS clinical trials group study. *Pharmacogenet Genomics*, **16**(**11**), 837–845.

70 Alonso-Villaverde C, Coll B, Gomez F, Parra S, Camps J, Joven J, *et al.* (2005) The efavirenz-induced increase in HDL-cholesterol is influenced by the multidrug resistance gene 1 C3435T polymorphism. *AIDS*, **19**(**3**),341–342.

71 Patel SM, Johnson S, Belknap SM, Chan J, Sha BE, Bennett C. (2004) Serious adverse cutaneous and hepatic toxicities associated with nevirapine use by non-HIV-infected individuals. *J Acquir Immune Defic Syndr*, **35**(**2**), 120–125.

72 Stern JO, Robinson PA, Love J, Lanes S, Imperiale MS, Mayers DL. (2003) A comprehensive hepatic safety analysis of nevirapine in different populations of HIV infected patients. *J Acquir Immune Defic Syndr*, **34**(**Suppl.1**), S21–S33.

73 Vitezica ZG, Milpied B, Lonjou C, Borot N, Ledger TN, Lefebvre A, *et al.* (2008) HLA-DRB1*01 associated with cutaneous hypersensitivity induced by nevirapine and efavirenz. *AIDS*, **22**(**4**), 540–541.

74 Martin AM, Nolan D, James I, Cameron P, Keller J, Moore C, *et al.* (2005) Predisposition to nevirapine hypersensitivity associated with HLA-DRB1*0101 and abrogated by low CD4 T-cell counts. *AIDS*, **19**(**1**),97–99.

75 Chantarangsu S, Mushiroda T, Mahasirimongkol S, Kiertiburanakul S, Sungkanuparph S, Manosuthi W, *et al.* (2009) HLA-B*3505 allele is a strong predictor for nevirapine-induced skin adverse drug reactions in HIV-infected Thai patients. *Pharmacogenet Genomics*, **19**(**2**), 139–146.

76 Littera R, Carcassi C, Masala A, Piano P, Serra P, Ortu F, *et al.* (2006) HLA-dependent hypersensitivity to nevirapine in Sardinian HIV patients. *AIDS*, **20**(**12**), 1621–1626.

77 Gatanaga H, Yazaki H, Tanuma J, Honda M, Genka I, Teruya K, *et al.* (2007) HLA-Cw8 primarily associated with hypersensitivity to nevirapine. *AIDS*, **21**(**2**), 264–265.

78 Ciccacci C, Borgiani P, Ceffa S, Sirianni E, Marazzi MC, Altan AM, *et al.* (2010) Nevirapine-induced hepatotoxicity and pharmacogenetics: a retrospective study in a population from Mozambique. *Pharmacogenomics*, **11**(**1**), 23–31.

79 Haas DW, Bartlett JA, Andersen JW, Sanne I, Wilkinson GR, Hinkle J, *et al.* (2006) Pharmacogenetics of nevirapine-associated hepatotoxicity: an Adult AIDS Clinical Trials Group collaboration. *Clin Infect Dis*, **43**(**6**),783–786.

80 Ritchie MD, Haas DW, Motsinger AA, Donahue JP, Erdem H, Raffanti S, *et al.* (2006) Drug transporter and metabolizing enzyme gene variants and nonnucleoside reverse-transcriptase inhibitor hepatotoxicity. *Clin Infect Dis*, **43**(**6**), 779–782.

81 Frohlich M, Hoffmann MM, Burhenne J, Mikus G, Weiss J, Haefeli WE (2004) Association of the CYP3A5 A6986G (CYP3A5*3) polymorphism with saquinavir pharmacokinetics. *Br J Clin Pharmacol*, **58**(**4**), 443–444.

82 Mouly SJ, Matheny C, Paine MF, Smith G, Lamba J, Lamba V, *et al.* (2005) Variation in oral clearance of saquinavir is predicted by CYP3A5*1 genotype but not by enterocyte content of cytochrome P450 3A5. *Clin Pharmacol Ther*, **78**(**6**), 605–618.

83 Bertrand J, Treluyer JM, Panhard X, Tran A, Auleley S, Rey E, *et al.* (2009) Influence of pharmacogenetics on indinavir disposition and short-term response in HIV patients initiating HAART. *Eur J Clin Pharmacol*, **65**(**7**), 667–678.

84 Anderson PL, Aquilante CL, Gardner EM, Predhomme J, McDaneld P, Bushman LR, *et al.* (2009) Atazanavir pharmacokinetics in genetically determined CYP3A5 expressors versus non-expressors. *J Antimicrob Chemother*, **64**(**5**), 1071–1079.

85 Wedlund PJ (2000) The CYP2C19 enzyme polymorphism. *Pharmacology*, **61**(**3**), 174–183.

86 Hirt D, Mentre F, Tran A, Rey E, Auleley S, Salmon D, *et al.* (2008) Effect of CYP2C19 polymorphism on nelfinavir to M8 biotransformation in HIV patients. *Br J Clin Pharmacol*, **65**(**4**), 548–557.

87 Damle BD, Uderman H, Biswas P, Crownover P, Lin C, Glue P (2009) Influence of CYP2C19 polymorphism on the pharmacokinetics of nelfinavir and its active metabolite. *Br J Clin Pharmacol*, **68**(5), 682–689.

88 Saitoh A, Capparelli E, Aweeka F, Sarles E, Singh KK, Kovacs A, *et al.* (2010) CYP2C19 genetic variants affect nelfinavir pharmacokinetics and virologic response in HIV-1-infected children receiving highly active antiretroviral therapy. *J Acquir Immune Defic Syndr*, **54**(3), 285–289.

89 Hennessy M, Clarke S, Spiers JP, Kelleher D, Mulcahy F, Hoggard P, *et al.* (2004) Intracellular accumulation of nelfinavir and its relationship to P-glycoprotein expression and function in HIV-infected patients. *Antivir Ther*, **9**(1), 115–122.

90 Zhu D, Taguchi-Nakamura H, Goto M, Odawara T, Nakamura T, Yamada H, *et al.* (2004) Influence of single-nucleotide polymorphisms in the multidrug resistance-1 gene on the cellular export of nelfinavir and its clinical implication for highly active antiretroviral therapy. *Antivir Ther*, **9**(6), 929–935.

91 Hartkoorn RC, Kwan WS, Shallcross V, Chaikan A, Liptrott N, Egan D, *et al.* (2009) HIV protease inhibitors are substrates for OATP1A2, OATP1B1 and OATP1B3 and lopinavir plasma concentrations are influenced by SLCO1B1 polymorphisms. *Pharmacogenet Genomics*, **20**(2),112–120.

92 Kohlrausch FB, de Cassia Estrela R, Barroso PF, Suarez-Kurtz G (2010) The impact of SLCO1B1 polymorphisms on the plasma concentration of lopinavir and ritonavir in HIV-infected men. *Br J Clin Pharmacol*, **69**(1), 95–98.

93 Handschin C, Meyer UA (2003) Induction of drug metabolism: the role of nuclear receptors. *Pharmacol Rev*, **55**(4), 649–673.

94 Chen Y, Ferguson SS, Negishi M, Goldstein JA (2004) Induction of human CYP2C9 by rifampicin, hyperforin, and phenobarbital is mediated by the pregnane X receptor. *J Pharmacol Exp Ther*, **308**(2), 495–501.

95 Goodwin B, Hodgson E, Liddle C (1999) The orphan human pregnane X receptor mediates the transcriptional activation of CYP3A4 by rifampicin through a distal enhancer module. *Mol Pharmacol*, **56**(6), 1329–1339.

96 Geick A, Eichelbaum M, Burk O (2001) Nuclear receptor response elements mediate induction of intestinal MDR1 by rifampin. *J Biol Chem*, **276**(18), 14581–14587.

97 Schipani A, Siccardi M, D'Avolio A, Baietto L, Simiele M, Bonora S, *et al.* (2008) Population pharmacokinetic modeling of the association between 63396C->T pregnane X receptor polymorphism and unboosted atazanavir clearance. *Antimicrob Agents Chemother*, **54**(12), 5242–5250.

98 Siccardi M, D'Avolio A, Nozza S, Simiele M, Baietto L, Stefani FR, *et al.* (2010) Maraviroc is a substrate for OATP1B1 in vitro and maraviroc plasma concentrations are influenced by SLCO1B1 521 T>C polymorphism. *Pharmacogenet Genomics*, **20**(12), 759–765.

99 Rotger M, Taffe P, Bleiber G, Gunthard HF, Furrer H, Vernazza P, *et al.* (2005) Gilbert syndrome and the development of antiretroviral therapy-associated hyperbilirubinemia. *J Infect Dis*, **192**(8), 1381–1386.

100 Lankisch TO, Behrens G, Ehmer U, Mobius U, Rockstroh J, Wehmeier M, *et al.* (2009) Gilbert's syndrome and hyperbilirubinemia in protease inhibitor therapy: an extended haplotype of genetic variants increases risk in indinavir treatment. *J Hepatol*, **50**(5),1010–1018.

101 Choe PG, Park WB, Song JS, Kim NH, Song KH, Park SW, *et al.* (2010) Incidence of atazanavir-associated hyperbilirubinemia in Korean HIV patients: 30 months follow-up results in a population with low UDP-glucuronosyltransferase1A1*28 allele frequency. *J Korean Med Sci*, **25**(10), 1427–1430.

102 Boyd MA, Srasuebkul P, Ruxrungtham K, Mackenzie PI, Uchaipichat V, Stek M, Jr., *et al.* (2006) Relationship between hyperbilirubinaemia and UDP-glucuronosyltransferase 1A1 (UGT1A1) polymorphism in adult HIV-infected Thai patients treated with indinavir. *Pharmacogenet Genomics*, **16**(5), 321–329.

103 Rodriguez-Novoa S, Martin-Carbonero L, Barreiro P, Gonzalez-Pardo G, Jimenez-Nacher I, Gonzalez-Lahoz J, *et al.* (2007) Genetic factors influencing atazanavir plasma concentrations and the risk of severe hyperbilirubinemia. *AIDS*, **21**(1), 41–46.

104 Foulkes AS, Wohl DA, Frank I, Puleo E, Restine S, Wolfe ML, *et al.* (2006) Associations among race/ethnicity, ApoC-III genotypes, and lipids in HIV-1-infected individuals on antiretroviral therapy. *PLoS Med*, **3**(3), e52.

105 Guardiola M, Ferre R, Salazar J, Alonso-Villaverde C, Coll B, Parra S, *et al.* (2006) Protease inhibitor-associated dyslipidemia in HIV-infected patients is strongly influenced by the APOA5-1131T->C gene variation. *Clin Chem*, **52**(10), 1914–1919.

106 Arnedo M, Taffe P, Sahli R, Furrer H, Hirschel B, Elzi L, *et al.* (2007) Contribution of 20 single nucleotide polymorphisms of 13 genes to dyslipidemia associated with antiretroviral therapy. *Pharmacogenet Genomics*, **17**(**9**), 755–764.

107 Wenning LA, Petry AS, Kost JT, Jin B, Breidinger SA, DeLepeleire I, *et al.* (2009) Pharmacokinetics of raltegravir in individuals with UGT1A1 polymorphisms. *Clin Pharmacol Ther*, **85**(**6**), 623–627.

108 Neely M, Decosterd L, Fayet A, Lee JS, Margol A, Kanani M, *et al.* (2010) Pharmacokinetics and pharmacogenomics of once-daily raltegravir and atazanavir in healthy volunteers. *Antimicrob Agents Chemother*, **54**(**11**), 4619–4625.

109 Tozzi V (2010) Pharmacogenetics of antiretrovirals. *Antiviral Res*, **85**(**1**), 190–200.

CHAPTER 9

Pharmacogenetics of Psychoactive Drugs

Jorge L. Sepulveda, MD, PhD
Philadelphia VA Medical Center and University of Pennsylvania

Introduction

The human brain is the most complex biological system known, with an estimated 100 billion (10^{11}) neurons connected by 10^{14} (adult) to 10^{15} (young child) synapses. Further complexity is achieved by the use of more than 100 different neurotransmitters, many of which interact with several different receptors with multiple anatomic locations and signaling pathways. In contrast with this complexity, a relatively small number of targets have been explored for therapy of mental illness, most commonly involving the serotonin-, dopamine-, norepinephrine-, or gamma-aminobutyric acid (GABA)-dependent pathways. While remarkable effectiveness has been achieved in several conditions, such as in schizophrenia or major depression, allowing a large number of affected individuals to lead nearly normal lives, there is wide variability in the effectiveness and tolerability of most psychotropic drugs. Given the complexity of brain biochemistry and signaling pathways, it is not surprising that broad-spectrum pharmacological interventions (e.g., generalized inhibition of serotonin reuptake at the synapses) are not universally effective and often have undesirable effects. Newer generation psychotropic drugs tend to have narrower targets and more specific actions, with fewer side effects. As an example, newer antidepressants targeting serotonin uptake lack the anticholinergic effects mediated by inhibition of muscarinic acetylcholine receptors in brain and intestine by older tricyclic antidepressants. However, even for newer drugs,

predictability of therapeutic effectiveness and tolerability remains difficult. It is likely that reliable, personalized pharmacotherapy of mental disease will require understanding of all the important pathways involved in disease causation and modification, therapeutic and off-target drug effects (pharmacodynamics), and drug pharmacokinetics (absorption, distribution, metabolism, and elimination, or ADME).

The discipline of pharmacogenomics is focused on understanding how genetic variation affects pharmacotherapy, while pharmacogenetics (PGx) can be more narrowly defined as the study of variation in specific genes in relation to their effect on drugs. In the case of psychotropic drugs, the number of pharmacogenetic studies has been exponentially growing, even though it is certain that given the complexity of brain biochemistry, pathology, and pharmacology, current knowledge is only beginning to evolve and no definite recommendations for the use of PGx testing to guide therapy can currently be made. This chapter focuses on some examples on the effect of genetic variation on the pharmacodynamics (PD) and pharmacokinetics (PK) of psychotropic drugs.

Genetic versus environmental factors in mental health

Mental illness is undoubtedly influenced by many environmental factors, including parenting, socioeconomic stressors, social networks, infections,

Pharmacogenomics in Clinical Therapeutics, First Edition. Edited by Loralie J. Langman and Amitava Dasgupta.
© 2012 John Wiley & Sons, Ltd. Published 2012 by John Wiley & Sons, Ltd.

climate, nutrition, and so on. An interaction between genetic and environmental factors has been observed in several mental disorders, including schizophrenia (1), major depression (2), bipolar disease (3), panic disorder (4), and attention-deficit/hyperactivity disorder (ADHD) (5). A meta-analysis of twin studies concluded that the genetic suscepti-bility for schizophrenia averaged 81% (95% confidence interval of 73–90%), while environmental factors accounted for about 11% of the risk (1). In the case of major depression, heritability accounted for 37% (CI = 31–42%) of liability, while individual-specific environmental factors accounted for 63% of the risk (2). The role of environmental factors compared to genetic predisposition is higher for less severe behavioral illnesses, including personality (6), anxiety (7), and addictive (8) disorders.

Compared to the complexity of genetic and environmental factors affecting causation and development of the mental illness, genetic predis-position plays a significant role in drug metabo-lism. For example, twin studies of antipyrine disposition demonstrated that 70–88% of the var-iability in the drug half-life is genetically deter-mined (9). The discovery and cloning of the genes responsible for AMDE mechanisms, in particular the cytochrome P450 enzymes, have elucidated many of the genetic and biochemical bases for hereditability of drug disposition. With the com-pletion of the Human Genome Project and the development of genome-wide association studies (GWAS), together with progress in affordable full genome sequencing platforms and bioinformatics, the knowledge in pharmacogenomics is exponen-tially expanding, and it is expected that in the future the genetic basis for drug action will be comprehensively understood and used routinely for truly personalized prescribing.

Antidepressant and antipsychotic drugs

Depression affects about 17.6 million Americans annually and can cause major disability, including death. Depression is estimated to be the leading cause of disability in the developed world, costing an estimated $83 billion in direct and indirect costs in 2000 in the United States (10). Suicide frequently associated with depressive disorders now ranks eighth as a cause of death, and may be a conse-quence of antidepressant treatment in children. Pharmacotherapy can make a significant positive impact in the prognosis of patients with major depression by improving their quality of life. How-ever, only a relatively small number of patients with depression receive appropriate treatment, including antidepressants (11). Various antidepressant drugs are listed in Table 9.1.

The costs of antidepressant therapy are signifi-cant. According to the IMS National Prescription Audit (www.imshealth.com), in 2008, 164 million prescriptions in the United States were for newer antidepressants (SSRIs and SNRIs), ranking third among all drug classes below lipid regulators and codeine analgesics, and were responsible for US$9.6 billion in sales. A major problem with antidepressant therapy is that approximately 40–50% of patients do not respond to therapy and only about two thirds eventually achieve remis-sion after long-term therapy. Moreover, the improvement usually is not seen for 2–6 weeks, and patients often undergo several cycles of drug and dose change trials. Discontinuation rates approach 15% even with the newer SSRIs, due to intolerable side effects (12). Therefore, it is critical to understand the mechanistic pathways of drug action, as well as the individual factors, including pharmacogenetic variation, that affect antidepressant response in a particular patient.

Neuroleptics, or antipsychotic drugs, are pre-scribed to patients with schizophrenia and other schizophrenia-related disorders. Schizophrenia is a chronic, debilitating mental illness characterized by deficits in cognition, perception, and emotivity, affecting about 1.1% of the U.S. adult population. The development of antipsychotic treatment in the mid-1950s is considered the single greatest advance-ment in psychiatry as it transformed the natural history of schizophrenia and allowed patients to live relatively normal lives. According to the IMS National Prescription Audit (www.imshealth.com),

Table 9.1 Antidepressants

Drug Class	Individual Drug
Monoamine Oxidase (MAO) Inhibitors	
Nonselective MAO-A/MAO-B Inhibitors	
Hydrazine	Phenelzine
Nonhydrazine	Isocarboxazid, Tranylcypromine
Selective MAO-A inhibitors	Moclobemide
Selective MAO-B inhibitors (dopamine)	Selegiline
Tricyclic Antidepressants (TCAs)	
Tertiary amines	Amitriptyline, Clomipramine Doxepin, Imipramine, Trimipramine
Secondary amines	Desipramine, Nortriptyline, Protriptyline
Serotonin and catecholamine inhibitors	
Selective serotonin reuptake inhibitors (SSRIs)	Citalopram, Escitalopram, Fluoxetine, Fluvoxamine, Paroxetine, *Dapoxetine*, Sertraline, Vilazodone
Serotonin-norepinephrine reuptake inhibitors (SNRIs)	Desvenlafaxine, Duloxetine, *Milnacipran*, Venlafaxine
Selective serotonin reuptake enhancers	*Tianeptine*
Serotonin antagonist and reuptake inhibitors	Nefazodone, Trazodone
Noradrenergic and specific serotoninergic	
Tetracyclic Antidepressants	Mianserin, Mirtazapine
Norepinephrine reuptake inhibitors (NRIs)	Maprotiline, *Reboxetine*, Viloxazine
Norepinephrine-dopamine disinhibitors	*Agomelatine*
Norepinephrine-dopamine reuptake inhibitors	Bupropion

Note: Drugs in *italic* are currently unavailable in the United States.

antipsychotics accounted for US$14.6 billion in sales in 2008, topping the rank of all therapeutic drug classes, and accounted for 32 million prescriptions in the United States to about 4 million Americans. A significant number of neuroleptics are currently prescribed to children.

Neuroleptics include the first-generation antipsychotics (FGAs), also known as *typical antipsychotics*, of which the phenotiazines and butyrophenones are still commonly used, and the atypical or second-generation antipsychotics (SGAs), which continue to grow and include a large number of drugs (Table 9.2). The development of SGAs aimed at improved effectiveness and decreased adverse drug reactions (ADRs), in particular the development of extrapyramidal side effects, including akathisia, dystonias, tardive dyskinesia, and overt parkinsonism, which is 10 times more frequent in FGAs than in SGAs, is possibly due to the wider therapeutic window and less reliance on antidopaminergic activity of SGAs. Other undesirable antidopaminergic effects of FGAs include hypotension, QT prolongation, and increased hypothalamic prolactin release. On the other hand, SGAs have higher rates (up to 40%) of metabolic disturbance leading to insulin resistance, metabolic syndrome, hyperlipemia, obesity, and diabetes.

A large National Institutes of Health (NIH)-funded trial (Clinical Antipsychotic Trials of Intervention Effectiveness, or CATIE) compared FGA perphenazine with the new SGAs and concluded that perphenazine was no less effective and more cost-effective for some patients. Moreover, there were no significant differences in the rates of ADRs (including extrapyramidal effects) and discontinuation between perphenazine and SGAs, suggesting that the choice between FGAs and SGAs should be a matter of careful evaluation of patient characteristics. Other trials have similar concluded that SGAs are not generally more effective than FGAs, although

Table 9.2 Neuroleptics

Drug Class	Individual Drug
First Generation (Typical)	
Butyrophenones	Haloperidol, Droperidol, Benperidol, Triperidol
Phenothiazines	Chlorpromazine, Fluphenazine, Perphenazine, Prochlorperazine, Thioridazine (Mellaril, Trifluoperazine, Mesoridazine, *Periciazine*, *Promazine*, Triflupromazine, Methotrimeprazine, Promethazine, Pimozide
Thioxanthenes	Chlorprothixene, Clopenthixol, Flupentixol, Thiothixene, Zuclopenthixol
Dibenzoxazeplnes	Loxapine
Second Generation (Atypical)	Aripiprazole, *Amisulpride*, Asenapine, *Blonanserin*, *Clotiapine*, Clozapine, Iloperidone, Lurasidone, *Mosapramine*, Olanzapine, Paliperidone, *Perospirone*, Quetiapine, *Remoxipride*, Risperidone, *Sertindole*, *Sulpiride*, Ziprasidone (Geodon), *Zotepine*

Note: Drugs in *italic* are currently unavailable in the United States.

these conclusions have been criticized, especially because of methodological weaknesses in the published studies (13). In any case, pharmacogenetics may play an important role in selecting patients for more cost-effective FGA therapy.

Application of pharmacogenomics in treating patients with mental illness

Factors contributing to difficulties in prescribing psychotropic drugs include the following:

1 Unpredictable efficacy: for example, the STAR*D trial of citalopram for major depression demonstrated that only about one third of patients achieved remission in one year, and more than 90% of these patients continued to experience selected residual depressive symptoms, associated with a higher probability of relapse (14).

2 Time lag to assess efficacy: many psychotropic drugs require several weeks of treatment to achieve full therapeutic effect. For example, the American Psychiatric Association 2010 practice guidelines for major depressive disorder state that while improvement can be observed as early as the first 1–2 weeks, full benefit at a given dose may not be achieved in less than 4–8 weeks and may continue for up to 12 weeks (15). Similarly, patients with schizophrenia may take 3 to 4 months to achieve full remission, and

lack of therapeutic efficacy is the major cause for antipsychotic drug discontinuation (16).

3 Adverse drug reactions: ADRs are a major cause of morbidity, mortality, and excessive health care costs. With psychotropic drugs, ADRs are often a reason for discontinuation (16), and therefore may affect response rates. The most severe side effects include suicide ideation in antidepressants, agranulocytosis, extrapyramidal syndromes, and the neuroleptic malignant syndrome. Interestingly, about 60% of all ADRs are associated with drugs that are metabolized by enzymes with genetic variability, in contrast with 7–22% of randomly selected drugs (17).

4 Lack of objective, reliable clinical assessment tools and biomarkers of drug action: because clinical assessment is variable and subjective, extensive research efforts are placed into finding precisely defined measurable psychological, physiological, or biochemical traits that correlate with clinical endpoints, sometimes called *intermediate phenotypes* or *endophenotypes* (18). Examples include serotonin in platelets (19), position emission tomography (PET) scans to measure brain serotonin and dopamine receptor distribution, and functional magnetic resonance tools to correlate brain activity and serotoninergic drug activity (20). However, none of these tools is ready for use in routine clinical practice.

5 Lack of good correlation between drug dosage, drug and metabolite plasma and brain levels, and efficacy for several psychotropic drugs, notably the antidepressants. This may relate to nonlinear pharmacokinetics of several psychotropic drugs, as well as the complexity of intermediate factors affecting the efficacy of treatment. A nonlinear relationship between drug dosage and drug levels is common in drugs that inhibit their own metabolism, such as paroxetine and fluoxetine inhibiting CYP2D6; drugs that stimulate their own elimination, such as carbamazepine; and saturation of protein binding or of ADME pathways. Similarly, receptor desensitization and tolerance can cause nonlinearity of dose:effect ratios.

6 Trial-and-error approach to dosing: for both antidepressants and antipsychotics it is recommended to start with lower doses and progressively increase if full effectiveness is not achieved, and patients often undergo several cycles of trial and error before a therapeutic benefit is achieved.

Pharmacogenetics offers the promise of addressing many of these issues by determining the role of genetic variation in causing variability in drug response. However, clinicians are reluctant to use PGx in their routine practice. In part, their lack of use of PGx relates to the absence of clear clinical guidelines for PGx-guided prescription and with several problems plaguing current knowledge in psychiatric PGx, including:

1 Complexity and heterogeneity of psychiatric disorders.

2 Inconsistency in psychiatric diagnostic classifications, especially in early stages.

3 Inconsistency in the definitions of treatment responses and use of nonquantitative (e.g., responder vs. nonresponder) outcomes that miss quantitative differences attributable to PGx genotypes.

4 Population selection and ethnic biases may result in the correlation of certain genetic polymorphisms with a phenotype, which derive from the different prevalence of the polymorphism in each population. Examples are the CYP450 enzymes such as CYP2D6 and CYP2C19, which show markedly different prevalence of poor metabolizer and ultra-metabolizer genotypes in different ethnic groups.

5 Small sample size causes poor statistical confidence, especially when a large number of genotypes or hypotheses are being tested, resulting in numerous false positive findings; on the other hand, heterogeneity of the phenotype classification can result in false negatives. Small population size often derives from the difficulty in acquiring uniform populations with defined diagnoses undergoing monotherapy.

6 Another problem of small studies is that rare genotypes are not included.

7 Interpretation of complex data, especially with large-scale or genome-wide association studies, requires sophisticated bioinformatics approaches including novel statistical approaches and neural networks.

8 Except for common polymorphisms in widely studied genes, such as CYP2D6 and the SLC2A6 serotonin transporter, genetic variants often are poorly characterized in terms of functional significance; without this knowledge, it is difficult to interpret the significant of a positive association. Positive correlation with a phenotype can be due to a functional effect on gene activity, can be highlighted by linkage disequilibrium with a functional polymorphism, or simply can be a statistical false positive. Without substantial replicability and mechanistic studies, it is difficult to distinguish between these possibilities. Unfortunately, most published PGx studies show poor replicability.

9 Inclusion of different alleles in one group without consideration for allele dominance and allelic interactions may obscure positive correlations.

10 Healthy volunteers and low drug doses do not reproduce naturalistic conditions, with patients often taking higher doses for prolonged periods.

11 Lack of a placebo control population to account for interaction between genetics and the placebo response; this is most notable in studies of antidepressant effects, which are indistinguishable from placebo in cases of mild depression (21).

12 Incomplete accounting of environmental factors, including diet, beverages, smoking, drug abuse, herb supplements, socioeconomic, parent involvement, and so on.

13 Publication bias of positive findings.

14 Lack of control for compliance and incomplete accounting of pharmacokinetics, including measurement of all relevant metabolites.

15 Methodological issues: failure to account for all relevant alleles, such as inversions, translocations, deletions and duplications (copy number variations), as well as epigenetic changes that may be of relevance to drug action and tolerance.

16 No adjustment for interaction between genes. Analysis of marker combinations appears more powerful than single-gene studies.

For all of these reasons, PGx-guided prescription of psychotropic drugs has not yet garnered wide acceptance. On the other hand enough, PGx information is available in selected areas to contribute to the variety of considerations used to prescribe psychotropic drugs, and the use of currently available PGx information may be better than ignoring it completely. Often physicians use pharmacokinetic or biological information on drug disposition (e.g., the effects of liver or renal failure) to make dose adjustments, even though for many drugs there are no outcome studies showing the reliability of this approach. The point is that PGx information showing significant effects of polymorphisms on drug ADME should be used as another piece of information, in addition to age, sex, body mass, liver and renal function, history and risk of ADRs, and other patient-specific clinical parameters, to achieve optimal individualized drug prescription. These factors include the following:

1 Disease variables: precise diagnosis, disease onset, duration, presentation, and manifestations

2 Patient variables: age, sex, body mass, comorbidities, history of drug effectiveness, tolerance, and allergies, susceptibility and risk of adverse effects, and personal preferences

3 Treatment variables: drug choice, pharmacokinetics and pharmacodynamics, therapeutic window, duration, and concomitant drugs

4 Environment: diet, herbs, smoking, beverages, and socioeconomic conditions, including affordability of treatment

Genetic testing has the potential to further define categories 1, 2, and 3, but clearly many nongenetic considerations need to be taken into account. Currently, the best options for PGx testing in psychiatry are (a) to help exclude drugs in selected patients like CYP2D6 poor metabolizers, (b) to guide personalized dosing for narrow window drugs like TCAs, and (c) to explain cases of unexpected ineffectiveness or ADRs.

Important psychopharmacodynamic genes

There are demonstrated associations between certain psychiatric disease and psychotropic drug response. A selection of these genes is likely to become part of comprehensive panels for PGx evaluation. However, the knowledge is currently incomplete, and practical applications of PGx testing for PD genes cannot be generally recommended. There are several comprehensive reviews available on this topic (3, 4, 22–26).

Most PGx studies addressing psychotropic pharmacodynamics have focused on genes belonging to one of three categories:

1 Neurotransmitter pathways, including biosynthetic and degradation enzymes, neurotransmitter receptors, and neurotransmitter transporters

2 Signal transduction genes more or less clearly related to neurotransmitter pathways

3 Other disease modifier genes, involved in pathogenesis or expression of psychopathological diseases

Neurotransmitter pathways

Neurotransmitters are chemicals involved in transmission or modification of the synaptic signals, and their action, whether excitatory or inhibitory, is dependent on the type of receptor they bind to. The most common neurotransmitters are glutamate, and GABA, which are released by more than 90% of neurons in the brain. In general, GABA interacts with inhibitory receptors, while glutamate mostly binds to excitatory receptors, with the exception of the inhibitory metabotropic glutamate receptors. Other common neurotransmitters include acetylcholine, which in the spinal cord binds to excitatory nicotinic receptors, and glycine, which generally binds to inhibitory receptors. Most important for the action of psychotropic drugs are the monoaminergic pathways involving dopamine, norepinephrine, and serotonin. Dopaminergic pathways have been related to cognition, mood, motivation, reward, sleep, fine motor control, and inhibition of prolactin release. Increased dopaminergic activity, especially in the mesolimbic pathway involved in motivation and reward, is found in schizophrenia, addiction, and depressive disorders. Serotoninergic activity generally improves cognition, memory, mood, satiety, introversion, and sleep, and decreases nociception. As a stress hormone, norepinephrine is involved in the fight-or-flight response, stimulating focused attention and increasing the cardiovascular tone and the brain's blood supply.

Serotinergic genes

Serotonin, also known as 5-hydroxy-tryptamine, is synthesized from the amino acid tryptophan by the action of tryptophan hydroxylase, which is encoded by TPH1 and TPH2 genes, with TPH1 being ubiquitous, while TPH2 is brain specific. Interestingly polymorphisms in the TPH1 gene have been related to the risk of schizophrenia (27), and both TPH1 and TPH2 appear to influence the response to antidepressants in major depression (24, 28, 29). The TPH2 gene has also been implicated in susceptibility to suicide in depression and bipolar disease (30–32), in addition to anxiety, panic, ADHD, obsessive-compulsive disorder (OCD), opioid addiction, and eating disorders.

The serotonin transporter, encoded by the SLC6A4 gene, is involved in serotonin reuptake and is the target of SSRI antidepressant drugs. Inhibition of SLC6A4-mediated serotonin reuptake results in increased synaptic serotonin concentration with consequent enhancement of serotoninergic signaling. Not surprisingly, many studies have demonstrated a correlation between SLC6A4 polymorphisms and response to SSRI treatment. For example, a meta-analysis of nine PGx studies of antidepressant response showed that the serotonin transporter promoter polymorphism (5-HTTLPR) correlated with SSRI side effects, while another polymorphism in the same gene (sTin2) was associated with better response in Asians in 5 studies (24). Another recent study using 811 patients showed that an interaction between SLC6A4 polymorphisms and stressful life events was predictive of the response to SSRIs (22). In addition to modulating antidepressant responses, the SLC6A4 gene has been associated with schizophrenia risk (27) and response to antipsychotics (33). Similar to the TPH2 gene, associations have been described between SLC6A4 and anxiety, panic,

autism, ADHD, OCD, substance addiction, and eating disorders.

Serotonin receptors can be classified in (a) G-protein coupled receptors, encoded by HTR1A to HTR1F, HTR2A to HTR2C, HTR4, HTR5A, HTR6, and HTR7; and (b) ligand-gated cation channels, encoded by HTR3A to HTR3E. The HTRA2A receptor has been the most extensively studied, and has been implicated in antidepressant (24, 34) and antipsychotic response (35). Several of the other serotonin receptor genes have polymorphisms correlating with antipsychotic response, including HTR2C (36), HTR3A (37, 38), HTR3B (37), and HTR3E (39). The risk for bipolar disorder appears affected by variation in HTR2A (40), HTR2C (41), HTR3B (42), and HTR5A (43). The HTR2A gene also has been associated with impulsive suicidal behavior (44, 45), and inactivation of HTR2B in mice or in humans was associated with severe impulsivity (46).

Dopaminergic genes

Dopamine is synthesized from L-tyrosine by the successive action of tyrosine hydroxylase (TH), forming L-DOPA, and DOPA decarboxylase (DDC), which converts L-DOPA to dopamine. Genetic variation in both of these genes may be associated with suicidal behavior (47). Furthermore, DDC polymorphisms were strongly associated with ADHD in both children and adults (48). The specific dopamine transporter is encoded by SLC6A3, a highly polymorphic gene, subjected to complex regulation which possibly includes epigenetic mechanisms (49). Interestingly variation in this gene has also been associated with ADHD and methylphenidate response (50) and with various behavioral traits, including nicotine dependence (51).

The dopamine receptors are expressed from five genes, from DRD1 to DRD5, and signal through G-protein-dependent pathways. First-generation antipsychotics appear to act through DRD2 inhibition, while newer antipsychotics also inhibit DRD1, DRD3, and DRD4; therefore these genes are of considerable PGx interest. Polymorphisms in all five dopamine receptor genes have been associated with psychopathology, with DRD1 and DRD2 being the most studied. For example, a comprehensive study using meta-analyses (118 different reports) concluded that DRD1, DRD2, and DRD4 had significant association with schizophrenia risk, with DRD1 showing the strongest effect (27). Correlations with antipsychotic response have been observed for DRD2 (52), DRD3 (53), and DRD4 variants (54). These three genes also have shown significant associations with the development of extrapyramidal symptoms in patients taking antipsychotics, including the SGA risperidone (55–58). DRD2 variants also demonstrated potential predictive value for antipsychotic-induced weight gain (59). All five DRD genes have been implicated in ADHD, with DRD2 showing significant association in a genome-wide screening of 600,000 SNPs (60). Given the functions of dopamine in the pleasure and reward system, it is interesting that polymorphisms in all dopaminergic receptors have been associated with alcohol, tobacco, or drug addiction, with DRD2 showing a significant effect in a meta-analysis study (25). A practical pyrosequencing assay for DRD2 variants for psychiatric PGx has been recently proposed (61).

Adrenergic genes

The dopamine beta-hydroxylase (DBH) catalyzes the conversion of dopamine to norepinephrine, therefore controlling the balance between dopaminergic and adrenergic pathways. Polymorphism in this gene have been related to impulsiveness (62), neuroleptic response in schizophrenia (63), and risk of ADHD (64, 65). The specific norepinephrine transporter SLC6A2 is involved in its reuptake and is a target of some antidepressants. A review of GWAS showed significant association of several polymorphisms in SLC6A2 with major depressive disorder (66), and a weak association with antidepressant response (67). A number of studies have also related this gene with ADHD and response to atomoxetine and amphetamine (68–70).

The adrenergic receptors can be classified into (a) alpha 1, encoded by ADRA1A to ADRA1C; (b) alpha 2, encoded by ADRA2A to ADRA2C; and (c) beta 1 (ADRB1), beta 2 (ADRB2) and beta 3 (ADRB3). ADRA1A, ADRA2A, and ADRA2C correlate with the therapeutic response in ADHD (23, 71, 72),

while ADRA1A, ADRA2A and ADRB3 variants have been linked to antipsychotic-induced weight gain (73–75).

Other monoaminergic genes

Genes coding for enzymes involved in monoamine degradation have been associated with various psychiatric disorders which may response to psychotropic drugs. The L-monoamine oxidase enzyme is encoded by two genes, MAOA and MAOB, and is responsible for the oxidative deamination of dopamine (MAOA and MAOB), norepinephrine (MAOA), and serotonin (MAOA). MAO enzymes are the targets of an older class of antidepressants, the MAO inhibitors (Table 9.1). Low activity of MAO presumably leads to higher synaptic levels of monoamines and increased monoaminergic activity. Congruently, both MAOA and MAOB polymorphisms have been correlated with impulsivity, suicidal ideation, and antisocial behavior, especially in combinations with other monoaminergic genes (76–78).

Another gene of major significance in modulating monoamine levels is the catechol-O-methyltransferase (COMT), which catalyzes the inactivation of catecholamines (dopamine and norepinephrine) in the postsynaptic neurons. The COMT gene is prevalent in the frontal cortex and appears to regulate cognition and higher executive functions by modulating dopaminergic activity in the frontal lobes in both normal individuals and schizophrenic patients (79, 80). A common polymorphism, Val158Met, leads to reduced activity of COMT and increased catecholaminergic signaling. An effect on antidepressant response in major depression has been observed in several studies (81–83). COMT polymorphisms also affect pain perception and emotional awareness (84–86), have been associated with schizophrenia risk (87–90), and appear to influence the response to risperidone (91).

The vesicular monoamine transporters, encoded by SLC18A1 and SLC18A2, are involved in presynaptic packaging of norepinephrine into synaptic vesicles. It is also involved in packaging of dopamine and serotonin, and appears to be the main target of methamphetamine, which inhibits its activity, resulting in uncontrolled release of the monoamines independently of synaptic activity. The large-scale trial of antipsychotic effectiveness (CATIE) showed some weak association of a SLC18A1 polymorphism with cognitive responses to antipsychotics (92). This gene has also been associated with schizophrenia, bipolar disorder, and anxiety disorders (93).

Cholinergic genes

Acetylcholine is a predominant neurotransmitter involved in motor synapses, parasympathetic system, and central neurons, and acts through nicotinic and muscarinic receptors. The nicotinic receptors are ligand-gated channels controlling permeability to sodium, potassium, and chloride ions. Muscle nicotinic receptors include CHRNA1, CHRNB1, CNRND, CHRNE, and CHRND; parasympathetic ganglia contain CHRNA3 and CHRNB4; and brain nicotinic receptors include CHRNA2-CHRNA10, and CHRNB2-CHNRB4. Polymorphisms in CHRNA2 to CHRNA5 and in all CHRNB genes have been associated with nicotine addiction (94–96). Interestingly, the CHRNA7 has been associated with schizophrenia (92), bipolar disorder (97), and delusional symptoms in Alzheimer's disease (98). The other acetylcholine receptors are the muscarinic receptors, which couple through G-proteins and are encoded by CHRM1 to CHRM5 genes. Variation in the CHRM2 gene has been associated with depressive and bipolar disease (99), and decreased cortical CHRM1 receptors have been associated with schizophrenia (100).

Another gene of interest involved in cholinergic pathways is the choline acetyltransferase gene (CHAT) responsible for acetylcholine biosynthesis, which shows significant association with nicotine addiction, depression, and Alzheimer's disease (101, 102).

Glutamatergic genes

The aminoacid glutamate is the most abundant neurotransmitter in the brain, and is involved in synaptic plasticity and consequently in learning and memory. The aging process involves considerable loss of glutamatergic neurons, and understanding this process and the complex neuropharmacology of glutamatergic pathways is a major goal of neuroscience and dementia research. Glutamate is easily synthesized from other aminoacids such as alanine by transamination, and degraded in the brain by glutamate dehydrogenase (GLUD1), but polymorphisms in glutamate metabolic genes have not been associated with psychopathology. Glutamate transport genes include (a) the vesicular glutamate transporters (SLC17A6, SLC17A7, and SLC17A8), which pack glutamate into presynaptic vesicles for controlled release; and (b) the excitatory amino acid transporters (SLC1A1, SLC1A2, SLC1A3, SLC1A6, and SLC1A7), which capture glutamate into storage vesicles. SLC1A7 is present in retina, and SLC1A6 in central neurons, while the other SLC1A genes code for glial and endothelial glutamate transporters. In particular, SLC1A2 is considered to be responsible for 90% of the regulation of extracellular glutamate concentration. Accordingly, polymorphisms in this gene have been associated with schizophrenia susceptibility and response to antipsychotics (92, 103). In contrast, the SLC1A1 gene has been associated with autistic and OCD disorders (104, 105), including the risk of OCD symptoms induced by atypical antipsychotics (106).

Glutamate receptors are encoded by numerous genes, which can be classified as follows:
1 Ionotropic (ligand-gated ion channel) receptors
    A AMPA: GRIA1 to GRIA4
    B Kainate: GRIK1 to GRIK4
    C NMDA: GRIN1, GRIN2A to GRIN2D, GRIN3A and GRIN3B
2 Metabotropic (G-protein coupled) receptors
    A Group 1: GRM1, GRM5
    B Group 2: GRM2, GRM3
    C Group 3: GRM4, 6, 7, 8
Polymorphisms in several of the glutamatergic receptors have been associated with major depression, bipolar disorder, schizophrenia, and mental retardation. For example, the large CATIE schizophrenia treatment trial identified a positive correlation between various glutamate receptor polymorphisms and antipsychotic-induced cognitive improvement, with strongest hits in the GRM7 and GRM8 genes (92). In another example, the effectiveness of clozapine was correlated with variation in the GRIN2B gene in a Chinese population (107).The response to

antidepressants is also influenced by polymorphisms in the glutamatergic receptors. Examples include (a) GRIK4 in two large antidepressant trials (108, 109); (b) GRM3 and fluvoxamine response (110); (c) GRIK2 and GRIA3 association with suicidal ideation; and (d) GRIA1, GRIA3, GRIK2, and GRIN3A linkage to sexual dysfunction in the large STAR*D antidepressant trial (111, 112). Another potential clinically important observation from a GWAS in bipolar disease was that a polymorphism in the GRIA2 gene was associated with more than doubling of the time to recurrence of a mood episode in response to lithium therapy (113).

GABAergic genes

Glutamate is also a precursor of the gamma-aminobutyric acid, the most abundant inhibitory neurotransmitter in the brain. Stimulation of GABAergic pathways typically induces relaxing, anti-anxiety, and anticonvulsive effects. GABA is synthesized in the brain from glutamate via the action of L-glutamic acid decarboxylase (GAD1), and polymorphisms in GAD1 promoter possibly related to gene downregulation are associated with the risk of schizophrenia (114). GABA is degraded by 4-aminobutyrate-aminotransferase (ABAT), a target of the anticonvulsant vigabatrin, and polymorphisms in this gene have been associated with autistic disorder (115). The GABA transporters include (a) SLC6A1, SLC6A11, and SLC6A13, which remove GABA from the synaptic cleft; (b) SLC6A12, which transports both GABA and betaine; and (c) the vesicular inhibitory vesicular transporter, SLC32A1, which packages glycine and GABA into presynaptic vesicles.

The GABA receptors genes include (a) the G-protein coupled metabotropic receptor subunits GABBR1 and GABBR2; and (b) the ionotropic receptors subunits GABRA1-6, GABRB1-3, GABRG1-3, GABRD, GABRE, GABRP, and GABRR1-3. Interestingly, the development of neuroleptic-induced extrapyramidal symptoms has been associated with several GABAergic genes, including ABAT, SLC6A11, GABRA3, GABRA4, GABRB2, GABRB3, GABRG1, GABRG2, and GABRG3 (116), suggesting that GABAergic inhibition of extrapyramidal dopaminergic pathways is important in preventing this complication of antipsychotic treatment.

Endocannabinoid-associated genes

Recently the pathways involved in the response to cannabinoids have become better elucidated. The major endogenous cannabinoids appear to be the arachidonic acid derivatives, anandamide and 2-arachidonoyl glycerol, which bind to the central (CB1) and peripheral (CB2) cannabinoid receptors, respectively encoded by the CNR1 and CNR2 genes. Another gene of relevance in this pathway is the fatty acid amide hydrolase (FAAH), which rapidly degrades anandamide. The endocannabinoid system is involved in analgesia, memory extinction, and appetite. Polymorphisms in CNR1 have been linked to schizophrenia (117), anxiety, and depression (118, 119), and appear to influence antidepressant response and emotional processing in major depression (119). CNR1 variants also seem to affect the risk for neuroleptic-induced extrapyramidal effects (120) and weight gain (121). Variation in the FAAH gene seems to correlate with susceptibility to alcohol, cannabis, and other drug addictions (122, 123). Given that this enzyme is a promising target for analgesic therapy, it may become a gene of considerable PGx interest.

Other important psychopharmacodynamic genes

Other neurotransmitter and hormone-related genes of PGx interest include the glycine transporter SLC6A5 associated with haloperidol-induced tardive diskinesia (124), and the corticotropin releasing hormone (CRH) and its receptors CRHR1 and CRHR2, linked to the response to antidepressants (125, 126). In addition to the ligand-gated ionotropic receptors mentioned above, several voltage-gated ion channels have shown variation correlating with major depression, antidepressant response, and bipolar disease, including the calcium channels CACNA1C and CACNG2 (127, 128), and the potassium channels KCNJ6, KCNK2, and KCNQ2 (129–131).

A number of signal transduction genes, possibly involved in neurotransmitter pathways, have been linked to antidepressant and antipsychotic response, including kinases GSK3B (132) and AKT1 (133), the phosphodiesterases PDE9A and PDE11A (134, 135), the calcineurin inhibitor FKBP5 (136), the cGTP hydrolase feedback regulator GCHFR (137), and G-protein subunit beta 3 (GNB3) (138, 139). The methyl-tetrahydrofolic acid reductase (MTHR), is essential to regenerate 5-methyl-tetrahydrofolic acid, a carbon donor for important metabolic pathways such as conversion of homocysteine to methionine, pyrimidine synthesis, and epigenetic DNA methylation. Various meta-analyses of several studies confirmed the association of polymorphisms in this gene with depression, schizophrenia, and bipolar disease, which may be mechanistically related to epigenetic changes in DNA methylation during brain development (27, 140, 141).

Genomic and genetic association studies with schizophrenia are tracked by the SzGene database (www.szgene.org), which ranks schizophrenia susceptibility genes according to the strength of association evidence (142). Today (May, 2011), the top 10 schizophrenia susceptibility genes are:

1 PRSS16 (serine protease 16)
2 PGBD1 (piggyBac transposable element derived 1)
3 NRGN (neurogranin)
4 NOTCH4 (a transmembrane receptor)
5 HIST1H2BJ (H2B histone family, member R)
6 PDE4B (phosphodiesterase 4b, cAMP specific)
7 TCF4 (transcription factor 4)
8 GWA_16p13.12 (unknown)
9 ZNF804A (zinc finger protein 804A)
10 DRD4 (dopamine receptor 4)

Interestingly, most of the genes in the list are related to brain developmental pathways rather than neurotransmitters, indicating a possible strong contribution of structural defects in the pathogenesis of schizophrenia. Other genes presumably involved in neurodevelopment and implicated by multiple genomic association studies in schizophrenia include dystrobrevin-binding protein 1 or dysbindin (DTNBP1), disrupted in schizophrenia 1 (DISC1), brain-derived neurotropic factor (BDNF) and its receptor (NTRK2), neuroregulins (NRG1 and NRG3), neurexin-1 (NRXN), chitinase (CHI3L1), the engrailed transcription factor (EN1), tumor protein 53 (TP53), neurofilament 3 (NEFM), neuronal adhesion protein (ASTN2), connexin 50 (GJA8), and synaptic protein (SNAP25), among others. It is possible that genotyping of these genes will contribute to individualization of antipsychotic therapy.

Table 9.3 Major Genes Involved in Antidepressant Pharmacodynamics

Effectiveness	Suicide Risk	Sexual Dysfunction
BDNF	GRIA3	GRIA1
CACNA1C	GRIK2	GRIA3
CANG2	GRIK4	GRIK2
COMT	HTR2A	GRIN3A
CRHR1-2	TPH1-2	
GRIK4		
GRM3		
HTR2A		
SLC6A4		
TPH1		
TPH2		

Note: Genes in **bold** show higher replicability or magnitude of the effect.

Other genes of potential relevance to antipsychotic pharmacodynamics include RIMS1, strongly associated with discontinuation of quetiapine, and the adenylcyclase gene ADCY1, strongly associated with cognitive improvement in the large CATIE trial (92). A selection of genes of relevance in antidepressant pharmacodynamics is illustrated in Table 9.3, and for antipsychotics is summarized on Table 9.4. Although a large number of genes show polymorphisms that were associated with various psychiatric disorders and may modulate the susceptibility for development of the disease and/or the effectiveness and tolerability of psychotropic drug therapy, most of the findings show weak effects and poor replicability. Nevertheless, these genes may be important, and further studies should be conducted in order to establish how polymorphisms of these genes can be incorporated into pharmacogenomics algorithms.

Important psychopharmacokinetic genes

Xenobiotic metabolism has traditionally been classified in three phases, consisting of (a) Phase I enzymes, typically the cytochrome P-450-dependent mixed-function oxidases (CYP), which add polar radicals, such as hydroxyl group, to the xenobiotic; (b) Phase II enzymes, which conjugate the

Table 9.4 Major Genes Involved in Antipsychotic Pharmacodynamics

Effectiveness	Extrapyramidal	Metabolic	NMS
ADCY1	ABAT	ADRA1A	**DRD2**
COMT	BDNF	**ADRA2A**	
DBH	CNR1	ADRAB3	
DRD1	CNR1	ADRB3	
DRD2	DRD2	APOE	
DRD3	**DRD3**	CNR1	
DRD4	DRD4	DRD2	
GNB3	GABRA3	GNB3	
GRM7-8	GABRA4	HTR2A	
GRIN2B			
HTR2A	GABRB2	HTR2C	
HTR2C	GABRB3	**Leptin**	
RIMS1	GABRG1	SNAP25	
SLC18A1	GABRG2		
SLC1A2	GABRG3		
	GNB3		
	GSTM1		
	HTR2A		
	HTR2C		
	NOS3		
	SLC6A11		
	SLC6A5		
	SOD2		

Note: Genes In **bold** show higher replicability or magnitude of the effect.
NMS = Neuroleptic malignant syndrome.

modified xenobiotic with glucuronidate, sulfate, or acetate to make it more polar and hydrophilic; and (c) Phase III enzymes, which includes further metabolism and elimination from the cells by xenobiotic transporters. Examples relevant to psychotropic drugs include the following:

Phase 1: CYP2A1, 2C19, 2D6, 3A4 are the major metabolizing enzymes for psychotropic drugs. In addition CYP2A6, 2B6, 2C8, 2C9, 2E1, and 3A5 are minor contributors to the metabolism of psychotropic drugs and will not be further discussed.

Phase 2: UGT2B7, UGT1A4; these glucuronidyl-transferases do not appear to be major sources of interindividual variation in antidepressant or antipsychotic response. UGT2B7 polymorphisms may have some minor influence in the variability of opioid response and UGT1A4 polymorphisms

have some influence in the pharmacokinetics of clozapine and imipramine (143).

Phase III: Drug Transporters: P-glycoprotein ABCB1, which contributes to exclusion of many drugs from the brain.

CYP2D6

The highly polymorphic cytochrome P450 enzyme CYP2D6 accounts for only 2–4% of hepatic P450 activity, but is involved in the metabolism of about 25% of current drugs (144). Currently, there are 126 allelic variations that have been acknowledged by the Human Cytochrome P450 Allele Nomenclature Committee (http://www.cypalleles.ki.se/cyp2a6.htm), which can be classified into (a) null alleles, with no enzymatic activity (*3–8, *11–16, *18–21, *38, *40, *42, *44, *56, and *62); (b) partial functional alleles (*9, *10, *17, *29, *36 and *41); and (c) fully functional alleles (*1, *2, and *35). Some alleles, like *17, are fully active against some drugs but partially active against others. Individuals can be classified by their CYP2D6 enzymatic activity into (a) poor metabolizers (PMs), which have no active alleles; (b) intermediate metabolizers (IMs), with one or two partially active alleles; (c) extensive metabolizers (EMs), with one or two active alleles; and (d) ultra-rapid metabolizers (UMs), with more than two active alleles. Different ethnic populations vary significantly in the prevalence of the various alleles, resulting in marked differences in the frequency of CYP2D6 PMs, IMs, EMs, and UMs (Table 9.5). Note that some authors classify individuals with only one active allele as IMs, as the enzymatic activity may be reduced compared to EMs. Strong inhibitors of CYP2D6 include quinidine, cinacalcet, and the SSRIs citalopram, fluoxetine, paroxetine, and bupropion; and moderate inhibitors include sertraline (in high doses only) and duloxetine. In contrast to other CYP450 enzymes, such as CYP1A2, CYP2C19, and CYP3A4, CYP2D6 is not significantly inducible.

Interestingly, in addition to the liver, CYP2D6 localizes to several areas of the brain, particularly in regions associated with reward, alertness and serotoninergic activity, and polymorphisms in CYP2D6 have been associated with brain function, personality traits, and psychopathology (145, 146). The CYP2D6 poor metabolizers have higher

Table 9.5 Distribution of CYP2D6 Genotypes According to Resulting Enzymatic Activity (245)

CYP2D6 Activity	Caucasians	African Americans	North Africans and Middle Easterners	East Asians	Pacific Islander
None (PM)	5–10%	5%	2%	1–2%	<1%
Reduced (IM)	2%	2%	5–10%	30–50%	<1%
Normal (EM)	80–94%	>90%	50–80%	45–65%	70–80%
Increased (UM)	1–10%	5%	10–40%	0–2%	20–30%

impulsiveness and perfectionism-related anxiety (146). Possible biologic bases for these correlations include the enzymatic activity of CYP2D6 on (a) tyramine to form dopamine (147), (b) the regeneration of serotonin from 5-methoxytryptamine (19, 148), and (c) the metabolism of the endocannabinoid anandamide (149).

Similarly, a direct effect of CYP2C19 genotype on psychopathology is also suggested by the observation that 2C19 poor metabolizers have significantly less depressive symptoms than extensive metabolizers, independently of antidepressant therapy (150). These direct effects of CYP450 enzymes generally considered to be involved exclusively in drug PK may complicate the interpretation of PGx studies examining the response to psychotropic drugs.

CYP2C19

CYP2C19 is another significantly polymorphic enzyme of interest in psychotropic drug PGx, with 35 allelic variants described in the Human Cytochrome P450 Allele Nomenclature Committee website (http://www.cypalleles.ki.se/cyp2c19.htm). However, only the *1 (normal activity), *2 and *3 (null activity), and *17 (increased activity) are common. Poor metabolizers are homozygous for *2 or *3 alleles, while individuals carrying at least one *1

allele are considered EMs. The *17 allele is associated with increased enzyme activity, and individuals homozygous for *17 can be considered ultra-rapid metabolizers, causing reduced levels of drugs such escitalopram (151), although the effects appear too small to be of clinical significance (152). For other drugs metabolized by CYP2C19, such as sertraline, the *17 allele does not appear to affect drug or metabolite levels (153). Heterozygous *1/*17, *2/*17, or *3/*17 individuals behave mostly as EMs (154). Poor metabolizers are found in high frequencies only in certain Asian populations and Pacific Islander ethnicities (Table 9.6).

CYP2C19 is potently inhibited by fluvoxamine, moclobemide, chloramphenicol and curcumin (from turmeric), while rifampicin, carbamazepine, artemisin, norethindrone, and St. John's wort (an antidepressant herbal supplement) are significant inducers. As a result of the accumulation of evidence involving CYP2D6 and CYP2C19 in the metabolism of psychotropic drugs, in 2005 the FDA has described CYP2D6 as a "valid biomarker" for psychotropic drug submissions, recommended voluntary PGx data submission, and also approved the Roche AmpliChip CYP 450 for determination of CYP2D6 and CYP2C19 genotypes. Recently, other platforms for CYP2D6 and CYP2C19 genotyping have become

Table 9.6 Distribution of CYP2C19 Genotypes According to Resulting Enzymatic Activity

CYP2C19 Activity (x = any allele)	Caucasians	African Americans	East Asians	Pacific Islander*
None (PM) (*2/*2, *3/*3, *2/*3)	1–4%	1–5%	10–25%	36–49%
Normal (EM) (*17/x, *1/x)	91–95%	90–96%	80–90%	51–64%
Increased (UM) (*17/*17)	4–5%	3–4%	0–0.2%	0%

*From Papua New Guinea.

commercially available at considerably lower costs (see Chapter 11), and may make it cost-effective to perform PGx genotyping for selected psychiatric indications.

The long-term future of CYP2D6 and CYP2C19 PGx testing is uncertain since pharmaceutical companies are trending to eliminate CYP2D6 and CYP2C19 metabolized drugs from their pipelines in an attempt to simplify prescription and widen the market. However, these newer generation drugs are typically several times more costly than similarly effective drugs which could be effectively used with currently available PGx testing, while it is certain that polymorphisms in other genes will continue to affect drug response and tolerability such that universally effective psychotropic drugs are unlikely to be developed.

CYP3A4/CYP3A5

These enzymes together account for the metabolism of about 50% of the drugs which are metabolized by CYP450. The activities of CYP3A4 and 3A5 appear to overlap, such that when one of the genes is impaired by genetic variation, the other is generally able to compensate. In addition, the enzymes are easily induced on exposure to substrates, therefore compensating for lower expression alleles. Therefore, in general, genetic polymorphisms do not appear to be clinically significant. However, CYP3A4 is potently inhibited by grapefruit juice and drugs such as nefazodone, protease inhibitors (ritonavir, indinavir, and nelfinavir), macrolides such as erythromycin, chloramphenicol, azole antifungals, aprepitant, cimetidine, diltiazem, and verapamil. Potent inducers appear to be pregnane X receptor (PXR) ligands, which include a large variety of substances, including steroids, bile acids, St. John's wort, rifampicin, phenytoin, carbamazepine, barbiturates, nonnucleoside reverse transcriptase inhibitors such as efavirenz and nevirapine, and modafinil. Psychotropic drug substrates include the antidepressants amitriptyline, citalopram, escitalopram, fluoxetine, norfluoxetine, sertraline, and venlafaxine, and the antipsychotics aripiprazole, haloperidol, risperidone, ziprazidone, quetiapine, and clozapine (when CYP1A2 is inhibited), as well as various opiates, benzodiazepines, trazodone, and nefazodone.

CYP1A2

Major substrates of CYP1A2 include steroids, fatty acids, caffeine, some tricyclic antidepressants, and the antipsychotics clozapine, olanzapine, and mirtazapine. Potent inhibitors include fluvoxamine, fluoroquinolone antimicrobials such as ciprofloxacin, and verapamil. CYP1A2 is potently induced by polycyclic aromatic hydrocarbons, some which are present in tobacco and inhaled by smoking. Forty-one alleles are recognized (http://www.cypalleles.ki.se/cyp1a2.htm), some of which decreasing enzymatic activity (*1C, *1K, *3, *4, *6–8, *11, *15, *16), while the *1F allele, containing a C > A transversion at the -163 position in the promoter results in high inducibility. In Caucasians, only the *1F (30–50%) and the *1D allelic variants have frequencies above 2%, and genotyping for 1A2 does not appear to be clinically relevant for psychotropic drugs, although one study indicated that the *1F homozygotes had on average 22% lower concentration of olanzapine, independently of smoking or other inducers, and olanzapine levels correlated with clinical response in schizophrenic patients (155). In any case, independently of CYP1A2 genotype, smoking does influence CYP1A2 activity and should be considered for 1A2 metabolized drugs, particularly the antipsychotic clozapine and olanzapine.

ABCB1

This gene codes for the P-glycoprotein transporter also known as multidrug resistance protein (MDR). MDR is an ATP-binding cassette (ABC) transporter responsible for the efflux of several hydrophobic drugs and xenobiotics across the cell membrane, playing an important role in their absorption, distribution and elimination. For example, ABCB1 catalyzed efflux into the intestinal lumen affects absorption while in the brain capillaries ABCB1 is involved in exclusion of drugs from the brain, therefore contributing to the blood–brain barrier. The latter is of importance to psychotropic drugs since pharmacodynamic actions in the brain are complicated by the need of the drugs to cross the blood–brain barrier. Consequently, changes in ABCB1 activity may lead to different concentrations of active drugs or metabolites at the brain targets. For example, common intronic SNPs in ABCB1 were correlated to treatment outcome of the ABCB1 substrates citalopram, venlafaxine, and paroxetine but not of nonsubstrates such as mirtazapine, fluoxetine or bupropion (156, 157). In another study a SNP in the third exon (3435C > T) correlated with nortriptyline-induced postural hypotension (158). Despite these positive studies, there is not a clear consensus on genotype–phenotype correlation for most of the ABCB1 haplotypes. In addition, the activity of ABCB1 is subject to a multitude of inducers and repressors, which complicates the interpretation of genotyping findings (159).

Pharmacogenomics of antidepressants

Pharmacogenomics may aid in pharmacotherapy of several antidepressants. In this section these drugs are summarized along with how pharmacogenomics may aid in drug therapy.

Monoamine oxidase inhibitors (MAO)

MAO inhibitors (MAOIs) are not commonly used as first-line therapy due to their significant side effects, although newer MAOI selegiline and moclobemide have less adverse effects, albeit with lower potency. However, they can be used in refractory depression, and recently the FDA approved a transdermal patch form of selegiline, which bypasses dietary interactions in the gastrointestinal tract, for treatment of major depression. Selegiline is metabolized by CYP2B6 (160), and can also be inactivated by CYP2C19, with CYP2C19 PMs having higher average levels (161). However, it is not clear if polymorphisms in any CYP450 genes correlate to efficacy or tolerability of MAOI. On the other hand, MAOIs such as moclobemide are potent inhibitors of CYP2C19 (162), which should be considered when co-prescribing CYP2C19 metabolized drugs, such as some SSRIs. Selegiline is also considered a potent inhibitor of CYP2B6, and weak inhibitor of CYP2C19 (163).

Tricyclic antidepressants (TCAs)

Most TCAs are inactivated by hydroxylation mediated by CYP2D6, and 2D6 PMs achieve concentration-to-dose (C/D) ratios of 4 to 6, whereas CYP2D6 EMs have C/D ratios of 0.5 to 1.5 (164). CYP2D6 PMs on TCA therapy are more likely to switch to an SSRI because of side effects (165). Therefore, lower doses of TCAs are recommended in CYP2D6 poor metabolizers, while increased dosing may be necessary in CYP2D6 UMs (Table 9.8). Tricyclic antidepressants are also demethylated by CYP2C19 to their respective desmethyl metabolites, which retain some pharmacologic activity. Examples include the conversion of amitriptyline to nortriptyline, imipramine to desipramine, and clomipramine and trimipramine to their respective desmethyl metabolites. The CYP2C19 genotype is a major determinant of the parent/desmethyl metabolite ratio, which is relevance because the spectrum of activity is different between parent and desmethyl metabolites (Table 9.7). For example, nortriptyline is sevenfold more potent than amitriptyline as an NRI, while amitriptyline is 10-fold more potent as an SRI. The ratio of nortriptyline to amitriptyline levels is 0.8 in CYP2C19 EMs, but changes to 0.3 in PMs and 0.6 in EMs (166). Therefore, to maintain a similar activity profile, dose adjustment is recommended in accordance to CYP2C19 genotyping. The CYP2C19*17 allele is associated with increased activity and may result in small increases in desmethyl metabolite levels, but that effect does not appear clinically significant for amitriptyline, imipramine, or clomipramine (167, 168). All the desmethyl metabolites can be subsequently inactivated by hydroxylation from CYP2D6. Trimipramine follows similar metabolism, with CYP2D6 genotypes affecting levels of active metabolites, while CYP2C19 is involved in conversion to the desmethyl metabolite (169).

Doxepin is a more recent TCA antidepressant with anxiolytic and hypnotic properties. It is mainly metabolized to N-desmethyldoxepin (nordoxepin) by CYP2D6, and variation in the activity of this enzyme strongly affects the parent:metabolite ratio, with PMs having lower nordoxepin and UMs having higher nordoxepin levels. The sum of doxepin and nordoxepin remains relatively constant, but tends to be lower in CYP2D6 UMs (19), and one forensic

Table 9.7 Metabolite rates and Serotoninergic (SRI) versus Noradrenergic (NRI) Activities of Antidepressants (Based on 168, 171)

| Metabolic Conversion | Metabolite:Parent Activity | | Metabolite:Parent Ratio | | | | | | |
| | | | CYP2C19 | | | CYP2D6 | | | |
	NRI	SRI	PM	IM	EM	PM	IM	EM	UM
Amitriptyline → Nortriptiline	7.0	0.1	0.3	0.6	0.8				
Imipramine → Desipramine	23.3	0.2	0.3	0.7	1.2				
Clomipramine → Desmethyl-Clomipramine	27.2	0.15	0.7	0.9	1.2				
Doxepin → Nordoxepin	n/a	n/a	2.2	6.9	8.0	7.4	5.0	8.0	n/a
Fluoxetine → Norfluoxetine	–	1.8	0.6	2.1	4.3	0.4	1.1	1.3	4.2
Venlafaxine → O-Desmethylvenlafaxine	0.6	1.1				0.1	2.0	3.9	14.6

report of a fatal doxepin poisoning in an individual with CYP2D6 PM genotype showed high levels of doxepin with a low doxepin:nordoxepin ratio (170). While nordoxepin is considered an active metabolite, changes in the ratio to nordoxepin may be relevant since brain penetration is 3.5-fold higher for doxepin compared to its metabolites (166).

Other enzymes with minor effect on TCA levels include CYP1A2 and CYP3A4 (171, 172), which may become significant only when high doses are used in CYP2D6 PMs. Additionally, the ABCB1 transporter is involved in efflux of amitriptyline from the brain, and a common polymorphism resulting in decreased ABCB1 activity correlated with increased hypotensive ADRs in patients treated with nortriptyline, but not fluoxetine, which is unaffected by ABCB1 (158).

In general, it has been recommended that TCA doses should be reduced by about 50% in CYP2D6 or CYP2C19 PMs and CYP2D6 UMs may need higher doses (173). Pharmacokinetically corrected doses for the various TCAs in patients with variant CYP2D6 genotypes are displayed in Table 9.8.

Tetracyclic antidepressants

This class includes maprotiline, mianserin, and mirtazapine. Maprotiline is primarily inactivated by CYP2D6 with a minor contribution from CYP1A2 (174). Mianserin has been largely replaced by its analogue mirtazapine, which, because its metabolism is shared by CYP2D6, 1A2, and 3A4, should be less susceptible to polymorphisms in these genes (175).

However, caution should be applied in co-treatment with fluvoxamine, since this drug inhibits all three enzymes, and can cause significant elevations in mirtazapine levels (176). In patients on long-term therapy with mirtazapine, CYP2D6 PM genotypes, as well as smoking, presumably through induction of CYP1A2, result in elevated levels of mirtazapine, although it is unclear if this is clinically significant (177). Concurrent with the notion that CYP2D6 genotypes contribute minimally to the response to mirtazapine, CYP2D6 PMs and UMs showed only mild changes in mirtazapine blood levels, and no correlation with cardiovascular effects (178).

Selective serotonin reuptake inhibitors (SSRIs)

These drugs in general have a wider therapeutic window than TCAs, and fewer adverse drug reactions (ADR), especially cardiovascular side effects. Moreover, the frequency of ADRs does not appear to be generally associated with higher plasma levels, therefore pharmacokinetic modeling using PGx data is unlikely to contribute to the prevention of ADRs (179). On the other hand, awareness of SSRI pharmacokinetics may be important to prevent ineffectiveness due to lower levels of the active drug and may explain some ADRs related to toxicity (180). For example, in a PGx study of patients taking a variety of antidepressants, five of the six CYP2D6 PMs had side effects, even though they did not correlate with drug levels (180).

Table 9.8 Spectrum of Activity of CYP450 Enzymes Involved in Psychotropic Drug Metabolism and Suggested Dose Adjustments Based on Pharmacokinetic Parameters in CYP2D6 and 2C19 Variants (166, 173, 179, 233, 238, 246)

Drug	CYP2D6			CYP2C19		CYP1A2	CYP3A4	Other
	Activity	PM	UM	Activity	PM			
Tricyclic Antidepressants								
Amitriptyline	+ +	70–75	130	+ + +	60	+	+	2C9 +
Nortriptyline	+ + +	50	155	+ + +	60	+	+	
Clomipramine	+ + +	60	145	+ + +	60	+	+	
Imipramine	+ + +	30	180	+ +	70	+	+	
Desipramine	+ + +	40	170	+ + +	50	+	+	
Trimipramine	+ + +	40	180	+ + +	40	+	+	
Doxepin	+ + +	35	170	+ + +	50	+	+	
Newer Antidepressants								
Maprotiline	+ + +	35	170	–	=	+		
Mirtazapine	+	=	=	–	=	+	+	
Paroxetine	+ + + ⇓	20–60	140	–	=	+ +		
Fluoxetine	+ + ⇓	70	?	+ + + ↓	40		+	2C9 + ⇓
Fluvoxamine	+ + +	60	?	– ⇓	=	+ + ⇓	+ ↓	
Citalopram	+	=	=	+ +	60		+	
Escitalopram	+	=	=	+ +			+	
Sertraline	+ ↓	=	=	+ +	75		+	2C9 +
Venlafaxine	+ + +	30–70	130	+	=		+	
Desvenlafaxine	–	=	=	+	=		+	UGT + + +
Duloxetine	+ ↓	=	=	–	=	+ + +		
Bupropion	– ⇓	=	=	–	=			2B6 + +
Trazodone	+	75	125	–	=		+ +	
Nefazodone	–	=	=	–	=		+ + ⇓	
First-Generation Antipsychotics								
Phenothiazines	+ + +	30–50	140–180	–	=			
Haloperidol	+ +	75	=	–	=	+	+	
Second-Generation Antipsychotics								
Clozapine	+	=	=	+ +	80	+ + +	+	
Risperidone	+ + +	50	120	–	=		+ +	
Paliperidone	–	=	=	–	=			
Ziprasidone	–	=	=	–	=		+ +	AOX1 + + +
Aripriprazole	+ + +	70	140	–	=		+ +	
Olanzapine	+	=	=	–	=	+ + +	+	UGT + + +
Quetiapine	–	=	=	–	=		+ + +	

Note: Numbers indicate suggested dose as a percentage of the standard dose. = No dose change suggested. + + + The enzyme plays a major role in the metabolism of the drug, usually of clinical significance. + + The enzyme has partial activity on the drug. + The enzyme has a minor role. ⇓ The drug is a strong inhibitor of the enzyme (>150%). ⇓ The drug is a moderate inhibitor (50–150%). UGT: Glucuronyl transferase; AOX1: Aldehyde oxidase.

Fluvoxamine, fluoxetine, and paroxetine

All three of these SSRIs are significantly metabolized by CYP2D6, and polymorphisms in this enzyme affect blood levels and parent drug to metabolite ratios (181).

Fluoxetine is demethylated to the active metabolite norfluoxetine by CYP2D6, with a minor contribution from CYP2C9 (182, 183), and is additionally metabolized to the inactive p-trifluoromethylphenol metabolite by CYP2C19, which may be clinically significant only at high doses (184). Since CYP2D6 PMs do not have higher blood levels of fluoxetine plus norfluoxetine (182), the FDA labeling information for fluoxetine states that pharmacodynamic activities are essential the same in CYP2D6 PMs and does not recommended dose changes in these patients. However, norfluoxetine is about twofold more potent as an SSRI than the parent drug (Table 9.7), and while both S- and R-enantiomers of fluoxetine are active, the S-enantiomer of norfluoxetine is 20-fold more potent than the R-enantiomer (182); therefore, differential metabolism of S- and R- enantiomers by CYP2D6 and CYP2C9 and changes in the fluoxetine:norfluoxetine ratio may affect the effectiveness and tolerability of therapy.

Most SSRI antidepressants have some inhibitory effect on CYP2D6, but fluoxetine and paroxetine are particularly potent inhibitors, converting about 66% of EMs to functional PMs. This inhibition results in nonlinear pharmacokinetics and increased half-life (about 4–6 days after prolonged use of fluoxetine and about 24 hours for paroxetine, which is 6 to 14 times higher than observed with a single dose), as well as the potential for clinically significant interactions with CYP2D6 metabolized drugs. It is conceivable that individuals with <2 functional alleles (IMs) may show higher degree of inhibition than EMs and UMs, but this has not been definitively demonstrated. Interestingly, a study of 365 psychiatric inpatients on antidepressant or antipsychotic therapy showed that IMs receiving higher doses (above the median) had three times more ADRs than EMs or IMs on lower doses, possibly resulting in lower clinical response (185). This study suggests that IMs have a clinically significant effect on psychotropic drugs and CYP2D6 genotyping may be cost-effective for this population to reduce ADRs and perhaps improve effectiveness with decreased hospital length of stay. This is especially important if there are other factors contributing to CYP2D6 inactivation. For example, an anecdotal report described life-threatening serotonin toxicity in a CYP2D6 IM (*1/*5) patient with worsening liver function treated with paroxetine (186), illustrating the notion that genetics, drug inhibition, and liver function all contribute to CYP2D6 function.

In addition to CYP2D6, CYP1A2 appears to have a small effect on the metabolism of fluvoxamine and paroxetine. In one report, some CYP1A2 polymorphisms correlated with dose and response to paroxetine at week 4 of treatment (187), while two studies showed that smoking, but not CYP1A2 genotype, influenced fluvoxamine blood levels (188, 189).

Citalopram and escitalopram

Both citalopram and escitalopram are metabolized by CYP2D6, CYP2C19, and CYP3A4, therefore inactivation of one of the enzymes is unlikely to result in marked changes in pharmacokinetics. However, in the case of escitalopram, one study showed that CYP2D6 IMs had a higher frequency of remission, and CYP2C19 PMs had high blood levels (190). Other studies confirmed that CYP2C19 PMs had impaired clearance of escitalopram (191, 192). A case of life-threatening serotonin toxicity in a patient treated with citalopram due to presumed inhibition of CYP2C19 by fluconazole has been described (193). In general, CYP2C19 genotype alone may not justify dose adjustment, given the wide therapeutic range of these drugs.

In the case of citalopram, CYP2C19 genotypes were correlated with tolerance and rate of remission of depressive symptoms (194), and with higher frequency of ADRs (195). A pharmacokinetically adjusted dose of citalopram for CYP2C19 PMs should be about 60% of the average dose (179), while UMs may need higher doses (173) (Table 9.7). CYP2D6 appears to be a minor contributor, and CYP2D6 genotype may be relevant only in CYP2C19 PMs (196). ABCB1 polymorphisms also may affect brain levels of citalopram (196). The large STAR*D trial of antidepressants did not reveal any significant association of CYP2C19, CYP2D6, CYP3A4, CYP3A5, or ABCB1 polymorphisms with tolerance or response to citalopram (197), and at this point, it is unclear that routine genotyping for any of these genes will improve therapy. However, knowledge of CYP2C19 and 2D6 activity may help determine the cause of significant ADRs and prevent unfavorable drug interactions with citalopram and escitalopram.

Sertraline

Sertraline is metabolized by at least by five CYP450 enzymes (CYP2B6, 2C19, 2C9, 2D6, and 3A4), as well as by glucuronyl-transferases (198), and shows a unimodal distribution of plasma concentrations, suggesting that PMs and UMs are unlikely to result in clinically significant effects. CYP2C19 appears to have the highest N-demethylation activity on sertraline (199), and CYP2C19 PMs (but not *17 UMs) have dose-adjusted blood levels increased by about 4.5-fold compared to EMs (153), although the clinically relevance of this finding has not been established. Kircheiner *et al.* did suggest a 25% reduction of sertraline dose in CYP2C19 PMs (179) (Table 9.8).

Venlafaxine

Venlafaxine is an inhibitor of both serotonin (SRI) and norepinephrine (NRI) reuptake, and it is mainly metabolized by CYP2D6 to N-desmethyl-venlafaxine, an active metabolite also clinically available under the name desvenlafaxine. Since CYP2D6 does not appear to affect the sum of venlafaxine and metabolite, the FDA labeling does not recommend dose adjustments based on CYP2D6 genotype. However, similarly to fluoxetine and some TCAs, the ratio of SRI to NRI activity is significantly different between venlafaxine and desvenlafaxine (Table 9.7). Additionally, venlafaxine brain penetration is about four times higher than desvenlafaxine (166). Since the levels of desvenlafaxine are reduced about 3–6-fold in CYP2D6 PMs compared to EMs, these considerations may explain the increased incidence of ADRs in PM patients taking doses higher than 75 mg in a randomized crossover study (200). Other studies have shown increased incidence of ADRs in CYP2D6 PMs treated with venlafaxine, including hyponatremia (201), and a fourfold increase in cardiovascular toxicity (202). Interestingly, in contrast to desvenlafaxine, venlafaxine was no more effective than placebo in CYP2D6 PMs in at least four trials (203), despite similar discontinuation and ADR rates. Whether desvenlafaxine brain concentration, increased NRI activity, or some other factor is responsible for these observations is unknown. In contrast to venlafaxine, desvenlafaxine does not depend on CYP2D6, but is eliminated mostly by

glucuronidation and renal excretion, with a 5% contribution from CYP3A4 (204). Therefore, CYP2D6 genotyping and, perhaps more importantly, evaluation for CYP2D6 inhibitors (205), with switching to alternative drug or dose reduction in case of genotypic or phenotypic PM, is recommended for venlafaxine, but not for desvenlafaxine (204).

Minor pathways for venlafaxine metabolism include demethylation to N-desmethyl-venlafaxine by CYP3A4, and CYP2C19 EMs were associated with lower venlafaxine levels compared to PMs, without affecting desvenlafaxine metabolite levels (206). Conversely, CYP2C19 PMs are associated with higher venlafaxine levels (207). These effects do not appear significant enough to recommend dose adjustments in CYP2C19 variants, but may become significant in rare (0.05–0.10%) patients with inactivation of both CYP2D6 and 2C19, especially if CYP3A4 is also inhibited by co-prescribed drugs.

Other antidepressants

Duloxetine is primarily eliminated by CYP1A2 and secondarily by CYP2D6. Smoking or CYP1A2 inhibitors such as fluvoxamine result in significant changes in duloxetine blood levels, while CYP2D6 inhibitors or PMs show lesser changes in pharmacokinetics that do not require dose adjustment (208). Duloxetine does inhibit CYP2D6 and should be considered for possible drug interactions.

Bupropion is not significantly metabolized by either CYP2C19 or 2D6, making it a good alternative choice especially in patients with inactivation of both enzymes. CYP2B6 is involved in the activation of bupropion to its 4-hydroxy-metabolite (209), and CYP2B6 polymorphisms affect the ratio of bupropion to hydroxybupropion but the effect is minor (210). An important consideration is that bupropion is a strong inhibitor of CYP2D6, converting about 50% of CYP2D6 EMs to the PM phenotype.

Trazodone and nefazodone are minimally affected by CYP2D6 or CYP2C19, but they are both converted to m-chlorophenylpiperazine (mCPP) by the enzymatic activity of CYP3A4 (211). This metabolite has significant pharmacologic activity, including induction of depressive, anxiogenic, and obsessive-compulsive symptoms and may also be activated by CYP2D6 and other enzymes into glutathione-adducts possibly involved in liver toxicity (212). Therefore, CYP2D6 PMs may indirectly contribute to liver toxicity of these drugs.

Pharmacogenetics of antipsychotics

In this section genetic variants affecting the pharmacokinetics of antipsychotics are discussed. The readers are referred to the section on important pharmacodynamic genes for examples of gene variants affecting neuroleptic PD, summarized on Table 9.4.

Phenothiazines
Phenothiazines are older antipsychotic drugs with narrow therapeutic windows and significant risk of adverse effects, including anticholinergic effects such as constipation, sedation, and hypotension, and antidopaminergic effects such as prolactin release and extrapyramidal symptoms. These drugs are significantly metabolized by CYP2D6 and PMs for this enzyme are at higher risk of ADRs, such as cardiotoxicity and hyperprolactinemia (213). Dose reduction by about 50% is recommended in CYP2D6 PMs, while increased dosing by about 40–80% may be necessary for effectiveness in UMs (173). Given their effectiveness and lower costs, prescription of phenotiazines to certain patients may be appropriate, and PGx testing for CYP2D6 may be helpful in individualizing therapy and avoid ADRs.

Haloperidol
Haloperidol has pharmacological actions similar to the phenothiazines, but with a higher potency, stronger anti-hallucinogenic efficacy, and weaker anticholinergic effects. However, it has an increased risk for development of the malignant neuroleptic syndrome, characterized by acute increase in temperature, rhabdomyolysis, and autonomic instability, and genetic predictors of this severe complication would be of major interest. Like the phenothiazines, haloperidol is significantly metabolized by CYP2D6 and also functions as a moderate inhibitor of its activity (214). CYP2D6 PMs have higher levels of haloperidol and increased incidence of QT prolongation (215) and extrapyramidal symptoms (216), but explained only 1/20 of all haloperidol-related ADRs (216). Dose adjustments may be indicated in CYP2D6 PMs and UMs (173). In addition to CYP2D6, 2A1 and 3A4 have some effect of haloperidol disposition, and both smoking and inhibition of CYP3A4 have been shown to affect haloperidol clearance (217, 218).

Clozapine
Clozapine is the first SGA to be introduced in the market, and was soon withdrawn due to the risk of agranulocytosis. However, it has been used as a second line of therapy because of its superior effectiveness as an antipsychotic. Patients on clozapine are required to have weekly blood neutrophil counts in the first 6 months of treatment to screen for neutropenia. In contrast to carbamazepine, no specific PGx test can predict this ADR, although a screen of 74 candidate genes has identified HLA-DBQ1 has having 17 times higher odds of developing agranulocytosis (219). The major metabolizing enzyme for clozapine is CYP1A2 (220), with minor contributions from CYP2C19, 2D6, and 3A4. Induction of CYP1A2 by smoking is more significant than genetic polymorphisms (221), and smokers with the highly induced CYP1A2*1F allele are at higher risk for nonresponse to clozapine therapy (222). Conversely, CYP1A2 inhibitors, such as ciprofloxacin, result in higher levels of clozapine (223).

As for the other metabolizing enzymes, CYP2C19 can also affect clozapine levels, and in one study, 2C19 PMs had 2–3 times higher levels than EMs (220). CYP2D6 genotypes do not significantly influence clozapine levels or therapeutic response (224).

Risperidone and paliperidone
Risperidone is a widely used SGA with a narrow therapeutic window that is metabolized primarily by CYP2D6, with a contribution from CYP3A4. CYP2D6 converts risperidone to 9-hydroxy-risperidone, a metabolite also available under the name of paliperidone. Paliperidone retains 70% of anti-dopaminergic, 50% of the antiserotoni-

nergic, and only 20–30% of the anti-alpha-1- and anti-alpha-2-adrenergic activity of risperidone (225). Compared to risperidone, the relative levels of paliperidone in the brain are fivefold lower, possibly related to its higher hydrophilicity and affinity for ABCB1 (166), and this metabolite does not appear to be substantively metabolized by the P450 system (225, 226). Therefore, while CYP2D6 PMs do not significantly affect the total level of risperidone and metabolites (227, 228), the pharmacodynamics of the treatment may be affected. For example, CYP2D6 UMs have a four-fold higher risk of prolactin release in children, an effect associated with increased 9-hydroxyrisperidone levels but not with risperidone concentrations (229). In a separate study, CYP2D6 PMs had no effect on clinical response or prolactin release (230, 231), but had higher rates of ADRs and discontinuation than EMs, despite similar total risperidone plus metabolite concentrations (232). A 2.5 fold increase in the frequency of ADRs was seen in PMs but this genotype explained only 10–20% of all ADRs (233). In a different study, CYP2D6 PMs were associated with higher dose-corrected levels of risperidone, higher risperidone/paliperidone and risperidone plus paliperidone levels, and increased corrected QT interval (234).

CYP3A4 has a partial effect on risperidone metabolism, but inducers such as carbamazepine, phenytoin, phenobarbital, and rifampin can result in a functional UM phenotype for risperidone (164, 225). Conversely, CYP3A4 inhibitors can decrease risperidone 9-hydroxylation and a 50% reduction in dosage is recommended if these drugs are concurrently prescribed. Fluoxetine, in particular, can have a severe impact since it potently inhibits CYP2D6 and its metabolite, norfluoxetine, inhibits CYP3A4 (225).

Since ABCB1 is involved in brain distribution of risperidone, researchers have examined the association of polymorphisms in this gene and risperidone therapy. Two studies showed no effect on the frequency of ADRs (232, 235) while two other studies uncovered an effect of ABCB1 on the response to risperidone in autism (36), and schizophrenia (236). ABCB1 also appears to influence peripheral pharmacokinetics, since inhibition of this gene with verapamil resulted in increased risperidone blood levels (237).

Guidelines for personalized prescription of risperidone have been published (238), suggesting a 50% dose reduction in CYP2D6 PMs and a 20% increase in UMs. However, the cost effectiveness of CYP2D6 PGx to personalize risperidone treatment remains undetermined (239). For concomitant therapy with potent CYP3A4 inducers a doubling of the dose is recommended and conversely, a 25% reduction should be used with potent 3A4 inhibitors (Table 9.8).

Aripiprazole

Aripiprazole is significantly metabolized by CYP2D6 and CYP3A4. CYP2D6 hydroxylates aripiprazole to its active metabolite dehydroaripiprazole. PMs have higher levels of aripiprazole (240) and a twofold increase in its half-life (241). CYP3A4 is involved in aripiprazole inactivation by N-dealkylation, dehydrogenation, and hydroxylation and becomes clinically relevant with CYP3A4 inducers. The FDA labeling for aripiprazole recommends a 50% reduction in dose in the presence of strong CYP3A4 or 2D6 inhibitors, while doubling is recommend with 3A4 inducers.

Other antipsychotics

Olanzapine is metabolized primarily by direct glucuronidation and by CYP1A2 to 4′-N-desmethylolanzapine. Polymorphisms in CYP1A2 correlate with blood levels and therapeutic response of olanzapine, while the frequency of ADRs correlates only with 5HTR2A polymorphisms (155). CYP3A4 and 2D6 have minor roles in the metabolism of olanzapine, while ABCB1 polymorphisms may affect its therapeutic levels in the brain and the clinical response (242).

Quetiapine is mainly metabolized by CYP3A4 while ziprasidone is mostly metabolized by aldehyde oxidase with some contribution from CYP3A4 (226). Both of these drugs are unaffected by polymorphisms in CYP2D6 or 2C19 (226, 243). ABCB1 polymorphisms have been shown to predict plasma levels and response to quetiapine (244).

Conclusions

The field of psychiatric pharmacogenomics is growing fast. Many genes have been implicated in the pharmacodynamics of psychotropic drugs, with relevance for genes involved in the serotoninergic pathways induced by most antidepressants (Table 9.3) and dopaminergic pathways inhibited by antipsychotics (Table 9.4). However, the effects are often small and poorly replicable and generally cannot be used to guide current clinical practice. Pharmacokinetic interindividual variation is more clearly associated with genetic variants in polymorphic drug metabolizing enzymes, with particular emphasis on CYP2D6 and CYP2C19. Moreover, knowledge of psychotropic drug metabolism is essential to avoid significant drug interactions caused by inhibitors or inducers of the various CYP450 enzymes. Individualized prescription of psychotropic drugs should optimally take into consideration all the genetic and nongenetic factors relevant for each drug and each patient, and educated dose adjustment or drug selection can currently be made in several cases of psychotropic drugs clearly affected by CYP2D6 or CYP2C19 polymorphisms (Table 9.8). It is expected that future developments in pharmacogenomics will lead to a more comprehensive view of all the genetic factors involved in drug action, and PGx-assisted individualized prescription will become routine clinical practice in psychiatry.

References

1 Sullivan, P.F., Kendler, K.S., Neale, M.C. (2003) Schizophrenia as a complex trait: evidence from a meta-analysis of twin studies. *Arch Gen Psychiatry*, **60**(12),1187–1192.

2 Sullivan, P.F., Neale, M.C., Kendler, K.S. (2000) Genetic epidemiology of major depression: review and meta-analysis. *Am J Psychiatry*, **157**(10), 1552–1562.

3 Craddock, N., Sklar, P. (2009) Genetics of bipolar disorder: successful start to a long journey. *Trends Genet*, **25**(2), 99–105.

4 Maron, E., Hettema, J.M., Shlik, J. (2010) Advances in molecular genetics of panic disorder. *Mol Psychiatry*, **15**(7),681–701.

5 Burt, S.A. (2009) Rethinking environmental contributions to child and adolescent psychopathology: a meta-analysis of shared environmental influences. *Psychol Bull*, **135**(4), 608–637.

6 Rhee, S.H., Waldman, I.D. (2002) Genetic and environmental influences on antisocial behavior: a meta-analysis of twin and adoption studies. *Psychol Bull*, **128**(3),490–529.

7 Hettema, J.M., Neale, M.C., Kendler, K.S. (2001) A review and meta-analysis of the genetic epidemiology of anxiety disorders. *Am J Psychiatry*, **158**(10), 1568–1578.

8 Agrawal, A., Prescott, C.A., Kendler, K.S. (2004) Forms of cannabis and cocaine: a twin study. *Am J Med Genet B Neuropsychiatr Genet*, **129B**(1), 125–128.

9 Penno, M.B., Dvorchik, B.H., Vesell, E.S. (1981) Genetic variation in rates of antipyrine metabolite formation: a study in uninduced twins. *Proc Natl Acad Sci U S A*, **78**(8), 5193–5196.

10 Wang, P.S., Simon, G., Kessler, R.C. (2003) The economic burden of depression and the cost-effectiveness of treatment. *Int J Methods Psychiatr Res*, **12**(1), 22–33.

11 Gonzalez, H.M., *et al.* (2010) Depression care in the United States: too little for too few. *Arch Gen Psychiatry*, **67**(1), 37–46.

12 EGAPP Working Group (2007) Recommendations from the EGAPP Working Group: testing for cytochrome P450 polymorphisms in adults with nonpsychotic depression treated with selective serotonin reuptake inhibitors. *Genet Med*, **9**(12), 819–825.

13 Agius, M., *et al.* (2010) What do large scale studies of medication in schizophrenia add to our management strategies? *Psychiatr Danub*, **22**(2), 323–328.

14 Nierenberg, A.A., *et al.* (2010) Residual symptoms after remission of major depressive disorder with citalopram and risk of relapse: a STAR*D report. *Psychol Med*, **40**(1), 41–50.

15 American Psychiatric Association (2010) *Treatment of Patients with Major Depressive Disorder*, 3rd ed. [WWW document] URL http://www.psychiatryonline.com/pracGuide/pracGuideTopic_7.aspx [accessed on 28 June 2011].

16 McEvoy, J.P., *et al.* (2006) Effectiveness of clozapine versus olanzapine, quetiapine, and risperidone in patients with chronic schizophrenia who did not respond to prior atypical antipsychotic treatment. *Am J Psychiatry*, **163**(4), 600–610.

17 Phillips, K.A., *et al.* (2001) Potential role of pharmacogenomics in reducing adverse drug reactions: a systematic review. *JAMA*, **286**(**18**), 2270–2279.

18 Puls, I., Gallinat, J. (2008) The concept of endophenotypes in psychiatric diseases meeting the expectations? *Pharmacopsychiatry*, **41**(**Suppl. 1**), S37–S43.

19 Kirchheiner, J., *et al.* (2005) Impact of the CYP2D6 ultra-rapid metabolizer genotype on doxepin pharmacokinetics and serotonin in platelets. *Pharmacogenet Genomics*, **15**(**8**), 579–587.

20 Rabl, U., *et al.* (2010) Imaging genetics: implications for research on variable antidepressant drug response. *Expert Review of Clinical Pharmacology*, **3**(**4**), 471–489.

21 Kirsch, I., *et al.* (2008) Initial severity and antidepressant benefits: a meta-analysis of data submitted to the Food and Drug Administration. *PLoS Med*, **5**(**2**), e45.

22 Keers, R., Aitchison, K.J. (2011) Pharmacogenetics of antidepressant response. *Expert Rev Neurother*, **11**(**1**), 101–125.

23 Kieling, C., *et al.* (2010) A current update on ADHD pharmacogenomics. *Pharmacogenomics*, **11**(**3**), 407–419.

24 Kato, M., Serretti, A. (2010) Review and meta-analysis of antidepressant pharmacogenetic findings in major depressive disorder. *Mol Psychiatry*, **15**(**5**), 473–500.

25 Le Foll, B., *et al.* (2009) Genetics of dopamine receptors and drug addiction: a comprehensive review. *Behav Pharmacol*, **20**(**1**), 1–17.

26 de Leon, J. (2009) The future (or lack of future) of personalized prescription in psychiatry. *Pharmacol Res*, **59**(**2**), 81–89.

27 Allen, N.C., *et al.* (2008) Systematic meta-analyses and field synopsis of genetic association studies in schizophrenia: the SzGene database. *Nat Genet*, **40**(**7**),827–834.

28 Anttila, S., *et al.* (2009) TPH2 polymorphisms may modify clinical picture in treatment-resistant depression. *Neurosci Lett*, **464**(**1**), 43–46.

29 Tsai, S.J., *et al.* (2009) Tryptophan hydroxylase 2 gene is associated with major depression and antidepressant treatment response. *Prog Neuropsychopharmacol Biol Psychiatry*, **33**(**4**), 637–641.

30 Lopez de Lara, C., *et al.* (2007) Effect of tryptophan hydroxylase-2 gene variants on suicide risk in major depression. *Biol Psychiatry*, **62**(**1**), 72–80.

31 Roche, S., McKeon, P. (2009) Support for tryptophan hydroxylase-2 as a susceptibility gene for bipolar affective disorder. *Psychiatr Genet*, **19**(**3**), 142–146.

32 Campos, S.B., *et al.* (2010) Association of polymorphisms of the tryptophan hydroxylase 2 gene with risk for bipolar disorder or suicidal behavior. *J Psychiatr Res*, **44**(**5**), 271–274.

33 Wang, L., *et al.* (2007) Response of risperidone treatment may be associated with polymorphisms of HTT gene in Chinese schizophrenia patients. *Neurosci Lett*, **414**(**1**), 1–4.

34 Kishi, T., *et al.* (2010) HTR2A is associated with SSRI response in major depressive disorder in a Japanese cohort. *Neuromolecular Med*, **12**(**3**), 237–242.

35 Benmessaoud, D., *et al.* (2008) Excess of transmission of the G allele of the -1438A/G polymorphism of the 5-HT2A receptor gene in patients with schizophrenia responsive to antipsychotics. *BMC Psychiatry*, **8**,40.

36 Correia, C.T., *et al.* (2010) Pharmacogenetics of risperidone therapy in autism: association analysis of eight candidate genes with drug efficacy and adverse drug reactions. *Pharmacogenomics J*, **10**(**5**), 418–430.

37 Souza, R.P., *et al.* (2010) Influence of serotonin 3A and 3B receptor genes on clozapine treatment response in schizophrenia. *Pharmacogenet Genomics*, **20**(**4**), 274–276.

38 Gu, B., *et al.* (2008) Association between a polymorphism of the HTR3A gene and therapeutic response to risperidone treatment in drug-naive Chinese schizophrenia patients. *Pharmacogenet Genomics*, **18**(**8**),721–727.

39 Schuhmacher, A., *et al.* (2009) Influence of 5-HT3 receptor subunit genes HTR3A, HTR3B, HTR3C, HTR3D and HTR3E on treatment response to antipsychotics in schizophrenia. *Pharmacogenet Genomics*, **19**(**11**),843–851.

40 McAuley, E.Z., *et al.* (2009) Association between the serotonin 2A receptor gene and bipolar affective disorder in an Australian cohort. *Psychiatr Genet*, **19**(**5**), 244–252.

41 Mazza, M., *et al.* (2010) Further evidence supporting the association between 5HTR2C gene and bipolar disorder. *Psychiatry Res*, **180**(**2–3**), 151–152.

42 Meineke, C., *et al.* (2008) Functional characterization of a -100_-102delAAG deletion-insertion polymorphism in the promoter region of the HTR3B gene. *Pharmacogenet Genomics*, **18**(**3**), 219–230.

43 Yosifova, A., *et al.* (2009) Case-control association study of 65 candidate genes revealed a possible association of a SNP of HTR5A to be a factor susceptible to bipolar disease in Bulgarian population. *J Affect Disord*, **117**(**1–2**), 87–97.

44 Fanous, A.H., *et al.* (2009) Genetic variation in the serotonin 2A receptor and suicidal ideation in a sample of 270 Irish high-density schizophrenia families. *Am J Med Genet B Neuropsychiatr Genet*, **150B(3)**, 411–417.

45 Giegling, I., *et al.* (2006) Anger- and aggression-related traits are associated with polymorphisms in the 5-HT-2A gene. *J Affect Disord*, **96(1–2)**, 75–81.

46 Bevilacqua, L., *et al.* (2010) A population-specific HTR2B stop codon predisposes to severe impulsivity. *Nature*, **468(7327)**, 1061–1066.

47 Giegling, I., *et al.* (2009) Tyrosine hydroxylase and DOPA decarboxylase gene variants in personality traits. *Neuropsychobiology*, **59(1)**, 23–27.

48 Ribases, M., *et al.* (2009) Exploration of 19 serotoninergic candidate genes in adults and children with attention-deficit/hyperactivity disorder identifies association for 5HT2A, DDC and MAOB. *Mol Psychiatry*, **14(1)**, 71–85.

49 Shumay, E., Fowler, J.S., Volkow, N.D. (2010) Genomic features of the human dopamine transporter gene and its potential epigenetic states: implications for phenotypic diversity. *PLoS One,* **5(6)**, e11067.

50 Rohde, L.A., *et al.* (2003) Dopamine transporter gene, response to methylphenidate and cerebral blood flow in attention-deficit/hyperactivity disorder: a pilot study. *Synapse*, **48(2)**, 87–89.

51 Ma, J.Z., *et al.* (2005) Haplotype analysis indicates an association between the DOPA decarboxylase (DDC) gene and nicotine dependence. *Hum Mol Genet*, **14(12)**,1691–1698.

52 Lane, H.Y., *et al.* (2004) Effects of dopamine D2 receptor Ser311Cys polymorphism and clinical factors on risperidone efficacy for positive and negative symptoms and social function. *Int J Neuropsychopharmacol*, **7(4)**,461–470.

53 Adams, D.H., *et al.* (2008) Dopamine receptor D3 genotype association with greater acute positive symptom remission with olanzapine therapy in predominately caucasian patients with chronic schizophrenia or schizoaffective disorder. *Hum Psychopharmacol*, **23(4)**, 267–274.

54 Tsutsumi, A., *et al.* (2009) Genetic polymorphisms in dopamine- and serotonin-related genes and treatment responses to risperidone and perospirone. *Psychiatry Investig*, **6(3)**, 222–225.

55 Gasso, P., *et al.* (2009) A common variant in DRD3 gene is associated with risperidone-induced extrapyramidal symptoms. *Pharmacogenomics J*, **9(6)**, 404–410.

56 Tsai, H.T., *et al.* (2010) The DRD3 rs6280 polymorphism and prevalence of tardive dyskinesia: a meta-analysis. *Am J Med Genet B Neuropsychiatr Genet*, **153B(1)**,57–66.

57 Zai, C.C., *et al.* (2009) Association study of tardive dyskinesia and five DRD4 polymorphisms in schizophrenia patients. *Pharmacogenomics J*, **9(3)**, 168–174.

58 Zai, C.C., *et al.* (2007) Association study of tardive dyskinesia and twelve DRD2 polymorphisms in schizophrenia patients. *Int J Neuropsychopharmacol*, **10(5)**, 639–651.

59 Muller, D.J., *et al.* (2010) Systematic analysis of dopamine receptor genes (DRD1-DRD5) in antipsychotic-induced weight gain. *Pharmacogenomics J*, epub 17 August.

60 Lasky-Su, J., *et al.* (2008) Genome-wide association scan of quantitative traits for attention deficit hyperactivity disorder identifies novel associations and confirms candidate gene associations. *Am J Med Genet B Neuropsychiatr Genet*, **147B(8)**, 1345–1354.

61 Doehring, A., Kirchhof, A., Lotsch, J. (2009) Genetic diagnostics of functional variants of the human dopamine D2 receptor gene. *Psychiatr Genet*, **19(5)**, 259–268.

62 Hess, C., *et al.* (2009) A functional dopamine-beta-hydroxylase gene promoter polymorphism is associated with impulsive personality styles, but not with affective disorders. *J Neural Transm*, **16(2)**, 121–130.

63 Yamamoto, K., *et al.* (2003) Dopamine beta-hydroxylase (DBH) gene and schizophrenia phenotypic variability: a genetic association study. *Am J Med Genet B Neuropsychiatr Genet*, **117B(1)**, 33–38.

64 Kopeckova, M., Paclt, I., Goetz, P. (2006) Polymorphisms and low plasma activity of dopamine-beta-hydroxylase in ADHD children. *Neuro Endocrinol Lett*, **27(6)**, 748–754.

65 Faraone, S.V., Khan, S.A. (2006) Candidate gene studies of attention-deficit/hyperactivity disorder. *J Clin Psychiatry*, **67(Suppl. 8)**, 13–20.

66 Bosker, F.J., *et al.* (2010) Poor replication of candidate genes for major depressive disorder using genome-wide association data. *Mol Psychiatry*, epub 30 March.

67 Dong, C., Wong, M.L., Licinio, J. (2009) Sequence variations of ABCB1, SLC6A2, SLC6A3, SLC6A4, CREB1, CRHR1 and NTRK2: association with major depression and antidepressant response in Mexican-Americans. *Mol Psychiatry*, **14(12)**, 1105–1118.

68 Dlugos, A.M., *et al.* (2009) Further evidence of association between amphetamine response and

SLC6A2 gene variants. *Psychopharmacology (Berl)*, **206**(**3**), 501–511.

69 Ramoz, N., *et al.* (2009) A haplotype of the norepinephrine transporter (Net) gene Slc6a2 is associated with clinical response to atomoxetine in attention-deficit hyperactivity disorder (ADHD). *Neuropsychopharmacology*, **34**(**9**), 2135–2142.

70 Kim, J.W., *et al.* (2008) Further evidence of association between two NET single-nucleotide polymorphisms with ADHD. *Mol Psychiatry*, **13**(**6**), 624–630.

71 Polanczyk, G., *et al.* (2007) Association of the adrenergic alpha2A receptor gene with methylphenidate improvement of inattentive symptoms in children and adolescents with attention-deficit/hyperactivity disorder. *Arch Gen Psychiatry*, **64**(**2**), 218–224.

72 Comings, D.E., *et al.* (1999) Additive effect of three noradrenergic genes (ADRA2a, ADRA2C, DBH) on attention-deficit hyperactivity disorder and learning disabilities in Tourette syndrome subjects. *Clin Genet*, **55**(**3**), 160–172.

73 Liu, Y.R., *et al.* (2010) ADRA1A gene is associated with BMI in chronic schizophrenia patients exposed to antipsychotics. *Pharmacogenomics J*, **10**(**1**), 30–39.

74 Sickert, L., *et al.* (2009) Association of the alpha 2A adrenergic receptor -1291C/G polymorphism and antipsychotic-induced weight gain in European-Americans. *Pharmacogenomics*, **10**(**7**), 1169–1176.

75 Ujike, H., *et al.* (2008) Multiple genetic factors in olanzapine-induced weight gain in schizophrenia patients: a cohort study. *J Clin Psychiatry*, **69**(**9**), 1416–1422.

76 Zalsman, G., *et al.* (2011) Association of polymorphisms of the serotonergic pathways with clinical traits of impulsive-aggression and suicidality in adolescents: a multi-center study. *World J Biol Psychiatry*, **12**(**1**), 33–41.

77 Grigorenko, E.L., *et al.* (2010) Aggressive behavior, related conduct problems, and variation in genes affecting dopamine turnover. *Aggress Behav*, **36**(**3**), 158–176.

78 Kinnally, E.L., *et al.* (2009) Parental care moderates the influence of MAOA-uVNTR genotype and childhood stressors on trait impulsivity and aggression in adult women. *Psychiatr Genet*, **19**(**3**), 126–133.

79 Barnett, J.H., *et al.* (2009) Effects of catechol-O-methyltransferase on normal variation in the cognitive function of children. *Am J Psychiatry*, **166**(**8**), 909–916.

80 Liao, S.Y., *et al.* (2009) Genetic variants in COMT and neurocognitive impairment in families of patients with schizophrenia. *Genes Brain Behav*, **8**(**2**), 228–237.

81 Illi, A., *et al.* (2010) Catechol-O-methyltransferase val108/158met genotype, major depressive disorder and response to selective serotonin reuptake inhibitors in major depressive disorder. *Psychiatry Res*, **176**(**1**), 85–87.

82 Perlis, R.H., *et al.* (2009) Variation in catechol-O-methyltransferase is associated with duloxetine response in a clinical trial for major depressive disorder. *Biol Psychiatry*, **65**(**9**), 785–791.

83 Benedetti, F., *et al.* (2009) The catechol-O-methyltransferase Val (108/158)Met polymorphism affects antidepressant response to paroxetine in a naturalistic setting. *Psychopharmacology (Berl)*, **203**(**1**), 155–160.

84 Swart, M., *et al.* (2011) COMT Val158Met polymorphism, verbalizing of emotion and activation of affective brain systems. *Neuroimage*, **55**(**1**), 338–344.

85 Finan, P.H., *et al.* (2011) COMT moderates the relation of daily maladaptive coping and pain in fibromyalgia. *Pain*, **152**(**2**), 300–307.

86 Rakvag, T.T., *et al.* (2005) The Val158Met polymorphism of the human catechol-O-methyltransferase (COMT) gene may influence morphine requirements in cancer pain patients. *Piain*, **116**(**1–2**), 73–78.

87 Voisey, J., *et al.* (2010) HapMap tag-SNP analysis confirms a role for COMT in schizophrenia risk and reveals a novel association. *Eur Psychiatry*, epub 7 October.

88 Costas, J., *et al.* (2011) Heterozygosity at catechol-O-methyltransferase Val158Met and schizophrenia: new data and meta-analysis. *J Psychiatr Res*, **45**(**1**), 7–14.

89 Chien, Y.L., *et al.* (2009) Association of the 3′ region of COMT with schizophrenia in Taiwan. *J Formos Med Assoc*, **108**(**4**), 301–309.

90 Hoenicka, J., *et al.* (2010) Gender-specific COMT Val158Met polymorphism association in Spanish schizophrenic patients. *Am J Med Genet B Neuropsychiatr Genet*, **153B**(**1**), 79–85.

91 Gupta, M., *et al.* (2009) Association studies of catechol-O-methyltransferase (COMT) gene with schizophrenia and response to antipsychotic treatment. *Pharmacogenomics*, **10**(**3**), 385–397.

92 Need, A.C., *et al.* (2009) Pharmacogenetics of antipsychotic response in the CATIE trial: a candidate gene analysis. *Eur J Hum Genet*, **17**(**7**), 946–957.

93 Lohoff, F.W. (2010) Genetic variants in the vesicular monoamine transporter 1 (VMAT1/SLC18A1) and neuropsychiatric disorders. *Methods Mol Biol*, **637**, 165–180.

94 De Ruyck, K., *et al.* (2010) Genetic variation in three candidate genes and nicotine dependence, withdrawal

and smoking cessation in hospitalized patients. *Pharmacogenomics*, **11**(**8**), 1053–1063.

95 Thorgeirsson, T.E., *et al.* (2008) A variant associated with nicotine dependence, lung cancer and peripheral arterial disease. *Nature*, **452**(**7187**), 638–642.

96 Schlaepfer, I.R., *et al.* (2008) The CHRNA5/A3/B4 gene cluster variability as an important determinant of early alcohol and tobacco initiation in young adults. *Biol Psychiatry*, **63**(**11**), 1039–1046.

97 Ancin, I., *et al.* (2010) Evidence for association of the non-duplicated region of CHRNA7 gene with bipolar disorder but not with schizophrenia. *Psychiatr Genet*, **20**(**6**), 289–297.

98 Carson, R., *et al.* (2008) Genetic variation in the alpha 7 nicotinic acetylcholine receptor is associated with delusional symptoms in Alzheimer's disease. *Neuromolecular Med*, **10**(**4**), 377–384.

99 Cannon, D.M., *et al.* (2010) Genetic variation in cholinergic muscarinic-2 receptor gene modulates M (2) receptor binding in vivo and accounts for reduced binding in bipolar disorder. *Mol Psychiatry*, epub 30 March.

100 Scarr, E., *et al.* (2009) Decreased cortical muscarinic receptors define a subgroup of subjects with schizophrenia. *Mol Psychiatry*, **14**(**11**), 1017–1023.

101 Ray, R., *et al.* (2010) Convergent evidence that choline acetyltransferase gene variation is associated with prospective smoking cessation and nicotine dependence. *Neuropsychopharmacology*, **35**(**6**), 1374–1382.

102 Grunblatt, E., *et al.* (2009) Genetic risk factors and markers for Alzheimer's disease and/or depression in the VITA study. *J Psychiatr Res*, **43**(**3**), 298–308.

103 Deng, X., *et al.* (2004) Association study of polymorphisms in the excitatory amino acid transporter 2 gene (SLC1A2) with schizophrenia. *BMC Psychiatry*, **4**,21.

104 Gadow, K.D., *et al.* (2010) Glutamate transporter gene (SLC1A1) single nucleotide polymorphism (rs301430) and repetitive behaviors and anxiety in children with autism spectrum disorder. *J Autism Dev Disord*, **40**(**9**), 1139–1145.

105 Wendland, J.R., *et al.* (2009) A haplotype containing quantitative trait loci for SLC1A1 gene expression and its association with obsessive-compulsive disorder. *Arch Gen Psychiatry*, **66**(**4**), 408–416.

106 Kwon, J.S., *et al.* (2009) Association of the glutamate transporter gene SLC1A1 with atypical antipsychotics-induced obsessive-compulsive symptoms. *Arch Gen Psychiatry*, **66**(**11**), 1233–1241.

107 Chiu, H.J., *et al.* (2003) Association analysis of the genetic variants of the N-methyl D-aspartate receptor subunit 2b (NR2b) and treatment-refractory schizophrenia in the Chinese. *Neuropsychobiology*, **47**(**4**), 178–181.

108 Horstmann, S., *et al.* (2010) Polymorphisms in GRIK4, HTR2A, and FKBP5 show interactive effects in predicting remission to antidepressant treatment. *Neuropsychopharmacology*, **35**(**3**), 727–740.

109 Paddock, S., *et al.* (2007) Association of GRIK4 with outcome of antidepressant treatment in the STAR*D cohort. *Am J Psychiatry*, **164**(**8**), 1181–1188.

110 Tsunoka, T., *et al.* (2009) Association analysis of group II metabotropic glutamate receptor genes (GRM2 and GRM3) with mood disorders and fluvoxamine response in a Japanese population. *Prog Neuropsychopharmacol Biol Psychiatry*, **33**(**5**), 875–879.

111 Laje, G., *et al.* (2009) Pharmacogenetics studies in STAR*D: strengths, limitations, and results. *Psychiatr Serv*, **60**(**11**), 1446–1457.

112 Laje, G., *et al.* (2007) Genetic markers of suicidal ideation emerging during citalopram treatment of major depression. *Am J Psychiatry*, **164**(**10**), 1530–1538.

113 Perlis, R.H., *et al.* (2009) A genomewide association study of response to lithium for prevention of recurrence in bipolar disorder. *Am J Psychiatry*, **166**(**6**), 718–725.

114 Du, J., *et al.* (2008) Comprehensive analysis of polymorphisms throughout GAD1 gene: a family-based association study in schizophrenia. *J Neural Transm*, **115**(**3**), 513–519.

115 Barnby, G., *et al.* (2005) Candidate-gene screening and association analysis at the autism-susceptibility locus on chromosome 16p: evidence of association at GRIN2A and ABAT. *Am J Hum Genet*, **76**(**6**), 950–966.

116 Inada, T., *et al.* (2008) Pathway-based association analysis of genome-wide screening data suggest that genes associated with the gamma-aminobutyric acid receptor signaling pathway are involved in neuroleptic-induced, treatment-resistant tardive dyskinesia. *Pharmacogenet Genomics*, **18**(**4**), 317–323.

117 Chavarria-Siles, I., *et al.* (2008) Cannabinoid receptor 1 gene (CNR1) and susceptibility to a quantitative phenotype for hebephrenic schizophrenia. *Am J Med Genet B Neuropsychiatr Genet*, **147**(**3**), 279–284.

118 Juhasz, G., *et al.* (2009) CNR1 gene is associated with high neuroticism and low agreeableness and interacts with recent negative life events to predict current

depressive symptoms. *Neuropsychopharmacology*, **34**(8),2019–2027.

119 Domschke, K., *et al.* (2008) Cannabinoid receptor 1 (CNR1) gene: impact on antidepressant treatment response and emotion processing in major depression. *Eur Neuropsychopharmacol*, **18**(10), 751–759.

120 Tiwari, A.K., *et al.* (2011) Association study of Cannabinoid receptor 1 (CNR1) gene in tardive dyskinesia. *Pharmacogenomics J*, epub 25 January.

121 Tiwari, A.K., *et al.* (2010) A common polymorphism in the cannabinoid receptor 1 (CNR1) gene is associated with antipsychotic-induced weight gain in schizophrenia. *Neuropsychopharmacology*, **35**(6), 1315–1324.

122 Schacht, J.P., Selling, R.E., Hutchison, K.E. (2009) Intermediate cannabis dependence phenotypes and the FAAH C385A variant: an exploratory analysis. *Psychopharmacology (Berl)*, **203**(3), 511–517.

123 Flanagan, J.M., *et al.* (2006) The fatty acid amide hydrolase 385 A/A (P129T) variant: haplotype analysis of an ancient missense mutation and validation of risk for drug addiction. *Hum Genet*, **120**(4),581–588.

124 Giegling, I., *et al.* (2010) Glutamatergic gene variants impact the clinical profile of efficacy and side effects of haloperidol. *Pharmacogenet Genomics*, epub 18 September.

125 Lotrich, F.E., Pollock, B.G. (2005) Candidate genes for antidepressant response to selective serotonin reuptake inhibitors. *Neuropsychiatr Dis Treat*, **1**(1), 17–35.

126 Liu, Z., *et al.* (2007) Association study of corticotropin-releasing hormone receptor1 gene polymorphisms and antidepressant response in major depressive disorders. *Neurosci Lett*, **414**(2), 155–158.

127 Ferreira, M.A., *et al.* (2008) Collaborative genome-wide association analysis supports a role for ANK3 and CACNA1C in bipolar disorder. *Nat Genet*, **40**(9), 1056–1058.

128 Silberberg, G., *et al.* (2008) Stargazin involvement with bipolar disorder and response to lithium treatment. *Pharmacogenet Genomics*, **18**(5), 403–412.

129 Lazary, J., *et al.* (2011) Epistatic interaction of CREB1 and KCNJ6 on rumination and negative emotionality. *Eur Neuropsychopharmacol*, **21**(1), 63–70.

130 Liou, Y.J., *et al.* (2009) Support for the involvement of the KCNK2 gene in major depressive disorder and response to antidepressant treatment. *Pharmacogenet Genomics*, **19**(10), 735–741.

131 Borsotto, M., *et al.* (2007) PP2A-Bgamma subunit and KCNQ2 K+ channels in bipolar disorder. *Pharmacogenomics J*, **7**(2), 123–132.

132 Tsai, S.J., *et al.* (2008) Glycogen synthase kinase-3beta gene is associated with antidepressant treatment response in Chinese major depressive disorder. *Pharmacogenomics J*, **8**(6), 384–390.

133 Ikeda, M., *et al.* (2008) Variants of dopamine and serotonin candidate genes as predictors of response to risperidone treatment in first-episode schizophrenia. *Pharmacogenomics*, **9**(10), 1437–1443.

134 Luo, H.R., *et al.* (2009) Association of PDE11A global haplotype with major depression and antidepressant drug response. *Neuropsychiatr Dis Treat*, **5**,163–170.

135 Wong, M.L., *et al.* (2006) Phosphodiesterase genes are associated with susceptibility to major depression and antidepressant treatment response. *Proc Natl Acad Sci U S A*, **103**(41), 15124–15129.

136 Kirchheiner, J., *et al.* (2008) Genetic variants in FKBP5 affecting response to antidepressant drug treatment. *Pharmacogenomics*, **9**(7), 841–846.

137 McHugh, P.C., *et al.* (2010) A polymorphism of the GTP-cyclohydrolase I feedback regulator gene alters transcriptional activity and may affect response to SSRI antidepressants. *Pharmacogenomics J*, epub 30 March.

138 Kohlrausch, F.B., *et al.* (2008) G-protein gene 825C>T polymorphism is associated with response to clozapine in Brazilian schizophrenics. *Pharmacogenomics*, **9**(10), 1429–1436.

139 Zill, P., *et al.* (2000) Evidence for an association between a G-protein beta3-gene variant with depression and response to antidepressant treatment. *Neuroreport*, **11**(9), 1893–1897.

140 Peerbooms, O.L., *et al.* (2010) Meta-analysis of MTHFR gene variants in schizophrenia, bipolar disorder and unipolar depressive disorder: evidence for a common genetic vulnerability? *Brain Behav Immun*, epub 24 December.

141 Gilbody, S., Lewis, S., Lightfoot, T. (2007) Methylenetetrahydrofolate reductase (MTHFR) genetic polymorphisms and psychiatric disorders: a HuGE review. *Am J Epidemiol*, **165**(1), 1–13.

142 Stefansson, H., *et al.* (2009) Common variants conferring risk of schizophrenia. *Nature*, **460**(7256), 744–747.

143 Mori, A., *et al.* (2005) UDP-glucuronosyltransferase 1A4 polymorphisms in a Japanese population and

kinetics of clozapine glucuronidation. *Drug Metab Dispos*, **33**(**5**), 672–675.

144 Zhou, S.F. (2009) Polymorphism of human cytochrome P450 2D6 and its clinical significance: part I. *Clin Pharmacokinet*, **48**(**11**), 689–723.

145 Kirchheiner, J., *et al.* (2011) CYP2D6 in the brain: genotype effects on resting brain perfusion. *Mol Psychiatry*, **16**(**3**), 333–341.

146 Dorado, P., Penas-Lledo, E.M., Llerena, A. (2007) CYP2D6 polymorphism: implications for antipsychotic drug response, schizophrenia and personality traits. *Pharmacogenomics*, **8**(**11**), 1597–1608.

147 Bromek, E., Haduch, A., Daniel, W.A. (2010) The ability of cytochrome P450 2D isoforms to synthesize dopamine in the brain: an in vitro study. *Eur J Pharmacol*, **626**(**2–3**), 171–178.

148 Yu, A.M., *et al.* (2003) Regeneration of serotonin from 5-methoxytryptamine by polymorphic human CYP2D6. *Pharmacogenetics*, **13**(**3**), 173–181.

149 Sridar, C., Snider, N.T., Hollenberg, P.F. (2011) Anandamide oxidation by wild type and polymorphically expressed CYP2B6 and CYP2D6. *Drug Metab Dispos*, epub 24 February.

150 Sim, S.C., *et al.* (2010) Association between CYP2C19 polymorphism and depressive symptoms. *Am J Med Genet B Neuropsychiatr Genet*, **153B**(**6**), 1160–1166.

151 Rudberg, I., *et al.* (2008) Impact of the ultrarapid CYP2C19*17 allele on serum concentration of escitalopram in psychiatric patients. *Clin Pharmacol Ther*, **83**(**2**),322–327.

152 Ohlsson Rosenborg, S., *et al.* (2008) Kinetics of omeprazole and escitalopram in relation to the CYP2C19*17 allele in healthy subjects. *Eur J Clin Pharmacol*, **64**(**12**), 1175–1179.

153 Rudberg, I., *et al.* (2008) Serum concentrations of sertraline and N-desmethyl sertraline in relation to CYP2C19 genotype in psychiatric patients. *Eur J Clin Pharmacol*, **64**(**12**), 1181–1188.

154 Li-Wan-Po, A., *et al.* (2010) Pharmacogenetics of CYP2C19: functional and clinical implications of a new variant CYP2C19*17. *Br J Clin Pharmacol*, **69**(**3**),222–230.

155 Laika, B., *et al.* (2010) Pharmacogenetics and olanzapine treatment: CYP1A2*1F and serotonergic polymorphisms influence therapeutic outcome. *Pharmacogenomics J*, **10**(**1**), 20–29.

156 Uhr, M., *et al.* (2008) Polymorphisms in the drug transporter gene ABCB1 predict antidepressant treatment response in depression. *Neuron*, **57**(**2**), 203–209.

157 Rosenhagen, M.C., Uhr, M. (2010) Single nucleotide polymorphism in the drug transporter gene ABCB1 in treatment-resistant depression: clinical practice. *J Clin Psychopharmacol*, **30**(**2**), 209–211.

158 Roberts, R.L., *et al.* (2002) A common P-glycoprotein polymorphism is associated with nortriptyline-induced postural hypotension in patients treated for major depression. *Pharmacogenomics J*, **2**(**3**), 191–196.

159 Hodges, L.M., *et al.* (2011) Very important pharmacogene summary: ABCB1 (MDR1, P-glycoprotein). *Pharmacogenet Genomics*, *2011*. **21**(**3**), 152–61.

160 Watanabe, T., *et al.* (2010) Functional characterization of 26 CYP2B6 allelic variants (CYP2B6.2-CYP2B6.28, except CYP2B6.22). *Pharmacogenet Genomics*, **20**(**7**), 459–462.

161 Yu, K.S., *et al.* (2001) Effect of omeprazole on the pharmacokinetics of moclobemide according to the genetic polymorphism of CYP2C19. *Clin Pharmacol Ther*, **69**(**4**), 266–273.

162 Cho, J.Y., *et al.* (2002) Omeprazole hydroxylation is inhibited by a single dose of moclobemide in homozygotic EM genotype for CYP2C19. *Br J Clin Pharmacol*, **53**(**4**), 393–397.

163 Kamada, T., *et al.* (2002) Metabolism of selegiline hydrochloride, a selective monoamine b-type inhibitor, in human liver microsomes. *Drug Metab Pharmacokinet*, **17**(**3**), 199–206.

164 de Leon, J. (2007) The crucial role of the therapeutic window in understanding the clinical relevance of the poor versus the ultrarapid metabolizer phenotypes in subjects taking drugs metabolized by CYP2D6 or CYP2C19. *J Clin Psychopharmacol*, **27**(**3**), 241–245.

165 Bijl, M.J., *et al.* (2008) Influence of the CYP2D6*4 polymorphism on dose, switching and discontinuation of antidepressants. *Br J Clin Pharmacol*, **65**(**4**), 558–564.

166 Hendset, M., *et al.* (2006) The complexity of active metabolites in therapeutic drug monitoring of psychotropic drugs. *Pharmacopsychiatry*, **39**(**4**), 121–127.

167 de Vos, A., van der Weide, J., Loovers, H.M. (2010) Association between CYP2C19*17 and metabolism of amitriptyline, citalopram and clomipramine in Dutch hospitalized patients. *Pharmacogenomics J*, epub 6 June.

168 Schenk, P.W., *et al.* (2010) The CYP2C19*17 genotype is associated with lower imipramine plasma concentrations in a large group of depressed patients. *Pharmacogenomics J*, **10**(**3**), 219–225.

169 Kirchheiner, J., *et al.* (2003) Effects of polymorphisms in CYP2D6, CYP2C9, and CYP2C19 on trimipramine pharmacokinetics. *J Clin Psychopharmacol*, **23**(**5**), 459–466.

170 Koski, A., *et al.* (2007) A fatal doxepin poisoning associated with a defective CYP2D6 genotype. *Am J Forensic Med Pathol*, **28**(**3**), 259–261.

171 Venkatakrishnan, K., *et al.* (1998) Five distinct human cytochromes mediate amitriptyline N-demethylation in vitro: dominance of CYP 2C19 and 3A4. *J Clin Pharmacol*, **38**(**2**), 112–121.

172 Koyama, E., *et al.* (1997) Reappraisal of human CYP isoforms involved in imipramine N-demethylation and 2-hydroxylation: a study using microsomes obtained from putative extensive and poor metabolizers of S-mephenytoin and eleven recombinant human CYPs. *J Pharmacol Exp Ther*, **281**(**3**), 1199–1210.

173 de Leon, J., Arranz, M.J., Ruano, G. (2008) Pharmacogenetic testing in psychiatry: a review of features and clinical realities. *Clin Lab Med*, **28**(**4**), 599–617.

174 Brachtendorf, L., *et al.* (2002) Cytochrome P450 enzymes contributing to demethylation of maprotiline in man. *Pharmacol Toxicol*, **90**(**3**), 144–149.

175 Wolf, C.R., Smith, G., Smith, R.L. (2000) Science, medicine, and the future: Pharmacogenetics. *BMJ*, **320**(**7240**), 987–990.

176 Anttila, A.K., Rasanen, L., Leinonen, E.V. (2001) Fluvoxamine augmentation increases serum mirtazapine concentrations three- to fourfold. *Ann Pharmacother*, **35**(**10**), 1221–3.

177 Lind, A.B., *et al.* (2009) Steady-state concentrations of mirtazapine, N-desmethylmirtazapine, 8-hydroxy-mirtazapine and their enantiomers in relation to cytochrome P450 2D6 genotype, age and smoking behaviour. *Clin Pharmacokinet*, **48**(**1**), 63–70.

178 Kirchheiner, J., *et al.* (2004) Impact of the CYP2D6 ultrarapid metabolizer genotype on mirtazapine pharmacokinetics and adverse events in healthy volunteers. *J Clin Psychopharmacol*, **24**(**6**), 647–652.

179 Kirchheiner, J., *et al.* (2004) Pharmacogenetics of antidepressants and antipsychotics: the contribution of allelic variations to the phenotype of drug response. *Mol Psychiatry*, **9**(**5**), 442–73.

180 Grasmader, K., *et al.* (2004) Impact of polymorphisms of cytochrome-P450 isoenzymes 2C9, 2C19 and 2D6 on plasma concentrations and clinical effects of antidepressants in a naturalistic clinical setting. *Eur J Clin Pharmacol*, **60**(**5**), 329–336.

181 Charlier, C., *et al.* (2003) Polymorphisms in the CYP 2D6 gene: association with plasma concentrations of fluoxetine and paroxetine. *Ther Drug Monit*, **25**(**6**), 738–742.

182 Scordo, M.G., *et al.* (2005) Influence of CYP2C9, 2C19 and 2D6 genetic polymorphisms on the steady-state plasma concentrations of the enantiomers of fluoxetine and norfluoxetine. *Basic Clin Pharmacol Toxicol*, **97**(**5**),296–301.

183 Llerena, A., *et al.* (2004) Effect of CYP2D6 and CYP2C9 genotypes on fluoxetine and norfluoxetine plasma concentrations during steady-state conditions. *Eur J Clin Pharmacol*, **59**(**12**), 869–873.

184 Liu, Z.Q., *et al.* (2001) Effects of CYP2C19 genotype and CYP2C9 on fluoxetine N-demethylation in human liver microsomes. *Acta Pharmacol Sin*, **22**(**1**), 85–90.

185 Laika, B., *et al.* (2009) Intermediate metabolizer: increased side effects in psychoactive drug therapy. The key to cost-effectiveness of pretreatment CYP2D6 screening[quest]. *Pharmacogenomics J*, **9**(**6**), 395–403.

186 Sato, A., *et al.* (2004) Life-threatening serotonin syndrome in a patient with chronic heart failure and CYP2D6*1/*5. *Mayo Clin Proc*, **79**(**11**), 1444–1448.

187 Lin, K.M., *et al.* (2010) CYP1A2 genetic polymorphisms are associated with treatment response to the antidepressant paroxetine. *Pharmacogenomics*, **11**(**11**), 1535–1543.

188 Suzuki, Y., *et al.* (2010) CYP2D6 genotype and smoking influence fluvoxamine steady-state concentration in Japanese psychiatric patients: lessons for genotype-phenotype association study design in translational pharmacogenetics. *J Psychopharmacol*, epub 14 June.

189 Katoh, Y., *et al.* (2010) Effects of cigarette smoking and cytochrome P450 2D6 genotype on fluvoxamine concentration in plasma of Japanese patients. *Biol Pharm Bull*, **33**(**2**), 285–288.

190 Tsai, M.H., *et al.* (2010) Genetic polymorphisms of cytochrome P450 enzymes influence metabolism of the antidepressant escitalopram and treatment response. *Pharmacogenomics*, **11**(**4**), 537–546.

191 Jin, Y., *et al.* (2010) Effect of age, weight, and CYP2C19 genotype on escitalopram exposure. *J Clin Pharmacol*, **50**(**1**), 62–72.

192 Noehr-Jensen, L., *et al.* (2009) Impact of CYP2C19 phenotypes on escitalopram metabolism and an evaluation of pupillometry as a serotonergic biomarker. *Eur J Clin Pharmacol*, **65**(**9**), 887–894.

193 Levin, T.T., *et al.* (2008) Life-threatening serotonin toxicity due to a citalopram-fluconazole drug interaction: case reports and discussion. *Gen Hosp Psychiatry*, **30**(4), 372–377.

194 Mrazek, D.A., *et al.* (2011) CYP2C19 variation and citalopram response. *Pharmacogenet Genomics*, **21**(1), 1–9.

195 Yin, O.Q., *et al.* (2006) Phenotype-genotype relationship and clinical effects of citalopram in Chinese patients. *J Clin Psychopharmacol*, **26**(4), 367–372.

196 Fudio, S., *et al.* (2010) Evaluation of the influence of sex and CYP2C19 and CYP2D6 polymorphisms in the disposition of citalopram. *Eur J Pharmacol*, **626**(2–3), 200–204.

197 Peters, E.J., *et al.* (2008) Pharmacokinetic genes do not influence response or tolerance to citalopram in the STAR*D sample. *PLoS One*, **3**(4), e1872.

198 Obach, R.S., Cox, L.M., Tremaine, L.M. (2005) Sertraline is metabolized by multiple cytochrome P450 enzymes, monoamine oxidases, and glucuronyl transferases in human: an in vitro study. *Drug Metab Dispos*, **33**(2), 262–270.

199 Xu, Z.H., *et al.* (1999) Evidence for involvement of polymorphic CYP2C19 and 2C9 in the N-demethylation of sertraline in human liver microsomes. *Br J Clin Pharmacol*, **48**(3), 416–423.

200 McAlpine, D.E., *et al.* (2007) Cytochrome P450 2D6 genotype variation and venlafaxine dosage. *Mayo Clin Proc*, **82**(9), 1065–1068.

201 Shams, M.E., *et al.* (2006) CYP2D6 polymorphism and clinical effect of the antidepressant venlafaxine. *J Clin Pharm Ther*, **31**(5), 493–502.

202 Lessard, E., *et al.* (1999) Influence of CYP2D6 activity on the disposition and cardiovascular toxicity of the antidepressant agent venlafaxine in humans. *Pharmacogenetics*, **9**(4), 435–443.

203 Lobello, K.W., *et al.* (2010) Cytochrome P450 2D6 phenotype predicts antidepressant efficacy of venlafaxine: a secondary analysis of 4 studies in major depressive disorder. *J Clin Psychiatry*, **71**(11), 1482–1487.

204 Preskorn, S.H. (2010) Understanding outliers on the usual dose-response curve: venlafaxine as a way to phenotype patients in terms of their CYP 2D6 status and why it matters. *J Psychiatr Pract*, **16**(1), 46–49.

205 Launiainen, T., *et al.* (2010) Fatal venlafaxine poisonings are associated with a high prevalence of drug interactions. *Int J Legal Med*, epub 30 April.

206 McAlpine, D.E., *et al.* (2011) Effect of cytochrome P450 enzyme polymorphisms on pharmacokinetics of venlafaxine. *Ther Drug Monit*, **33**(1), 14–20.

207 Fukuda, T., *et al.* (2000) The impact of the CYP2D6 and CYP2C19 genotypes on venlafaxine pharmacokinetics in a Japanese population. *Eur J Clin Pharmacol*, **56**(2), 175–180.

208 Knadler, M.P., *et al.* (2011) Duloxetine: clinical pharmacokinetics and drug interactions. *Clin Pharmacokinet*, epub 2 March.

209 Foley, K.F., DeSanty, K.P., Kast, R.E. (2006) Bupropion: pharmacology and therapeutic applications. *Expert Rev Neurother*, **6**(9), 1249–1265.

210 Kirchheiner, J., *et al.* (2003) Bupropion and 4-OH-bupropion pharmacokinetics in relation to genetic polymorphisms in CYP2B6. *Pharmacogenetics*, **13**(10), 619–626.

211 Rotzinger, S., *et al.* (1998) Human CYP2D6 and metabolism of m-chlorophenylpiperazine. *Biol Psychiatry*, **44**(11), 1185–1191.

212 Wen, B., *et al.* (2008) Detection of novel reactive metabolites of trazodone: evidence for CYP2D6-mediated bioactivation of m-chlorophenylpiperazine. *Drug Metab Dispos*, **36**(5), 841–850.

213 Aklillu, E., *et al.* (2007) CYP2D6 and DRD2 genes differentially impact pharmacodynamic sensitivity and time course of prolactin response to perphenazine. *Pharmacogenet Genomics*, **17**(11), 989–993.

214 Llerena, A., *et al.* (2004) Relationship between haloperidol plasma concentration, debrisoquine metabolic ratio, CYP2D6 and CYP2C9 genotypes in psychiatric patients. *Pharmacopsychiatry*, **37**(2), 69–73.

215 Desai, M., *et al.* (2003) Pharmacokinetics and QT interval pharmacodynamics of oral haloperidol in poor and extensive metabolizers of CYP2D6. *Pharmacogenomics J*, **3**(2), 105–113.

216 Brockmoller, J., *et al.* (2002) The impact of the CYP2D6 polymorphism on haloperidol pharmacokinetics and on the outcome of haloperidol treatment. *Clin Pharmacol Ther*, **72**(4), 438–452.

217 Park, J.Y., *et al.* (2006) Combined effects of itraconazole and CYP2D6*10 genetic polymorphism on the pharmacokinetics and pharmacodynamics of haloperidol in healthy subjects. *J Clin Psychopharmacol*, **26**(2), 135–142.

218 Ohara, K., *et al.* (2003) Effects of smoking and cytochrome P450 2D6*10 allele on the plasma haloperidol concentration/dose ratio. *Prog Neuropsychopharmacol Biol Psychiatry*, **27**(6), 945–949.

219 Athanasiou, M.C., *et al.* (2010) Candidate gene analysis identifies a polymorphism in HLA-DQB1 associated with clozapine-induced agranulocytosis. *J Clin Psychiatry*.

220 Jaquenoud Sirot, E., *et al.* (2009) ABCB1 and cytochrome P450 polymorphisms: clinical pharmacogenetics of clozapine. *J Clin Psychopharmacol*, **29**(4), 319–326.

221 van der Weide, J., Steijns, L.S., van Weelden, M.J. (2003) The effect of smoking and cytochrome P450 CYP1A2 genetic polymorphism on clozapine clearance and dose requirement. *Pharmacogenetics*, **13**(3), 169–172.

222 Eap, C.B., *et al.* (2004) Nonresponse to clozapine and ultrarapid CYP1A2 activity: clinical data and analysis of CYP1A2 gene. *J Clin Psychopharmacol*, **24**(2), 214–219.

223 Brouwers, E.E., *et al.* (2009) Ciprofloxacin strongly inhibits clozapine metabolism: two case reports. *Clin Drug Investig*, **29**(1), 59–63.

224 Arranz, M.J., *et al.* (1995) Cytochrome P4502D6 genotype does not determine response to clozapine. *Br J Clin Pharmacol*, **39**(4), 417–420.

225 de Leon, J., Wynn, G., Sandson, N.B. (2010) The pharmacokinetics of paliperidone versus risperidone. *Psychosomatics*, **51**(1), 80–88.

226 Urichuk, L., *et al.* (2008) Metabolism of atypical antipsychotics: involvement of cytochrome p450 enzymes and relevance for drug-drug interactions. *Curr Drug Metab*, **9**(5), 410–418.

227 Yasui-Furukori, N., *et al.* (2003) Effects of CYP2D6 genotypes on plasma concentrations of risperidone and enantiomers of 9-hydroxyrisperidone in Japanese patients with schizophrenia. *J Clin Pharmacol*, **43**(2), 122–1227.

228 Scordo, M.G., *et al.* (1999) Cytochrome P450 2D6 genotype and steady state plasma levels of risperidone and 9-hydroxyrisperidone. *Psychopharmacology (Berl)*, **147**(3), 300–305.

229 Troost, P.W., *et al.* (2007) Prolactin release in children treated with risperidone: impact and role of CYP2D6 metabolism. *J Clin Psychopharmacol*, **27**(1), 52–57.

230 Riedel, M., *et al.* (2005) Risperidone plasma levels, clinical response and side-effects. *Eur Arch Psychiatry Clin Neurosci*, **255**(4), 261–268.

231 Huang, M.L., *et al.* (1993) Pharmacokinetics of the novel antipsychotic agent risperidone and the prolactin response in healthy subjects. *Clin Pharmacol Ther*, **54**(3), 257–268.

232 de Leon, J., *et al.* (2005) The CYP2D6 poor metabolizer phenotype may be associated with risperidone adverse drug reactions and discontinuation. *J Clin Psychiatry*, **66**(1), 15–27.

233 de Leon, J., Armstrong, S.C., Cozza, K.L. (2006) Clinical guidelines for psychiatrists for the use of pharmacogenetic testing for CYP450 2D6 and CYP450 2C19. *Psychosomatics*, **47**(1), 75–85.

234 Llerena, A., *et al.* (2004) QTc interval, CYP2D6 and CYP2C9 genotypes and risperidone plasma concentrations. *J Psychopharmacol*, **18**(2), 189–193.

235 Yasui-Furukori, N., *et al.* (2004) Effects of various factors on steady-state plasma concentrations of risperidone and 9-hydroxyrisperidone: lack of impact of MDR-1 genotypes. *Br J Clin Pharmacol*, **57**(5), 569–575.

236 Xing, Q., *et al.* (2006) Polymorphisms of the ABCB1 gene are associated with the therapeutic response to risperidone in Chinese schizophrenia patients. *Pharmacogenomics*, **7**(7), 987–993.

237 Nakagami, T., *et al.* (2005) Effect of verapamil on pharmacokinetics and pharmacodynamics of risperidone: in vivo evidence of involvement of P-glycoprotein in risperidone disposition. *Clin Pharmacol Ther*, **78**(1), 43–51.

238 Kirchheiner, J.S.A., Viviani, R., Hodgkinson, S. (2010) One tablet or two? Towards the development of pharmacogenomically informed drug dose individualization. In: K.W. Schwab & E. Spina (eds), *Pharmacogenomics in Psychiatry*, 1–11. Krager, Basel.

239 Rodriguez-Antona, C., *et al.* (2009) CYP2D6 genotyping for psychiatric patients treated with risperidone: considerations for cost-effectiveness studies. *Pharmacogenomics*, **10**(4), 685–699.

240 Suzuki, T., *et al.* (2011) Effects of the CYP2D6*10 allele on the steady-state plasma concentrations of aripiprazole and its active metabolite, dehydroaripiprazole, in Japanese patients with schizophrenia. *Ther Drug Monit*, **33**(1), 21–24.

241 Swainston Harrison, T., Perry, C.M. (2004) Aripiprazole: a review of its use in schizophrenia and schizoaffective disorder. *Drugs*, **64**(15), 1715–1736.

242 Lin, Y.C., *et al.* (2006) The relationship between P-glycoprotein (PGP) polymorphisms and response to olanzapine treatment in schizophrenia. *Ther Drug Monit*, **28**(5), 668–672.

243 Prior, T.I., Baker, G.B. (2003) Interactions between the cytochrome P450 system and the second-generation antipsychotics. *J Psychiatry Neurosci*, **28**(2), 99–112.

244 Nikisch, G., *et al.* (2010) Cytochrome P450 and ABCB1 genetics: association with quetiapine and norquetiapine plasma and cerebrospinal fluid concentrations and with clinical response in patients suffering from schizophrenia: a pilot study. *J Psychopharmacol*, epub 8 December.

245 Sistonen, J., *et al.* (2007) CYP2D6 worldwide genetic variation shows high frequency of altered activity variants and no continental structure. *Pharmacogenet Genomics*, **17**(**2**), 93–101.

246 Seeringer, A., Kirchheiner, J. (2008) Pharmacogenetics-guided dose modifications of antidepressants. *Clin Lab Med*, **28**(**4**), 619–626.

CHAPTER 10

Pharmacogenomic Aspects of Adverse Drug–Drug Interactions

Loralie J. Langman, PhD and Christine L.H. Snozek, PhD
Department of Laboratory Medicine and Pathology, Mayo Clinic Rochester, Minnesota

Introduction

Adverse drug reaction (ADR, or adverse drug effect) is a broad term referring to any unwanted, uncomfortable, or dangerous effect that a drug may have (1). ADRs, including drug–drug interactions, are the fourth leading cause of death in the United States; ADRs are the cause of 3–7% of all hospitalizations, and occur during 10–20% of hospitalizations due to other causes. Incidence of death due to ADRs is unknown; suggested rates of 0.5–0.9% may be falsely high because many of the patients included had serious and complex disorders (1). Patients receive, on average, 10 different drugs during each hospitalization. The more ill the patient, the more drugs are given, with a corresponding increase in the likelihood of ADRs. When <6 different drugs are given to hospitalized patients, the probability of an adverse reaction is ~5%, but if >15 drugs are given, the probability is >40%. Even in ambulatory patients, ADRs occur 20% of the time (2). Drug interactions can complicate therapy by increasing or decreasing the action of one or more prescribed agents, and must be considered in the differential diagnosis of any unusual response occurring during pharmacological therapy (2).

Most ADRs are dose related; others are allergic or idiosyncratic. Dose-related reactions are particularly a concern when drugs have a narrow therapeutic index, that is, when the drug levels associated with desired responses are close to those that induce toxicity. Dose-related effects are usually predictable; ADRs unrelated to dose are unpredictable. Prescribers should recognize that patients often come to them with a legacy of drugs acquired during previous medical experiences, often with multiple physicians who may not be aware of all the patient's medications. A meticulous drug history should include examination of the patient's medications. It should also address the use of agents not often volunteered during questioning, such as over-the-counter (OTC) medicines, health food supplements, topical agents, and illicit drugs. Serious adverse reactions have been recognized with "herbal" remedies and OTC compounds: examples include kava-associated hepatotoxicity, L-tryptophan-associated eosinophilia-myalgia, and phenylpropanolamine-associated stroke, each of which has caused fatalities. While it is unrealistic to expect the practicing physician to memorize the entire list of potentially toxic compounds, certain drugs consistently run the risk of generating interactions, often by inhibiting or inducing specific drug elimination pathways (2). A small group of widely used drugs accounts for a disproportionate number of reactions. Aspirin and other NSAIDs, acetaminophen, opioid analgesics, digoxin, anticoagulants, diuretics, antimicrobials, glucocorticoids, antineoplastics, and hypoglycemic agents account for 90% of reactions, although the specific drugs involved differ between ambulatory and hospitalized patients (2).

Types of drug interactions

Drug interactions are changes in a drug's effects due to recent or concurrent use of one or more other xenobiotic agents (drug–drug interactions) or due to ingestion of food (drug–nutrient interactions). A drug interaction may increase or decrease the effects of one or both drugs involved. One can describe drug–drug interactions based on the type of physiological response: the effect can be additive, synergistic, potentiating, or antagonistic (Table 10.1). An additive interaction is the most common, and occurs when the combined response to two chemicals is equal to the sum of the effects of each agent given alone (3, 4). For example, when exposure to two organophosphate pesticides occurs together, the degree of cholinesterase inhibition is roughly the sum of the inhibition that would have resulted from each agent alone. A synergistic interaction occurs when the combined effects of two chemicals are much greater than the sum of responses to each individual agent (3, 4). For example, both ethanol and carbon tetrachloride induce liver disease, but when they are co-ingested, the resulting hepatotoxicity is much more severe than the sum of each compound's effect in isolation (4). Potentiation reactions occur when one substance by itself does not have a significant effect on a given organ or system, but when combined with another agent, increase the response to the second compound (3). For example, isopropanol does not induce liver damage when taken in isolation, but when taken with carbon tetrachloride, the hepatotoxicity is greater than that expected from carbon tetrachloride alone.

Antagonism occurs when two substances interfere with each other's action, or one interferes with the action of the other. There are four types of antagonism: functional, chemical, dispositional, and receptor (3). Functional antagonism occurs when two drugs counterbalance each other by producing opposite effect of the same physiologic function. For example, when one drug produces seizures, it can be functionally antagonized by giving an anticonvulsant. Chemical antagonism (or inactivation) is simply a chemical reaction between two compounds that produces a less toxic compound. For example, in the presence of chelating agent, heavy metals are prevented from reaching target molecules, thus their toxic effects are reduced. Dispositional antagonism occurs when the pharmacokinetics (PK) of a drug are altered such that its concentration at the target site or duration of action is diminished. This could occur in any or all of the PK processes of absorption, distribution, metabolism, or elimination. Receptor antagonism occurs when two drugs with the same target receptor counteract the expected downstream pharmacodynamic (PD) responses to one or both agents. PK- and PD-based drug interactions, both antagonistic and agonistic, will be discussed in further detail below.

Pharmacogenetics of drug–drug interactions

Drugs interact with specific target molecules to produce their effects. The chain of events between drug administration and physiological response can be described as two series of processes, both of which contribute to variability in how a specific individual reacts to a given compound. The first series, PK, is composed of the processes that determine the rate at which the drug arrives at, and is removed from, molecular targets; in other words, PK describes the relationship between drug concentration and time (2). The second series of processes, PD, is the relationship between drug concentration and effect, and includes the description of variability in

Table 10.1 Classification of Drug Interactions

Type of Interaction	Magnitude of Effect of Drug 1	Magnitude of Effect of Drug 2	Net Effect
Additive	2	2	4
Synergistic	2	2	10
Potentiation	0	2	10
Antagonism	4	6	8
	4	−4	0
	4	0	1

physiological responses despite equivalent drug delivery to effector sites (2).

In PK-based drug interactions, one drug alters absorption, distribution, protein binding, metabolism, or excretion of another drug, and therefore, the amount and duration of available drug at receptor sites are affected (3, 4). PK interactions alter the magnitude and duration of a drug's effect, not its type. They are often predicted based on knowledge of the individual drugs, or detected by monitoring drug concentrations or clinical signs (1). In PD interactions, one drug alters the sensitivity or responsiveness of the body to another drug by having the same (agonistic) or a blocking (antagonistic) effect at the site of action. These effects usually occur at the receptor level but may occur intracellularly (1, 3, 4).

The incidence and severity of ADRs vary depending on patient characteristics (e.g., age, sex, ethnicity, coexisting disorders, and genetics) and drug factors (e.g., drug type, administration route, treatment duration, dosage, and co-prescribed medications) (1). Pharmacogenetics (PGx) is the study of the genetic contribution to variations in drug response. If PD is what a drug does to the body and PK is what the body does to the drug, then PGx can be viewed as the genetic driver that controls both. Select examples of PGx and its role in drug–drug interactions involving PK and PD will be discussed.

Pharmacokinetic interactions

All stages of PK can be influenced by the genetic makeup of the individual. Absorption, distribution, and elimination all may be influenced by genetic alterations in drug transporters, for example. However, the area of PK that is the most studied for genetic variability is metabolism. The activity of drug-metabolizing enzymes often differs widely among healthy people: drug elimination rates can vary up to 40-fold between individuals, even in the absence of confounding factors such as disease (1). Drugs can be metabolized by oxidation, reduction, hydrolysis, hydration, conjugation, condensation, or isomerization; whatever the process, the goal is to make the drug easier to excrete. As discussed throughout this book, variation in the rates at which these processes occur can have clinical consequences (1). Some

patients may metabolize a given drug so rapidly that therapeutically effective blood and tissue concentrations are not reached, while in others, metabolism may be so slow that usual doses have toxic effects.

The enzymes involved in metabolism are present in many tissues but generally are more concentrated in the liver (1). The most important family of Phase I (nonconjugation reactions) metabolic enzymes are the cytochromes P450 (CYPs), which are involved to varying degrees in the biotransformation of the vast majority of drugs. CYP activity is age dependent: children have the highest metabolic rates, whereas with aging, hepatic CYP function is reduced by $\geq 30\%$ because liver volume and hepatic blood flow are decreased. Thus, drugs that are metabolized through this system reach higher levels and have prolonged half-lives in the elderly, who are therefore at greater risk for PK drug interactions (1). In addition to age-related differences, CYP enzymes can be induced or inhibited by many drugs and other substances (1). Shared substrates of a single enzyme can compete for access to the active site of the protein; however, some drugs are especially potent as inhibitors or inducers of specific drug elimination pathways, of which they may or may not also be substrates (2). Genetics are an important aspect of CYP-mediated metabolism, as will be discussed below; wild-type alleles confer an extensive metabolizer (EM) phenotype, in contrast to alleles conferring severely reduced (poor metabolizer, PM), mildly reduced (intermediate metabolizer, IM), or enhanced (ultra-rapid metabolizer, UM) phenotypes.

An excellent example of a PK interaction involving enzyme inhibition is the role of CYP2D6 in tamoxifen therapy for breast cancer. The drug is extensively metabolized by CYP2D6 and other enzymes. Several metabolites possess equal or greater anti-estrogenic activity compared to tamoxifen, and one metabolite, endoxifen, is considered the primary active form of the drug (5, 6). The influence of *CYP2D6* genotype in tamoxifen metabolism and clinical response has been shown in a number of studies. During tamoxifen treatment, women with two or more fully functional copies of CYP2D6 have higher plasma endoxifen concentrations than patients with at least one null allele (3–7). The influence of *CYP2D6* variant alleles has also been documented in terms of side effects such as hot flashes (which appear to correlate with efficacy) and treatment outcome (8–11). *CYP2D6* PM cannot efficiently convert tamoxifen to endoxifen, and therefore have fewer hot flashes and less anticancer benefit than EM. A similar phenomenon occurs due to a drug–drug interaction between tamoxifen and inhibitors of CYP2D6 activity. In the presence of CYP2D6 inhibitors such as fluoxetine or other antidepressants (often given to reduce discomfort from hot flashes), endoxifen plasma concentrations are decreased (7, 9, 12, 13), which likely renders tamoxifen therapy less effective (14, 15). In fact, very potent CYP2D6 inhibitors have been shown to reduce endoxifen concentrations in EM to levels comparable to the endoxifen concentrations seen in PM (7). This is referred to as a *phenocopy*, that is, a phenotype induced by environmental factors (in this case, enzymatic activity reduced by co-medications) which mimics a different genotype.

A less well-studied question is what effect the presence of an enzyme inhibitor would have on an IM or PM genotype. Conceptually, someone with an IM phenotype would be at increased risk compared to an EM for PK drug interactions, because the IM would have less baseline metabolic activity to support, for example, addition of another drug metabolized by the same enzyme. However, the degree to which metabolism is impaired by IM variants may differ between substrates. With *CYP2D6*, it was found that the protein expressed from recombinant *CYP2D6*10* showed severely impaired demethylation of codeine and fluoxetine, and O-demethylation of dextromethorphan, but displayed only moderate impairment in N-demethylation of dextromethorphan (16). This suggests that IM variants may be more susceptible to interactions between certain combinations of drugs – those which display more severely altered metabolism – compared to substrates whose metabolism is less affected by the specific variant allele. Unfortunately, the process of detailing substrate-specific metabolism for the multitudes of IM alleles that have been described is still in its infancy.

In contrast to IM, PM genotypes may confer relative resistance to drug interactions involving the variant enzyme. It is unlikely that the presence of an inhibitor or inducer would have a significant influence on the enzymatic activity, since, simply put, there is no active enzyme to inhibit or induce. In the example of tamoxifen therapy, *CYP2D6* PM treated with fluoxetine would be expected to receive comparable (i.e., very little) clinical benefit to PM individuals who do not receive the antidepressant. However, it is possible that a drug may be shunted to alternate pathways of metabolism, which has the potential to cause unexpected drug–drug interactions due to the unusual reliance upon those pathways. UM individuals may also resistant to enzyme inhibitors, because the excess metabolic capacity could likely absorb a large degree of inhibition before clinical effects became noticeable. However, if dosage of a drug were increased to accommodate the UM's higher metabolism, it may be necessary to step down to a standard dose if enzyme inhibition results in a more EM-like phenotype.

Although metabolic interactions are currently the best studied, PK interactions can also occur during absorption, distribution, or excretion of a drug. Drug transport plays a vital role in most PK processes, and data are emerging regarding the influence of genetic variation in transporter proteins. One important transporter is P-glycoprotein (P-gp), which is a 170 kDa, 1280 amino acid transmembrane protein belonging to the ATP- binding cassette (ABC) superfamily of transport proteins. P-gp is encoded by the multidrug resistance gene (*MDR1* or *ABCB1*). In humans, two MDR genes, MDR1 and MDR3 (also called MDR2), have been described but only the *MDR1* gene product appears to be involved in drug transport (17). In the human gastrointestinal tract, P-gp is found in high concentrations on the apical surfaces of epithelial cells of the colon, distal small bowel, small biliary ductules, small ductules of the pancreas, proximal ductules of the kidneys, and adrenal glands (18). In the brain, P-gp is richly expressed on the subapical surface of the choroid plexus epithelium (which forms the blood–cerebrospinal fluid [CSF] barrier) as well as the luminal surfaces of capillary endothelial cells (which form the blood–brain barrier) (19–22). In blood, peripheral mononuclear cells, macrophages, natural killer cells, dendritic cells, and T and B lymphocytes all express P-gp at varying levels (23).

P-gp and other ABC transporters serve as barriers against entry of compounds into the body or into tissues. This has obvious implications in regulating the absorption and distribution of drugs and other xenobiotics, but can also indirectly affect metabolism by limiting the entry of a drug into hepatocytes. Furthermore, P-gp participates in removal of drugs by exporting them from cells, either out of tissues and into the blood for clearance, or out of the body at sites of elimination such as intestinal cells. Consequently, drug interactions or genetic variations that alter the function or expression of P-gp can substantially affect a large number of drugs (24). Because the specifics of PK may be different for various P-gp substrates, it is important to consider which process is the rate-limiting step, that is, whether drug transport is a bottleneck for absorption, distribution, metabolism, or elimination of the compound in question.

P-gp kinetics are saturable, therefore its role is most critical when the therapeutic concentration of the substrate drug is low (e.g., digoxin, fexofenadine, and talinolol) (25). Moreover, P-gp activity can influence the penetration of drugs not only into the blood, but also into compartments where the drug may have activity (24). Loperamide is an opioid antidiarrheal that is normally kept out of the brain due to P-gp-mediated export. However, when given with the P-gp inhibitor quinidine, loperamide is not effectively removed from the CSF; this leads to accumulation of the opioid in the brain and depression of the respiratory control center (26). Genetic variation in *MDR1* has been associated with similar effects on P-gp function. Numerous single-nucleotide polymorphisms (SNPs) have been identified, but a synonymous SNP in exon 26 (C3435T) was the first variant to be associated with altered protein expression. Although the SNP does not change the encoded amino acid isoleucine, it has been shown to decrease intestinal P-gp expression and thereby reduce plasma concentrations of substrate drugs such as digoxin (27). This genotype has also been shown to be a risk factor for the side effect of orthostatic hypotension with the P-gp substrate nortriptyline (28). P-gp is just the beginning of a much larger area of study: SNPs in other drug transporters such as the MDR-related proteins (MRP1, MRP2, etc.) are also emerging as regulators of PK in individual patients. Potential implications of genetic variants in metabolic enzymes and drug transporters as modulators of PK interactions will be discussed in a later section.

Pharmacodynamic interactions

PD interactions are less well characterized than PK interactions, they are but no less important. Many drugs interact with a receptor protein to initiate the steps leading to physiological response(s) to that particular compound. PD interactions are frequently due to effects at the site of action (i.e., the ninteraction of more than one drug with the same receptor or downstream effectors). This is analogous to the mechanism of action of a number of drugs. For example, tamoxifen interacts with the estrogen receptor in various tissues (e.g., breast and endometrial) to modulate the effects of endogenous estrogen (29, 30). This pharmacological activity is essentially an intentional PD interaction whereby tamoxifen diminishes the response of breast epithelial cells and breast cancers to estrogen. Some of the adverse effects of the drug, such as heightened risk for endometrial cancer, are also due to PD interactions; in this case, tamoxifen actually enhances endometrial cell response to endogenous estrogen, which can predispose a patient on tamoxifen therapy to increased likelihood of malignant transformation of this tissue (31).

In the case of opioid drugs, such as morphine, oxycodone, and fentanyl, the opioid receptor is the site of action. Endogenous receptors for opiates were reported in 1973 (32–34) and consist of the mu (MOR), delta (DOR), and kappa (KOR) receptors, encoded by *OPRM1*, *OPRD1*, and *OPRK1*, respectively. Endogenous ligands have been described, such as endorphins and enkephalins, polypeptides that are involved in innate responses to pain. The MOR is essential for morphine analgesia, physical dependence, and reward (35). Many variants, particularly SNPs, have been identified throughout *OPRM1* and tested for association with addiction to opiates, cocaine, and other substances. To date, the best-studied *OPRM1* polymorphism is a base change at position 118 from adenine to guanine (A118G) that alters the protein sequence at residue 40 from asparagine to aspartate (36, 37). The A118G substitution leads to the loss of a putative glycosylation site in the N-terminal domain of the receptor (36, 37). The glycosylation of G protein-coupled receptors such as the MOR is important in mediating appropriate protein conformation for receptor trafficking to the cell membrane (38–40).

Most studies of *OPRM1* to date have examined the functional consequences of the A118G SNP in vitro using cell culture systems. In these studies it was noted that the binding affinity for beta-endorphin was threefold higher in the G118 allele as compared to the A118 allele. However, this was not seen with exogenous ligands (37). Additional studies showed that both DAMGO ([D-Ala2, N-MePhe4, Gly-ol]-enkephalin) and morphine caused greater inhibition of Ca^{2+} current in neurons expressing the G118 variant (41). This allele-specific effect was not seen with morphine-6-glucuronide or endomorphin I, again suggesting enhanced response of the G118 receptor to some (but not all) exogenous and endogenous opioid compounds. These findings may contribute to the variability of responses to opiates observed with carriers of the mutant allele.

Opioid receptors mediate both the desired effects (e.g., analgesia) and ADRs such as constipation and drowsiness. Antidotes are frequently based on intentional drug–drug PD interactions; opioid antagonists have been used in the treatment of opioid-induced toxicity, especially central respiratory depression, which can be life-threatening (42). The prototypical opioid antagonist, naloxone, binds nonspecifically to all three receptor types, with the greatest effect at the MOR (42, 43). In the absence of an opioid agonist, typical doses of naloxone produce no discernible subjective effects in humans, but in the presence of an opioid agonist, naloxone can prevent or promptly reverse the effects (42). Because of its ability to block activation of opioid receptors, naloxone is used to treat opioid overdose and acts rapidly to reverse respiratory depression. However, it should be used cautiously because it also can precipitate withdrawal symptoms in opioid-dependent subjects and cause undesirable cardiovascular side effects.

One of the few pharmacogenetic evaluations of a drug–drug interaction demonstrated that, in neurons exposed chronically to morphine, naloxone-induced withdrawal was differentially regulated by the A118 and G118 receptor isoforms (44). Although this in vitro study has not been extended to animal models to define the in vivo implications, these findings support the hypothesis that genetic variation can regulate individual response to PD drug interactions. Given the large number of endogenous and exogenous opioid receptor ligands, it may be that other combinations of drugs interact differently at the MOR based on genotype, potentially leading to atypical and unpredictable PD interactions.

Conclusion and potential applications

In theory, knowledge of an individual's genotype for key PK- and PD-related molecules should allow for prediction of how that person will react to an administered drug, in terms of both overall exposure to the drug and physiological response. By extension, genotypic data could also provide information as to whether that individual is at risk for ADRs or undesirable drug interactions. However, few studies have actually been done to assess the utility of prospective analysis of polymorphic genes in predicting response to a single drug. The clinical trials of tamoxifen in CYP2D6 PM described above are excellent examples of prospective confirmation of hypothesis generated through retrospective analyses; most other areas of PGx lag behind this field (45). To the authors' knowledge, no clinical trials have been performed to date prospectively assessing genotype as a tool to predict risk for drug interactions.

As assays for pharmacogenetically relevant polymorphisms become more widespread, it is likely that prospective studies of the role of PGx in ADRs and drug interactions will become feasible. Warfarin is an interesting, if controversial, example of one of the first drugs that is approaching clinical utility. Polymorphisms in a metabolic enzyme (*CYP2C9*) and a drug target (*VKORC1*) have been associated with variability in response to warfarin therapy (46, 47), yet despite years of retrospective study, the first large, multicenter prospective trial assessing the utility of genotyping in avoiding ADRs was only recently published (48) The authors found that prospective genotyping prior to initiating warfarin therapy   successfully   reduced   hospitalization, especially for bleeding or thrombotic events. The economic impact of avoiding warfarin ADRs is likely to be large, given that it is one of the most commonly prescribed drugs in Western countries, and is associated with extremely high variability in patient response leading to significant morbidity and mortality.

The utility of PGx in predicting drug interactions has yet to be tested clinically, yet the combination of an aging population and increase in multidrug therapy indicates that this is a vitally important area of study. One would predict that greater knowledge of PK-relevant genetic variants would allow the normalization of individual patients' exposure to administered drugs, while PD-related polymorphisms may inform prediction of "unexpected" drug reactions during polypharmacy. The most promising targets for PGx in relation to drug interactions are likely the metabolic enzymes, particularly the CYPs: they are the best characterized to date as far as polymorphisms, with extensive knowledge of which drugs are major substrates for specific enzymes.

PK interactions are already being exploited clinically, for example with the use of ritonavir in highly active antiretroviral therapy (HAART) for treatment of HIV-positive patients. Ritonavir is active against HIV, but it is most commonly combined with other HAART agents because it is a potent inhibitor of CYP3A4, the enzyme that metabolizes several other HAART drugs (49). The inclusion of ritonavir therefore prolongs exposure to the second agent; this PK interaction is a potential cost-reducing means of using lower doses of the second agent without sacrificing efficacy (49). Similarly, determining the genotype of enzymes with clinically relevant polymorphisms and multiple substrates (e.g., CYP2D6) may allow patient-specific selection of drugs to avoid situations of likely PK interactions (e.g., two substrates given to an IM), or to intentionally create them (e.g., an inhibitor given to an EM to reduce the required dose of a second drug).

The study of PD-relevant genes lags somewhat behind that of PK-related genes. Treatment of drug addiction is one potential field where PGx may allow prediction of drug interactions. In the case of the A118G SNP in *OPRM1*, the difference in naloxone-precipitated withdrawal may be important in determining which patients can safely be treated with the antagonist during opioid overdose. Further, the polymorphism may affect the safety or efficacy of combined agents such as Suboxone, wherein buprenorphine is combined with naloxone (42): if Suboxone is taken properly, the naloxone is poorly absorbed, but if Suboxone is used inappropriately (e.g., injected), naloxone enters the body and induces withdrawal symptoms (50). This is an excellent example of intentional use of PD interactions for therapeutic purposes; however, the genetic understanding of individual responses to combined therapy requires a great deal of further study before PGx can be clinically useful to predict individual outcomes.

As pharmacogenetic knowledge grows, it is likely that its utility will eventually expand to encompass the PK and PD of multidrug therapy. The need for better individualization of pharmacological therapy is clear, even with monotherapy. It is usually the patients with the most severe medical conditions who require the largest number of drugs and are at the highest risk of ADRs and drug interactions; ironically, these are the exact patients who current PGx understanding is least able to accommodate because of the complexity of their treatment. As discussed throughout this book, the first inroads have been made into applications of PGx to predict and optimize outcomes with a single agent. The next steps forward must include consideration of multiple drugs and potential interactions.

References

1 Porter, R.S., Kaplan, J.L. (2011) Clinical pharmacology. In: R.S. Porter, and J.L. Kaplan (eds), *The Merck Manuals Online Library*. Merck Sharp & Dohme, New York.

2 Roden, D.M. (2008) Principles of clinical pharmacology. In: A. Fauci, E. Braunwald, D. Kasper, S. Hauser, D. Longo, J. Jameson, J. Loscalzo (eds.), *Harrison's Principles of Internal Medicine*, 17th ed. McGraw-Hill, New York.

3 Eaton, D.L., Gilbert, S.G. (2010) Principles of toxicology. In: J.B.I. Watkins and C. Klaassen (eds), *Essentials of Toxicology*, 2nd ed. McGraw-Hill, New York.

4 Eaton, D.L., Gilbert, S.G. (2007) Principles of toxicology. In: C. Klaassen (ed.), *Toxicology: The Basic Science of Poisons*, 7th ed. McGraw-Hill, New York.

5 Stearns, V., Johnson, M.D., Rae, J.M., *et al.* (2003) Active tamoxifen metabolite plasma concentrations after coadministration of tamoxifen and the selective serotonin reuptake inhibitor paroxetine. *Journal of the National Cancer Institute*, **95**, 1758–1764.

6 Lim, Y.C., Desta, Z., Flockhart, D.A., *et al.* (2005) Endoxifen (4-hydroxy-N-desmethyl-tamoxifen) has anti-estrogenic effects in breast cancer cells with potency similar to 4-hydroxy-tamoxifen. *Cancer Chemotherapy and Pharmacology*, **55**, 471–478.

7 Jin, Y., Desta, Z., Stearns, V., *et al.* (2005) CYP2D6 genotype, antidepressant use, and tamoxifen metabolism during adjuvant breast cancer treatment. *Journal of the National Cancer Institute*, **97**, 30–39.

8 Goetz, M.P., Rae, J.M., Suman, V.J., *et al.* (2005) Pharmacogenetics of tamoxifen biotransformation is associated with clinical outcomes of efficacy and hot flashes. *Journal of Clinical Oncology*, **23**, 9312–9318.

9 Borges, S., Desta, Z., Li, L., *et al.* (2006) Quantitative effect of CYP2D6 genotype and inhibitors on tamoxifen metabolism: implication for optimization of breast cancer treatment. *Clinical Pharmacology and Therapeutics*, **80**, 61–74.

10 Kiyotani, K., Mushiroda, T., Sasa, M., *et al.* (2008) Impact of CYP2D6*10 on recurrence-free survival in breast cancer patients receiving adjuvant tamoxifen therapy. *Cancer Science*, **99**, 995–999.

11 Xu, Y., Sun, Y., Yao, L., *et al.* (2008) Association between CYP2D6 *10 genotype and survival of breast cancer patients receiving tamoxifen treatment. *Annals of Oncology*, **19**, 1423–1429.

12 Lien, E.A., Solheim, E., Kvinnsland, S., *et al.* (1988) Identification of 4-hydroxy-N-desmethyltamoxifen as a metabolite of tamoxifen in human bile. *Cancer Research*, **48**, 2304–2308.

13 Loibl, S., Schwedler, K., von Minckwitz, G., *et al.* (2007) Venlafaxine is superior to clonidine as treatment of hot flashes in breast cancer patients: a double-blind, randomized study. *Annals of Oncology*, **18**, 689–693.

14 Bijl, M.J., van Schaik, R.H., Lammers, L.A., *et al.* (2009) The CYP2D6*4 polymorphism affects breast cancer survival in tamoxifen users. *Breast Cancer Research and Treatment*, **103**.

15 Goetz, M.P., Knox, S.K., Suman, V.J., *et al.* (2007) The impact of cytochrome P450 2D6 metabolism in women receiving adjuvant tamoxifen. *Breast Cancer Research and Treatment*, **101**, 113–121.

16 Yu, A., Kneller, B.M., Rettie, A.E., *et al.* (2002) Expression, purification, biochemical characterization, and comparative function of human cytochrome P450

2D6.1, 2D6.2, 2D6.10, and 2D6.17 allelic isoforms. *The Journal of Pharmacology and Experimental Therapeutics*, **303**, 1291–1300.

17 Fardel, O., Payen, L., Courtois, A., *et al.* (2001) Regulation of biliary drug efflux pump expression by hormones and xenobiotics. *Toxicology*, **167**, 37–46.

18 Thiebaut, F., Tsuruo, T., Hamada, H., *et al.* (1987) Cellular localization of the multidrug-resistance gene product P-glycoprotein in normal human tissues. *Proceedings of the National Academy of Sciences of the United States of America*, **84**, 7735–7738.

19 Wijnholds, J., Evers, R., van Leusden, M.R., *et al.* (1997) Increased sensitivity to anticancer drugs and decreased inflammatory response in mice lacking the multidrug resistance-associated protein. *Nature Medicine*, **3**, 1275–1279.

20 Rao, V.V., Dahlheimer, J.L., Bardgett, M.E., *et al.* (1999) Choroid plexus epithelial expression of MDR1 P glycoprotein and multidrug resistance-associated protein contribute to the blood-cerebrospinal-fluid drug-permeability barrier. *Proceedings of the National Academy of Sciences of the United States of America*, **96**, 3900–3905.

21 Cordon-Cardo, C., O'Brien, J.P., Casals, D., *et al.* (1989) Multidrug-resistance gene (P-glycoprotein) is expressed by endothelial cells at blood–brain barrier sites. *Proceedings of the National Academy of Sciences of the United States of America*, **86**, 695–698.

22 Zhao, J.Y., Ikeguchi, M., Eckersberg, T., *et al.* (1993) Modulation of multidrug resistance gene expression by dexamethasone in cultured hepatoma cells. *Endocrinology*, **133**, 521–528.

23 Klimecki, W.T., Futscher, B.W., Grogan, T.M., *et al.* (1994) P-glycoprotein expression and function in circulating blood cells from normal volunteers. *Blood*, **83**, 2451–2458.

24 Brinkmann, U., Eichelbaum, M. (2001) Polymorphisms in the ABC drug transporter gene MDR1. *The Pharmacogenomics Journal*, **1**, 59–64.

25 Marzolini, C., Paus, E., Buclin, T., *et al.* (2004) Polymorphisms in human MDR1 (P-glycoprotein): recent advances and clinical relevance. *Clinical Pharmacology and Therapeutics*, **75**, 13–33.

26 Sadeque, A.J., Wandel, C., He, H., *et al.* (2000) Increased drug delivery to the brain by P-glycoprotein inhibition. *Clinical Pharmacology and Therapeutics*, **68**, 231–237.

27 Hoffmeyer, S., Burk, O., von Richter, O., *et al.* (2000) Functional polymorphisms of the human multidrug-resistance gene: multiple sequence variations and correlation of one allele with P-glycoprotein expression

and activity in vivo. *Proceedings of the National Academy of Sciences of the United States of America*, **97**, 3473–3478.

28 Roberts, R.L., Joyce, P.R., Mulder, R.T., *et al.* (2002) A common P-glycoprotein polymorphism is associated with nortriptyline-induced postural hypotension in patients treated for major depression. *The Pharmacogenomics Journal*, **2**, 191–196.

29 Loose, D.S., Stancel, G.M. (2006) Estrogens and progestins. In: L.L. Brunton, J.S. Lazo, and K.L. Parker (eds.), *Goodman & Gilman's The Pharmacological Basis of Therapeutics*, 11th ed. McGraw-Hill, New York.

30 Osborne, C.K. (1998) Tamoxifen in the treatment of breast cancer. *The New England Journal of Medicine*, **339**, 1609–1618.

31 Lee, K.H., Ward, B.A., Desta, Z., *et al.* (2003) Quantification of tamoxifen and three metabolites in plasma by high-performance liquid chromatography with fluorescence detection: application to a clinical trial. *Journal of Chromatography*, **791**, 245–253.

32 Pert, C.B., Snyder, S.H. (1973) Opiate receptor: demonstration in nervous tissue. *Science*, **179**, 1011–1014.

33 Simon, E.J., Hiller, J.M., Edelman, I. (1973) Stereospecific binding of the potent narcotic analgesic (3H) Etorphine to rat-brain homogenate. *Proceedings of the National Academy of Sciences of the United States of America*, **70**, 1947–1949.

34 Terenius, L. (1973) Stereospecific interaction between narcotic analgesics and a synaptic plasm a membrane fraction of rat cerebral cortex. *Acta Pharmacologica et Toxicologica*, **32**, 317–320.

35 Becker, A., Grecksch, G., Brodemann, R., *et al.* (2000) Morphine self-administration in mu-opioid receptor-deficient mice. *Naunyn Schmiedebergs Archive of Pharmacology*, **361**, 584–589.

36 Bergen, A.W., Kokoszka, J., Peterson, R., *et al.* (1997) Mu opioid receptor gene variants: lack of association with alcohol dependence. *Molecular Psychiatry*, **2**, 490–494.

37 Bond, C., LaForge, K.S., Tian, M., *et al.* (1998) Single-nucleotide polymorphism in the human mu opioid receptor gene alters beta-endorphin binding and activity: possible implications for opiate addiction. *Proceedings of the National Academy of Sciences of the United States of America*, **95**, 9608–9613.

38 George, S.T., Ruoho, A.E., Malbon, C.C. (1986) N-glycosylation in expression and function of beta-adrenergic receptors. *Journal of Biological Chemistry*, **261**, 16559–16564.

39 Hughes, R.J., Pasillas, M., Saiz, J., *et al.* (1997) Decreased transcript expression coincident with

impaired glycosylation in the beta2-adrenergic receptor gene does not result from differences in the primary sequence. *Biochimica Biophysica Acta*, **1356**, 281–291.

40 Petaja-Repo, U.E., Hogue, M., Laperriere, A., *et al.* (2000) Export from the endoplasmic reticulum represents the limiting step in the maturation and cell surface expression of the human delta opioid receptor. *Journal of Biological Chemistry*, **275**, 13727–13736.

41 Margas, W., Zubkoff, I., Schuler, H.G., *et al.* (2007) Modulation of Ca2+ channels by heterologously expressed wild-type and mutant human micro-opioid receptors (hMORs) containing the A118G single-nucleotide polymorphism. *Journal of Neurophysiology*, **97**, 1058–1067.

42 Gutstein, H.B., Akil, H. (2006) Opioid analgesics. In: L. L. Brunton, J.S. Lazo, and K.L. Parker (eds), *Goodman & Gilman's The Pharmacological Basis of Therapeutics*, 11th ed. McGraw-Hill, New York.

43 Trescot, A.M., Datta, S., Lee, M., *et al.* (2008) Opioid pharmacology. *Pain Physician*, **11**, S133–S153.

44 Deb, I., Chakraborty, J., Gangopadhyay, P.K., *et al.* (2011) Single-nucleotide polymorphism (A118G) in exon 1 of OPRM1 gene causes alteration in downstream signaling by mu-opioid receptor and may contribute to the genetic risk for addiction. *Journal of Neurochemistry*, **112**, 486–496.

45 Goetz, M.P., Kamal, A., Ames, M.M. (2008) Tamoxifen pharmacogenomics: the role of CYP2D6 as a predictor of drug response. *Clinical Pharmacology and Therapeutics*, **83**, 160–166.

46 Gage, B.F., Eby, C., Johnson, J.A., *et al.* (2008) Use of pharmacogenetic and clinical factors to predict the therapeutic dose of warfarin. *Clinical Pharmacology and Therapeutics*, **84**, 326–331.

47 Gage, B.F., Lesko, L.J. (2008) Pharmacogenetics of warfarin: regulatory, scientific, and clinical issues. *Journal of Thrombosis and Thrombolysis*, **25**, 45–51.

48 Epstein, R.S., Moyer, T.P., Aubert, R.E., *et al.* (2009) Warfarin genotyping reduces hospitalization rates results from the MM-WES (Medco-Mayo Warfarin Effectiveness study). *Journal of the American College of Cardiology*, **55**, 2804–2812.

49 Charles, F. (2006) Antiretroviral agents and treatment of HIV infection. In: L.L. Brunton, J.S. Lazo, and K.L. Parker (eds), *Goodman & Gilman's The Pharmacological Basis of Therapeutics*, 11th ed. McGraw-Hill, New York.

50 SUBOXONE® (buprenorphine HCl/naloxone HCl dihydrate sublingual tablets) package insert. (2011) Reckitt Benckiser Pharmaceuticals, Richmond, VA.

CHAPTER 11

Microarray Technology and Other Methods in Pharmacogenomics Testing

Jorge L. Sepulveda, MD, PhD
Philadelphia VA Medical Center and University of Pennsylvania

Introduction

The completion of the first draft of the human genome in 2003 opened a new era of medicine, in which there would be increasing use of genetic information in order to estimate susceptibility to disease and probabilities of response to preventive or therapeutic interventions. In particular, the field of pharmacogenetics (PGx) studies the relationship of gene sequences with drug response. A wider definition of pharmacogenetics testing includes assays for phenotypic markers that closely correlate with pharmacogenetic changes. An early example is the measurement of erythrocyte glucose-6-phosphate dehydrogenase activity, which predicts susceptibility to hemolysis induced by primaquine and other drugs. This susceptibility of certain individuals to hemolysis was identified as early as 510 B.C. by Pythagoras, who described the adverse effects of eating fava beans (1), although the actual enzyme defect was discovered in 1956 (2), and the gene cloned in 1986 (3). Another example is measurement of thiopurine methyl transferase (TPMT) enzymatic activity in erythrocytes to screen for defective alleles of TPMT that decrease metabolism of thiopurine drugs (such as azathioprine and 6-mercaptopurine) and place the patients at high risk for toxicity (4). Another, phenotypic measurement of pharmacogenetic susceptibility is the ratio of N-acetyl-procainamide (NAPA) to procainamide,

both usually measured by an immunoassay, to define the activity of procainamide N-acetyl transferase (NAT2) (5, 6). Slow acetylators have low NAT2 activity, and are at higher risk for procainamide-induced lupus-like syndrome, while the rapid acetylators have higher serum levels of NAPA and are at higher risk for QT prolongation, torsades-de-pointes, and other arrhythmias (5). Another example is the measurement of cholinesterase activity in the serum to predict susceptibility to the muscle-relaxant succinylcholine induced-apnea, which is related to variation in the butyrylcholinesterase gene (BChE) (7). In all of these cases, the phenotypic assays were developed long before the respective genes were cloned and the mutations identified, and remain a cost-effective approach to predict drug toxicity.

More recent phenotypic assays for pharmacogenetic susceptibility include immunohistochemical analysis of Her2/Neu, estrogen and progesterone receptors in tumors, which are critical for determination of proper cancer therapy (e.g., Herceptin [trastuzumab] or Lapatinib for Her2/Neu positive cases, tamoxifen and aromatase inhibitors for estrogen-receptor positive tumors, and progestogens for progesterone receptor-positive tumors). In these cases, somatic genetics of tumor cells is indirectly assessed to predict response to therapy and prognosis. As described in Chapter 4, assays for direct somatic mutations in selected genes, such as EGFR,

Pharmacogenomics in Clinical Therapeutics, First Edition. Edited by Loralie J. Langman and Amitava Dasgupta.
© 2012 John Wiley & Sons, Ltd. Published 2012 by John Wiley & Sons, Ltd.

KRAS, and BRAF, are increasingly used to select pathway-targeted anticancer therapies. With the development of low-cost, higher throughput genomics, it is expected that the use of somatic pharmacogenetics of tumors will become increasingly critical to determine appropriate therapies.

Early genetic assays for detecting pharmacogenetic variation

In the early days of molecular biology, a variety of labor-intense techniques were used to visualize genetic changes. The first technique was described by Edwin Southern and became known as the Southern blot. It involves digestion of the DNA with site-specific restriction endonucleases, separation of the resulting DNA fragments by agarose gel electrophoresis, transfer of the separated DNA to a membrane, and probing the membrane with radiolabeled DNA (or RNA) probes complementary to the sequences of interest. The position of the radiolabeled bands is identified by autoradiography and is proportional to the size of the digested fragment. This technique can be used to identify deletions and insertions in the DNA sequence, as well as mutations that affect the restriction enzyme cleavage site, resulting in different fragment sizes. Variation in these restriction enzyme sites are known as restriction fragment-length polymorphisms (RFLP).

A variation of the Southern blot procedure without restriction digestion or electrophoresis involves spotting the DNA into dots or slots into a membrane. Polymorphisms can then be identified by stringent hybridization of labeled oligonucleotide probes specific to the polymorphisms of interest (allele-specific oligonucleotide hybridization). Chromogenic or chemiluminescent labels can be substituted for radioactivity, further simplifying the procedure.

With the advent of the polymerase chain reaction (PCR) amplification technique, specific regions of DNA can be amplified from small amounts of DNA using oligonucleotide primers complementary to the 5′ and 3′ ends of the region of interest. Most modern techniques available to identify genetic variation use PCR-amplified DNA to isolate the region of interest while massively increasing the number of target molecules for analysis. In a variation of the RFLP technique described above, PCR-amplified DNA is digested with restriction enzymes and the fragments separated by agarose gel electrophoresis and visualized with fluorescent dyes, such as ethidium bromide, that intercalate into the DNA. When alleles differ by a single base, the resulting polymorphism is defined as a single-nucleotide polymorphism (SNP). Allele-specific PCR uses primers with the bases at the 3′ end complementary to the different bases responsible for the SNP; only the primer with perfect complementary at the 3′ end is extended by the polymerase to generate enough amplified product for detection.

Initially, cytogenetic assays for the Philadelphia chromosome defined chronic myeloid leukemia, in which the Bcr-Abl translocation resulted in activation of the tyrosine kinase activity of the Abl protein. Inhibition of the Abl kinase by imatinib-mesylate (Gleevac) defined a breakthrough in targeted anticancer therapies, since very high remission rates can be achieved. For increased sensitivity, a PCR assay for Bcr-Abl translocation better defines candidates for imatinib treatment. However, due to possible development of resistance to imatinib, adequate prediction of response to imatinib may require assaying for ABL exon mutations, and also for cKIT, PDGFRA and PDGFRB mutations. These assays can be viewed as special group of pharmacogenetic assays, in which somatic mutations in the tumor are interrogated to predict the response to therapeutic agents, in contrast with classic pharmacogenetics which is concerned with germline polymorphisms.

Another set of techniques use physical properties of DNA molecules that depend on their structure. For example, single-stranded conformation polymorphisms (SSCP) rely on small changes in the electrophoretic mobility of single-stranded DNA, usually derived from asymmetric PCR or after denaturation and purification of a biotinylated DNA strand. With careful optimization of fragment size and nondenaturing polyacrylamide or capillary gel electrophoresis, the SSCP procedure can identify a single change in up to 90% of the bases in the fragment.

Another group of methods to identify polymorphisms rely on the different properties of homoduplexes versus heteroduplexes. The DNA is PCR amplified, heat-denatured to separate the two strands, and allowed to reanneal. If there are two alleles differing in one or more nucleotides, the resulting reannealed molecules will have perfectly matched homoduplexes as well as mismatched heteroduplexes. To identify heteroduplexes, denaturing gradient gel electrophoresis (DGGE) uses a gel containing progressively higher concentrations of a chemical denaturing agent so that heteroduplexes will denature at a lower concentration of the denaturant and migrate at a different position than a perfectly matched homoduplex. Modifications of this method include temperature gradient gel electrophoresis, where a temperature gradient is used in the same manner as the chemical gradient in DGGE, and denaturing high performance liquid chromatography (dHPLC), in which gel electrophoresis is replaced by HPLC performed at an appropriate column temperature such that heteroduplexes have a different retention time than homoduplexes. These methods have been largely replaced by real-time PCR coupled with high resolution melting curve analysis which can provide simple assays for known point mutations as well as for mutation scanning (see below).

Finally, the gold standard for detection of nucleotide polymorphisms is Sanger sequencing. The method is based on primer extension using DNA polymerase and a mix of deoxynucleotides, which are normally incorporated and extended, and dideoxynucleotides (ddNTP), which terminate the chain at the incorporation position, therefore generating different size fragments that are separated by gel or capillary electrophoresis. By labeling each ddNTP (A, C, T, or G) with a different label (or running in separate lanes), the sequence can be directly read from the order of the separated fragments. While this method accurately detects base substitutions in heterozygous alleles and in mutant DNA present at levels above 10–20%, it lacks sensitivity to pick up small amounts of mutated DNA and can miss gene duplication or deletions.

A variation of this method is the single-base primer extension. For example, the *SNaPshot*® system (Applied Biosystems) uses single-base primer extension and capillary electrophoresis to interrogate up to 10 SNPs at known locations. Basically, multiplex PCR is performed, DNA is purified from PCR primers and treated with alkaline phosphatase and exonucleotidase I to prevent template extension, primer extension oligonucleotides are added together with the SNaPshot® reaction mix, and the polymerase adds a single labeled ddNTP, which cannot be further extended. After another round of purification, the reaction is loaded on a capillary electrophoresis analyzer. Since each ddNTP can be labeled with a different fluorescent dye, the incorporated base in the SNP can be read directly on the electrophoretogram. Using different sized primers, multiplexing for various loci is possible in a single reaction without overlap of electrophoretic peaks. While costs are relatively low since no labeled primers or probes are required, the method is labor intensive and multiplexing is limited to about 10 loci per reaction.

Currently available commercial assays

The technology of genetic assays is rapidly evolving and commercially assays are constantly being introduced in the marketplace, although the pace of FDA approval for pharmacogenetic assays has been relatively slow. For example, by mid 2011, only nine pharmacogenetics assays were FDA approved, of which five are used for Warfarin PGx (Table 11.1). However, this number is expected to rapidly increase, given the pace of 510(K) submissions to the FDA for various genetic assays.

This section describes some currently available assays, with a focus on the technical principles and the advantages and disadvantages of each platform.

Real-time PCR assays
One the simplest assay for genetic variation is real-time PCR coupled with high resolution melting curve analysis (see below). The method employs thermocyclers with built-in fluorometers that can measure fluorescence generated in the PCR reaction vial, usually by an intercalating dye such as SYBR green, specific for double-stranded DNA. Since fluorescence is proportional the amount of double-stranded DNA

Table 11.1 FDA-Approved Pharmacogenetics Assays

Product	Company	Approval Date
INFINITI CYP2C19 assay	Autogenomics	10/25/10
XTAG CYP2D6 kit	Luminex	8/26/10
EQ-PRC LC Warfarin genotyping	Trimgen	2/6/09
ESENSOR Warfarin sensitivity	Osmetech/GenMark	7/17/08
CYP2C9 & VKORC1 genotyping	ParagonDx	4/28/08
INFINITI 2C9 & VKORC1 Warfarin	Autogenomics	1/23/08
VERIGENE Warfarin metabolism	Nanosphere	9/17/07
INVADER UGT1A1 molecular assay	Third Wave/Hologic	8/18/05
AMPLICHIP CYP450 test system	Roche	1/10/05, 12/17/04

present, a melting profile can be generated post-PCR cycles by slowly increasing the temperature and measuring the point at which fluorescence decreases significantly (Figure 11.1). Heteroduplexes formed between two heterozygous alleles will have a lower melting point than homoduplexes because of base pair mismatches. With careful control of well-to-well temperature uniformity and high-resolution melting curve analysis, homozygous alleles with different base composition forming homoduplexes can also be reliably differentiated due to small differences in their melting temperature profiles. The main advantage of this method is the lack of need for complex probes, simplifying workflow and reducing costs of the assay.

Instrumentation, software and/or reagents that can be used for PGx testing with high resolution melting curve analysis include

• 7500 or 7900HT Fast-Real Time PCR systems with HRM Software and MeltDoctor™ reagents by Applied Biosystems (Foster City, CA)
• CFX96 or CFX384™ by Bio-Rad (Richmond, CA)
• Eco Real-Time PCR system by Illumina (San Diego, CA)
• LightCycler 480 by Roche Molecular Systems (Indianapolis, IN)
• LightScanner system by Idaho Technology (Salt Lake City, UT)
• Rotor-Gene Q real-time cycler and Type-it HRM PCR Reagents by Qiagen (Valencia, CA)
• eQ-PCR™ LC Warfarin genotyping kit, FDA-cleared for clinical laboratory testing in the Roche LightCycler, by TrimGen (Sparks, MD)

The *Taqman method* (Applied Biosystems/Life Technologis, Carlsbad, CA) is based on the 5′ nuclease activity of Taq DNA polymerase. A PCR is performed using primers that will amplify the DNA region containing the SNP of interest. Included in the reaction are two allele-specific fluorogenic probes, each consisting of a different fluorescent reporter dye and a fluorescent quencher. In the intact probe, the proximity of the quencher to the fluorophore causes fluorescence resonance energy transfer (FRET), reducing the fluorescence from the reporter dye. During PCR, the 5′ nuclease activity of Taq digests the allele-specific probe bound to the region of the SNP, releasing the fluorescent dye from the quencher and allowing generation of a fluorescence signal. Mismatched probes have melting temperatures below the Taq polymerase extension temperature, and detach from the template before Taq 5′ nucleotidase releases the fluorophore from the quencher (Figure 11.2). Depending on which dye signal is generated, the SNP alleles are determined. If only one dye signal is detected, the SNP is homozygous for the allele corresponding to the allele-specific probe, and if both dyes are detected, then the SNP is heterozygous.

The company provides a Drug Metabolism Kit assaying over 2,700 polymorphisms in 220 drug metabolism and transport genes, as well as individual ordering of over 1.6 million pre-designed human SNPs or custom-designed assays when a pre-designed assay is not available. The assays can be easily automated and batch-analyzed in 96- or 384-well plates with real-time PCR instruments.

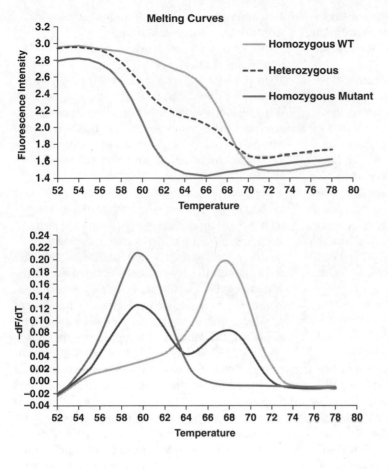

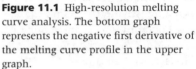

Figure 11.1 High-resolution melting curve analysis. The bottom graph represents the negative first derivative of the melting curve profile in the upper graph.

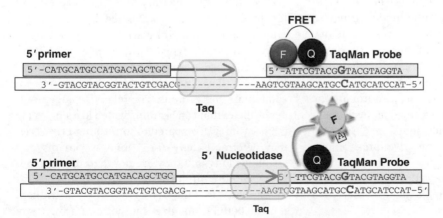

Figure 11.2 Taqman assay: F represents the fluorescent label and Q represents the quencher.

Disadvantages of this approach for clinical laboratories are the lack of FDA validation clearance at the time of this writing, and the need for separate reactions for each SNP.

In a slightly different approach, ParagonDx (Morrisville, NC) uses *molecular-beacon probes* with a fluorescent dye on the 5′-end and a quencher on the 3′-end. Upon hybridization, the quencher is separated from the fluorophore, and fluorescence can be measured during real-time PCR. Using two different fluorophores emitting at different wavelengths, two alleles can be discriminated in one tube. The assay can take as little as one hour from DNA extraction to results. The CYP2C9 and VKORC1 Rapid Genotyping assay has been FDA cleared for analysis with the SmartCycler® (Cepheid, Sunnyvale, CA). ParagonDx also provides a variety of SNP controls for several PGx genes.

Microarray assays

The *Roche AmpliChip® CYP450* is the first FDA-cleared assay for clinical pharmacogenetics use. The technology is based on microarrays manufactured by Affymetrix (Santa Clara, CA) using photolithography, a semiconductor manufacturing technique, to synthesize 25-mer oligonucleotides directly on the array surface. Hybridization to the target DNA is done under conditions that distinguish a single base-pair change in the immobilized probes, therefore allowing identification of SNPs. The CYP450 array contains probes that interrogate the major variants in the CYP2D6 and CYP2C19 genes, which play an important role in the metabolism of about 25% of all prescription drugs. A major advantage of the assay is that with one reaction, it provides a comprehensive survey of CYP2C19 (2 variants) and CYP2D6 (27 variants) and is able to detect deletions and duplications in both genes. Disadvantages of this platform are the elevated cost (≥$250) of the arrays and instrumentation (>$150,000 for the GeneChip® 3000Dx) and the relatively labor intensive pre-scanning steps, including:

1 DNA extraction and purification;
2 Multiplex long PCR amplification of the target genes;
3 Fragmentation using DNAse I;

4 Biotinylation of the PCR-amplified DNA using terminal deoxynucleotide transferase;
5 Hybridization to the array;
6 Washing of the array;
7 On chip labeling with streptavidin-coupled fluorescent dye (phycoerythrin).

The included software performs the data analysis, determines the genotype, and predicts the phenotype (CYP2D6: poor, intermediate, extensive, or ultra-rapid metabolizer; and CYP2C19: poor, or extensive metabolizer).

The *Infiniti*™ (Autogenomics, Carlsbad, CA) method involves multiplex amplification of the target DNA using primers specific for each gene of interest, followed by primer extension using SNP-specific oligonucleotides and labeled dCTP. After denaturation, the labeled DNA is captured on the microarray via a specific "zip code" sequence present in the 5′ region of each primer. The fluorescent signals are then read by a confocal scanning microscope, and the software determines whether a particular SNP is present or absent. The Infiniti microarrays (BioFilmChips™) are designed with a special coating to remove background fluorescence, and with several layers of a hydrogel providing a 3D matrix for incorporation of biological probes (DNA or protein arrays are available). "Zip-code" complementary probes are biotinylated and bound to the arrays by streptavidin trapped in the hydrogel in a maximum of 240 spots per array on standard arrays and 1024 spots on high density arrays. This approach provides a reliable process for attaching probes to the arrays. The complementary "zip-code" addresses of the probes allow DNA amplified by any custom primers to be captured by array probes, as long as the primers are designed with the appropriate "zip-code" sequence at their 5′-ends (Figure 11.3). This flexibility allows easy introduction of testing for additional gene variants. The relatively large number of alleles that can be interrogated in a single chip is an advantage compared to some other PGx assays that determine only the common variants and assume wild type if they are not detected. A disadvantage of the Infiniti system is the relatively large investment in the cost of the instrument (>$100,000), although it can perform a variety of genetic (and also proteomic) assays, and the reagent

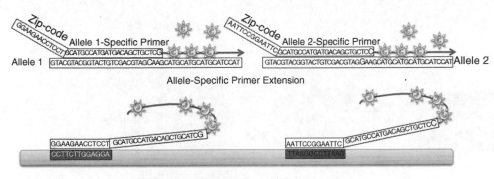

Figure 11.3 Autogenomics Infiniti™ technology.

and supply costs per assay are comparable to other platforms.

Currently, DNA extraction and the initial PCR reaction is performed offline, and all of the subsequent steps are carried automatically by the Infiniti analyzer:

1 All of the reagents and microarrays are supplied in kit form and can be pre-loaded in the instrument.

2 Sample pipetting is performed from 24-well plates with pre-loaded disposable pipette tips and robotic arm-driven probe.

3 Primer extension of PCR-amplified DNA is performed with loaded reagents and the built-in thermocycler and thermal stringency station.

4 The labeled DNA is then mixed with hybridization solution and loaded onto the microarrays.

5 Microarrays are incubated in the temperature controlled chamber to allow stringent hybridization to occur.

6 Automated washing of the microarrays is performed using robotic probes and pre-loaded wash buffer.

7 The arrays are moved to built-in confocal microscope with two lasers that read the fluorescence intensity of each spot.

8 Data are processed by the software, results are presented in graphical or numerical formats, and interpretative reports are produced for review on the screen or printed.

The time from DNA extraction to obtain the results is about 8 hours, which may be a limitation if rapid turnaround time is required before initiating therapy (e.g., with warfarin). Tests are performed in a random access mode (i.e., different tests can be intermixed in the same run). This is a helpful feature when one needs to characterize the pharmacogenetic profile of one sample with multiple arrays, such as CYP2D6 and CYP2C19. The throughput with the current instrument is up to 24 arrays per run, and depending on the assay, up to four samples per array. The new *Infiniti Plus* analyzer will be able to load 48 arrays in one run, effectively doubling the throughput, and provide results in less than 6 hours. While the system offers considerable improvement in labor requirements relative to other microarray platforms, it still requires offline DNA extraction and PCR amplification. The new *Infiniti Assist* instrument will be able to automate DNA extraction and amplification, so that there is no manual pipetting after sampling.

Other highly multiplexed assays

The *eSensor*® platform (Osmetech/Genmark Dx, Carlsbad, CA) uses electrochemical principles to detect DNA hybridization in a microfluidics cartridge. The method involves several offline steps, including DNA extraction, amplification, and preparation of single-stranded DNA. Single-stranded DNA can be prepared by using a 5′ phosphorylated primer in the PCR reaction and adding lambda exonucleotidase post PCR to digest the strand of the DNA extended from the phosphorylated primer. This latest step has the disadvantage of requiring opening of the tube post PCR, potentially creating a source of contamination. An alternative is to use asymmetric PCR with unequal primer concentrations. After the preparation

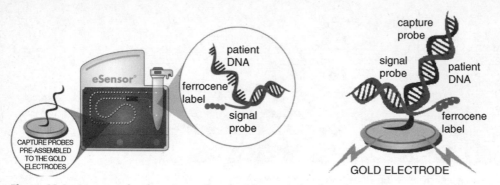

Figure 11.4 eSensor technology (reproduced with permission from http://www.genmarkdx.com/technology/ esensor.php).

steps, the DNA is mixed with ferrocene-labeled probes and loaded into the eSensor cartridge, which contains a microfluidic chamber directing the sample onto 72 gold electrode spots where different DNA capture probes have been immobilized (Figure 11.4). Typically, the capture probes are not SNP specific, allowing for capture of all alleles of interest in one spot. The allele specificity is conferred by the ferrocene probes, which contain a ferrous ion that upon close proximity to the gold electrode will undergo cycles of oxidation and reduction, releasing and accepting electrons and therefore create alternating currents at different redox potentials. Harmonic signal analysis is then used to distinguish signal from background current. Currently, up to four different ferrocene labels can be used simultaneously allowing the identification of up to four different alleles per spot.

eSensor cartridges are loaded into the XT-8 system, which has a modular design with one to three towers, each able to process eight cartridges, for a maximum of 24 independent, random-access assays at any one time. The entire procedure can be completed in 4 hours, which may be advantageous if initiation of therapy is dependent on test results. The online hybridization and detection take about 30 minutes, allowing a possible throughput of over 300 samples per 8-hour shift.

Verigene® technology (Nanosphere, Northbrook, IL) involves hybridization to gold nanoparticles, which have high stability and low background binding, and can scatter light with an intensity equivalent to 500,000 fluorophore molecules,

therefore providing increased signal-to-noise ratio and high sensitivity (Figure 11.5). Nonamplified DNA is sheared to a size of 300–500 bp by a proprietary sonication process, and hybridized to capture probes immobilized on specific spots on a slide array contained in a closed cartridge. Simultaneously, the target DNA is hybridized to gold

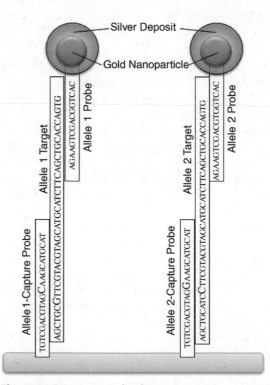

Figure 11.5 Verigene technology.

nanoparticle-labeled oligonucleotides complementary to a different region of the target. The target is therefore sandwiched between the capture and the gold particles. After washing of unbound gold nanoparticles, signal amplification is achieved by depositing elemental silver on the gold particles. After another wash, the strong light-scattering of silver-enhanced gold particles is measured by the Verigene ID image analyzer. If PCR amplification is not used, the amount of DNA required is higher than for other platforms (about 0.25 to 2 μg), although that amount is easily obtainable from blood samples. Turnaround time after DNA isolation for one sample is fast (about 1.5 hours), but additional samples add about 10 minute per sample (8). Due to its sensitivity the method can be applied to nonamplified DNA (9) and since only 2 pipetting steps are required, operator time and expertise required are minimal and therefore it may be amenable to point-of-care testing. The recently introduced Verigene® SP processor can perform DNA extraction, reverse transcription (for RNA targets), PCR amplification (if needed) and target identification and analysis in up to four cartridges, further simplifying the assay procedure to a sample-to-result workflow. The method has been FDA cleared for Warfarin PGx and is under development for clinical CYP2C19 genotyping.

The *xTAG*® assay (Luminex Corporation, Austin, TX, initially developed as Tag-It® at TmBioscience, Toronto, Canada) takes advantage of universal tag/antitag system consisting of 24-mer oligonucleotides with isothermal melting temperatures that have been designed to minimize nonspecific hybridization to genomic DNA and between each other, allowing high-level multiplexing to occur in a single tube (Figure 11.7). After multiplex PCR, allele-specific primer extension, similarly to the Infiniti™ procedure described above, generates single-stranded DNA containing the allele-specific tag in the 5′ region and incorporated biotinylated nucleotides. The biotin moieties allow for a streptavidin conjugated fluorophore (typically phycoerythrin) to bind to the tagged DNA, while the 5′-tag sequence allows the DNA to be captured by 5.6 micron polystyrene beads containing the corresponding antitag

probes. The beads are then read by the xMAP analyzer, which separates and identifies each bead by flow cytometry coupled with laser-induced fluorescence detection, since different types of beads are impregnated with a different ratio of two fluorophores, creating up to 100 different spectral addresses. Therefore, each allele, bound by a specific bead, can be identified and quantified, and up to 100 alleles or 50 bi-allelic variants can be analyzed simultaneously. A recent expansion of this technology uses three internal dyes to create up to 500 simultaneous unique assays using a single sample (FlexMap-3D®).

Other assays with low multiplexing

The *Invader*™ assay (Third Wave Technologies, Hologic, Bedford, MA) is a homogeneous, single-tube, single-addition assay that uses the thermostable flap endonuclease Cleavase™, which recognizes and cleaves hairpin and "flap" structures formed when a single-stranded oligonucleotide recognizes and binds to double-stranded DNA after denaturation and cooling (10) (Figure 11.6). The steps include:

A Standard PCR amplification of the target DNA;

B Inactivation of the DNA polymerase for - 10 minutes at 99C;

C Incubation at 63C for the Cleavase reaction:

1 Binding of the Invader oligonucleotide immediately 5′ of the polymorphic nucleotide (SNP). This oligonucleotide is designed to be stably bound to the target at the incubation temperature.

2 Binding of the allele-specific oligonucleotide probe #1 to the target DNA, with the SNP as the 5′ end of its recognition sequence.

3 5′ to the SNP, oligonucleotides #1 contains a defined sequence that does not hybridize to the target, therefore forming a single-stranded flap.

4 Cleavase recognizes the double-stranded plus flap structure and cleaves oligo # 1, releasing the flap. If the SNP is changed, a gap forms between oligo # 1 and the invader probe and no cleavage occurs.

5 The allele-specific probe is designed with a melting temperature close to the incubation temperature, resulting in constant annealing, cleavage, and detachment.

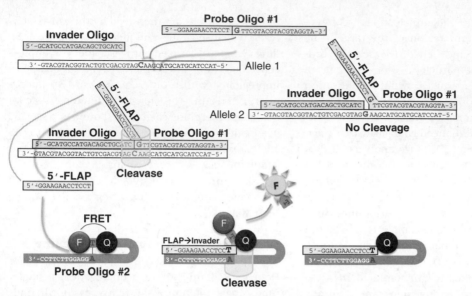

Figure 11.6 Invader reaction; F represents the fluorescent label and Q represents the quencher.

6 The released 5'-flap serves as a second invader oligonucleotide that binds to the hairpin-oligonucleotide probe # 2. This probe contains a fluorophore on the 5'-end of the single-stranded flap region, and a closely spaced quencher, resulting in little fluorescence in the basal state.

7 Upon binding of the released oligonucleotide from the first Cleavase reaction, the enzyme again recognizes the double-strand plus flap structure and cleaves the fluorophore containing single-stranded flap. Released from the proximity of the quencher, the fluorophore then increases several fold in fluorescence intensity.

Since binding, cleavage, and release of the 5' flaps occur repeatedly, a standard 4 hour reaction can result in more than 10-million-fold signals, allowing zeptomol (10^{-21} mol) quantities of DNA to be analyzed (10, 11). This corresponds to about 20–100 ng of genomic DNA, but with initial PCR amplification of the target, the Cleavase reaction incubation time can be reduced to 10 minutes with good sensitivity. A major advantage of this method is that universal fluorophore probes can be used (i.e., all SNP-detecting oligonucleotides contain the same 5'-flap region and therefore can invade one common probe). One disadvantage is that

each SNP requires a different reaction, which may lead to false calls of homozygosity if one reaction fails. To obviate this problem, two FRET detection probes are employed in current commercial duplex Invader™ assays, one with FAM and one with Redmond Red dyes. The fluorescence can be quantified by commonly available microtiter plate fluorometers, such as Tecan® GENios®, GENios® FL, or Infinite® and does not require additional expensive equipment. To further reduce hands-on time, the InPlex™ technology uses a microfluidic card to perform the multiplex Invader assays, which can be read in an inexpensive fluorometer. Further development of the technology (Invader-PLUS) uses a closed, single-tube system to perform PCR followed by heat denaturation, which destroys the polymerase but not the Cleavase, allowing the Invader® reaction to proceed. In addition to the commercially available assays using FRET probes, another detection approaches uses multiple fluorophores and fluorescence polarization detection, obviating the need for a quencher (12). However, even these approaches are limited by the number of non-overlapping fluorophores available, and high-level multiplexing is not possible with a homogeneous assay. Alternatively, high-level multiplexing can be

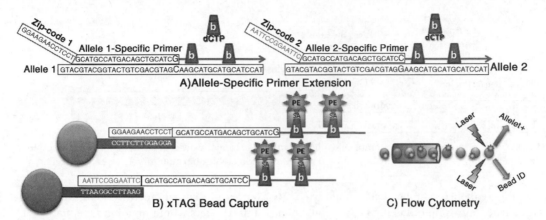

Figure 11.7 xMAP® technology; *b* represents biotinylated dCTP; *PE/SA* represents phycoerythrin-coupled streptavidin.

achieved by identifying the 5′-flap DNA by bead flow-cytometry (13), microarrays (14), or matrix-assisted laser desorption/ionization time-of-flight mass spectrometry (MALDI-TOF MS) (15), although none of these approaches has been widely used so far.

Pyrosequencing (Qiagen, Valencia, CA) is a sequencing technology developed by Biotage AB (Uppsala, Sweden) based on the release of pyrophosphate during nucleotide extension catalyzed by DNA polymerase. After initial PCR amplification with a biotinylated primer and purification of single-stranded DNA templates on streptavidin beads, the process uses specific sequencing primers to initiate the polymerase-catalyzed extension at specific DNA sites followed by serial addition of each of the 4 deoxynucleotide triphosphates (dNTP) and measuring of the pyrophosphate stoichiometrically released from each incorporated dNTP to derive the nucleotide sequence. The levels of released pyrophosphate are measured using sulfurylase to incorporate the pyrophosphate into adenosine-phosphosulfate and generate adenosine-triphosphate (ATP), which can easily be measured by chemiluminescence, using luciferase and luciferin to generate visible light proportional to the amount of ATP. Before adding the next base, remaining unincorporated deoxynucleotides are destroyed with apyrase. If the sequence has more than one nucleotide of the same type in a row, the signal will be proportional to the number of bases (e.g., the TT sequence will generate a signal twofold

higher when dATP is added) (Figure 11.8). With longer homopolymer tracts the signal is proportionally higher, but it becomes increasingly difficult to determine how many bases are present in homopolymers beyond seven or eight bases. This difficulty is obviated for known sequences with proper choice of primer sites. Major advantages of pyrosequencing are accurate sequence determination around the site of interest, sensitivity, ease of automation, and the quantitative nature of the measurement, allowing quick assessment of allele copy numbers and sensitive detection of mutations or reliable quantification of CpG methylation levels in tumor DNA contaminated with normal tissue DNA. High throughput, 96-well plate automated parallel processing of the PCR products to single-stranded DNA templates appropriate for Pyrosequencing is available (PyroMark workstation), but the method still requires offline DNA extraction and PCR amplification. Other disadvantages include the relatively high cost of biotinylated primers and the pyrosequencing instrument.

The Pyrosequencing technology has been adapted for large-scale genome sequencing by 454 Life Sciences (now owned by Roche Diagnostics) using parallel reactions in microarrays to generate about 400 million nucleotide data in a 10 hour run. Another derived technology (Ion Torrent, San Francisco, CA) detects the proton released when a nucleotide is incorporated during the polymerase extension reaction. By consecutively adding each of the

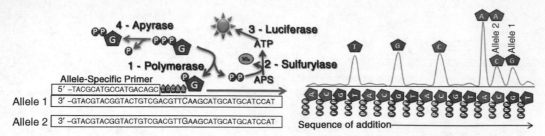

Figure 11.8 Pyrosequencing reaction; the template sequence can be read from the order and height of the pyrophosphate quantification peaks. In this example, two alleles are present in approximately equal amounts (heterozygous genotype).

four bases, the sequence can be read, similarly to pyrosequencing but using only polymerase and natural deoxynucleotides, without apyrase, luciferase, or sulfurylase enzymes, therefore improving speed and lowering costs.

Choice of assay

There have been a few studies comparing various platforms for PGx assays, mostly concentrating on warfarin PGx methods. In general, the agreement between platforms is 99–100% and the accuracy of the results is very high when compared to gold standard Sanger sequencing (8, 16–19). While generally accurate, no platform is ideal for all applications, and the choice of a platform for clinical PGx analysis may involve weighing the following variables (20):

1 FDA status of reagents and platforms (cleared, analytical-specific reagents or research use only reagents for laboratory-developed tests)

2 Analytical performance, including sensitivity and specificity for each allelic variant

3 Allelic coverage (i.e., how many alleles are interrogated for each loci)

4 Availability of user-definable assays and ease of introduction of new assays for genetic variants

5 Ability to detect copy number variations (deletions, duplications)

6 Multiplexing (i.e., the number of variants interrogated on a single reaction)

7 No-call rate (i.e., how often no result is called)

8 Complexity of procedure and amount of training required

9 Technologist hands-on time involved

10 Number of manual pipetting steps, tube openings, and transfers (contamination potential)

11 Turnaround time from sample to results, to include DNA extraction, PCR, and any other steps

12 Throughput, the number of assays per work session

13 General ability to use the platform for other assays

14 Random access versus batch processing of assays

15 Reagent stability, storage conditions, and onboard reagent management

16 Software user-friendliness, including data management and interpretative reports

17 Interfacing to laboratory information systems

18 Availability of proper quality control materials and onboard QC management

19 Availability of proficiency testing programs

20 Space and other facility requirements

21 Instrument maintenance requirements

22 Warranty and servicing costs

23 Initial equipment investment and cost per assay

One key aspect for the successful implementation of a clinical PGx assay is the quality of the reports issued to the clinical providers. In our experience, busy clinicians welcome comprehensive interpretative reports accompanying the raw PGx genotype results, which, in addition to the accurate description of the genetic variants interrogated and the assay methodology, include the following clinical points:

1 Summary of patient's clinical situation and indications for PGx testing

2 A list of laboratory results, medications and other possible environmental factors that may interact with each other and the genotype and influence a particular patient's response to therapy

3 A list of other common drugs potentially affected by the PGx genotype

4 Dosing recommendations, when available

5 A disclaimer stating that the recommendations should be used only as guidelines due to the limitations of genotyping in predicting phenotype, and that appropriate clinical evaluation and follow-up are recommended

While laboratory personnel can acquire sufficient expertise to produce appropriate interpretative reports for the medical record, in our opinion the best positioned professionals to do so are pharmacists who develop special interest and training in PGx and maintain good collaborative interactions with the clinical laboratory professionals.

Future of pharmacogenetic testing

Two trends are emerging in PGx assays. In one direction, companies are developing rapid, point-of-care (POC) assays for those drugs that have a limited number of associated PGx genes with relatively strong phenotypic association. Examples are CYP2C9 and VKORC1 for warfarin and CYP2C19 for clopidogrel. The goal is to provide information in a fast enough manner to optimize initial prescription. Although genetic analysis technologies that involve little manual intervention with automated DNA extraction, amplification, and SNP detection are available and adaptable for POC instrumentation (e.g., the Verigene system described above, the GeneXpert system by Cepheid, or the FilmArray system by Idaho Technology), expert software and PGx-guided dosing algorithms will need to be further developed and validated for these assays to become widely used at the point of care.

Another emerging trend involves more comprehensive analysis of a larger number of genes and gene variations with influence on drug response. While the few loci currently tested to predict drug response have moderately strong phenotypic associations, they have relatively low predictive value. For example, CYP2D6 PM genotype explains only 10–20% of adverse effects to risperidone, although, when present, has over 90% specificity of predicting risperidone adverse effects (21). Therefore, it is critical to identify the large number of possible genes with weaker phenotypic effects, which together explain the majority of the genetic influences on drug response. In the near future, easy-to-use platforms that interrogate a large number of genetic variations will become more commonly used for PGx assays. The trend started with platforms such as the Roche AmpliChip CYP450, the Autogenomics Infiniti, and the Luminex xMAP systems, with multiplexing limited to two orders of magnitude. New platforms for cost-effective higher level multiplexing are becoming available. For example, the MassARRAY® system (Sequenom, San Diego, CA) uses matrix-assisted laser desorption/ionization time-of-flight mass spectrometry (MALDI-TOF MS) to accurately measure the mass of DNA fragments, allowing genotyping by single base primer extension, since each different terminating nucleotide adds a unique mass. While the level of multiplexing is limited to 40 SNPs per well, the system is able to process up to 138,000 genotypes per day with a 384-well format. Another platform allowing higher level multiplexing is the VeraCode system (Illumina), which uses cylindrical glass micron microbeads embedded with high-density holographic bar codes that can be excited by a laser and imaged by the BeadXpress Reader system. By pooling microbeads with a variety of different codes, up to 384 SNPs can be interrogated in one well of a 96-well plate, allowing up to 300,000 genotypes generated in 6 hands-on hours. Another technology uses nanoliter reactions in nanofluidic Integrated Fluidic Circuit (IFC) chips (Fluidigm Corporation, San Francisco, CA) to process thousands of samples for 30–300 SNPs (22).

This trend to increased SNP multiplexing will continue to evolve, and eventually will be replaced with genome-wide scanning and sequencing (GWS) technologies. One important factor is that genome-wide association studies use SNPs that are present at relatively high frequencies and rare alleles (<5%) may not be represented in the platforms but may contribute significantly to the phenotype of interest (23). On the other hand, the cost of GWS has dropped exponentially from US$3 billion in 2003 to about $10,000 in 2010, and it is expected that in

2–10 years the cost of sequencing the entire human genome will be between $100 and $1,000. Currently available GWS technology is derived from the type of assays described above, and requires high-throughput detection of DNA modified with costly enzymes, reagents or probes. For example, the 454 Genome Sequencer (Roche), uses hundreds of thousands of beads coated with specific DNA probes for massive parallel pyrosequencing. The Illumina HiSeq 2000 sequencing system uses random primer extension of immobilized DNA fragments with reversible fluorescent terminators to visualize the DNA sequence in high density arrays and can provide 30-fold coverage of two human genomes for under US$10,000 in a single run. Ultimately, cost-effective GWS technology might involve either massive miniaturization to reduce costs of reagents or simple high-throughput scanning of DNA molecules by physical methods, such visualization by aberration corrected transmission electron microscopes (being developed by Halcyon Molecular, Redwood City, CA), or micro-impedance measurement of DNA molecules flowing in single file through a nanopore (24, 25).

With cost-effective high-throughput genomic technologies, testing will be shifted to elective timing, such as neonatal screening or the first clinical visit as an adult. It is likely that deep-sequencing technologies will obviate the need for specific SNP testing. When GWS becomes affordable, germ line genetic testing for specific mutations will become obsolete, and many phenotypic surrogate tests for genetic disease or predisposition will be unnecessary. For example, biochemical newborn screening will be significantly decreased. Fully understanding genetic risks for disease will shift the focus of preventive medicine from wide scale screening of populations for common diseases (e.g., glucose for diabetes, lipid profiles for dyslipidemias, and prostate-specific antigen for prostate cancer), to targeted screening approaches for all significant diseases that a particular individual is genetically predisposed. As part of the initial genetic profiling, traits predicting response to environmental factors, including microbes, toxins, and therapeutic and recreational drugs will be also determined. The combination of comprehensive genetic profiling and individualized screening, prevention, and therapeutics will result in significant enhancement of health care cost-effectiveness. This will be accomplished only with full understanding of the interplay between the genome, environmental factors, drug metabolism, and pharmacodynamics. It is possible that initial societal benefits of wide-scale population full genome sequencing will allow reinvestment of cost savings in improving the underlying science, therefore enabling a positive feedback loop where improved cost-effectiveness creates additional savings that can be reinvested in cost-effectiveness research. This process will be lengthy and will certainly require both large-scale genome-wide association studies (similar to HapMap but aimed at the full genome sequence (23, 26)) and a combination of hard-core reductionist science and systems biology to understand the mechanistic connections between genotypes and phenotypes.

Conclusions

The field of PGx testing is rapidly changing in various fronts, including technologic developments in assay methodology, knowledge of genomic associations and genotype–phenotype correlation, and, importantly, availability of well-validated assays of practical application in clinical practice with proper regulatory approval. The various assays described in this chapter illustrate some ingenious approaches to the problem of detecting genetic variation but are likely to rapidly undergo significant change and obsolescence. Manufacturers, consumers, and regulators of these technologies must be agile in adapting to this rapidly evolving environment in order for pharmacogenetics to realize its full potential to optimize health care for each individual. On the other hand, the optimum should not preclude the good, and many of the assays described have been successfully implemented in the clinical laboratory with a significant beneficial impact in health care. As with other laboratory tests, close attention to method performance, validation, quality assurance, and peer group proficiency testing, together with appropriate reporting and interaction with users, are keys to success.

References

1 Nebert, D.W. (1999) Pharmacogenetics and pharmacogenomics: why is this relevant to the clinical geneticist? *Clinical Genetics*, **56**, 247–258.

2 Alving, A.S., Carson, P.E., Flanagan, C.L., Ickes, C.E. (1956) Enzymatic deficiency in primaquine-sensitive erythrocytes. *Science*, **124**, 484–485.

3 Persico, M.G., Viglietto, G., Martini, G., Toniolo, D., *et al.* (1986) Isolation of human glucose-6-phosphate dehydrogenase (G6PD) cDNA clones: primary structure of the protein and unusual 5′ non-coding region. *Nucleic Acids Research*, **14**, 2511–2522.

4 Weinshilboum, R.M., Sladek, S.L. (1980) Mercaptopurine pharmacogenetics: monogenic inheritance of erythrocyte thiopurine methyltransferase activity. *American Journal of Human Genetics*, **32**, 651–662.

5 Okumura, K., Kita, T., Chikazawa, S., Komada, F., *et al.* (1997) Genotyping of N-acetylation polymorphism and correlation with procainamide metabolism. *Clinical Pharmacology & Therapeutics*, **61**, 509–517.

6 Olshansky, B., Martins, J., Hunt, S. (1982) N-acetyl procainamide causing torsades de pointes. *American Journal of Cardiology*, **50**, 1439–1441.

7 Levano, S., Ginz, H., Siegemund, M., Filipovic, M., *et al.* (2005) Genotyping the butyrylcholinesterase in patients with prolonged neuromuscular block after succinylcholine. *Anesthesiology*, **102**, 531–535.

8 Lefferts, J.A., Schwab, M.C., Dandamudi, U.B., Lee, H.K., *et al.* (2010) Warfarin genotyping using three different platforms. *American Journal of Translational Research*, **2**, 441–446.

9 Bao, Y.P., Huber, M., Wei, T.F., Marla, S.S., *et al.* (2005) SNP identification in unamplified human genomic DNA with gold nanoparticle probes. *Nucleic Acids Research*, **33**, e15.

10 Olivier, M. (2005) The Invader assay for SNP genotyping. *Mutation Research*, **573**, 103–110.

11 Hall, J.G., Eis, P.S., Law, S.M., Reynaldo, L.P., *et al.* (2000) Sensitive detection of DNA polymorphisms by the serial invasive signal amplification reaction. *Proceedings of the National Academy of Sciences of the United States of America*, **97**, 8272–8277.

12 Hsu, T.M., Law, S.M., Duan, S., Neri, B.P., Kwok, P.Y. (2001) Genotyping single-nucleotide polymorphisms by the invader assay with dual-color fluorescence polarization detection. *Clinical Chemistry*, **47**, 1373–1377.

13 Rao, K.V., Stevens, P.W., Hall, J.G., Lyamichev, V., *et al.* (2003) Genotyping single nucleotide polymorphisms directly from genomic DNA by invasive cleavage reaction on microspheres. *Nucleic Acids Research*, **31**, e66.

14 Lu, M., Shortreed, M.R., Hall, J.G., Wang, L., *et al.* (2002) A surface invasive cleavage assay for highly parallel SNP analysis. *Human Mutation*, **19**, 416–422.

15 Berggren, W.T., Takova, T., Olson, M.C., Eis, P.S., *et al.* (2002) Multiplexed gene expression analysis using the invader RNA assay with MALDI-TOF mass spectrometry detection. *Analytical Chemistry*, **74**, 1745–1750.

16 Babic, N., Haverfield, E.V., Burrus, J.A., Lozada, A., *et al.* (2009) Comparison of performance of three commercial platforms for warfarin sensitivity genotyping. *Clinica Chimica Acta: International Journal of Clinical Chemistry*, **406**, 143–147.

17 Toriello, M., Meccariello, P., Mazzaccara, C., Di Fiore, R., *et al.* (2006) Comparison of the TaqMan and Light-Cycler systems in pharmacogenetic testing: evaluation of CYP2C9*2/*3 polymorphisms. *Clinical Chemistry and Laboratory Medicine*, **44**, 285–287.

18 King, C.R., Porche-Sorbet, R.M., Gage, B.F., Ridker, P.M., *et al.* (2008) Performance of commercial platforms for rapid genotyping of polymorphisms affecting warfarin dose. *American Journal of Clinical Pathology*, **129**, 876–883.

19 Maurice, C.B., Barua, P.K., Simses, D., Smith, P., *et al.* (2010) Comparison of assay systems for warfarin-related CYP2C9 and VKORC1 genotyping. *Clinica Chimica Acta: International Journal of Clinical Chemistry*, **411**, 947–954.

20 Di Francia, R., Frigeri, F., Berretta, M., Cecchin, E., *et al.* (2010) Decision criteria for rational selection of homogeneous genotyping platforms for pharmacogenomics testing in clinical diagnostics. *Clinical Chemistry and Laboratory Medicine*, **48**, 447–459.

21 de Leon, J., Armstrong, S.C., Cozza, K.L. (2006) Clinical guidelines for psychiatrists for the use of pharmacogenetic testing for CYP450 2D6 and CYP450 2C19. *Psychosomatics*, **47**, 75–85.

22 Wang, J., Lin, M., Crenshaw, A., Hutchinson, A., *et al.* (2009) High-throughput single nucleotide polymorphism

genotyping using nanofluidic Dynamic Arrays. *BMC Genomics*, **10**, 561.

23 Kim, S.Y., Li, Y., Guo, Y., Li, R., *et al.* (2010) Design of association studies with pooled or un-pooled next-generation sequencing data. *Genetic Epidemiology*, **34**, 479–491.

24 Stoddart, D., Heron, A.J., Mikhailova, E., Maglia, G., Bayley, H. (2009) Single-nucleotide discrimination in immobilized DNA oligonucleotides with a biological

nanopore. *Proceedings of the National Academy of Sciences of the United States of America*, **106**, 7702–7707.

25 ten Bosch, J.R., Grody, W.W. (2008) Keeping up with the next generation: massively parallel sequencing in clinical diagnostics. *Journal of Molecular Diagnostics*, **10**, 484–492.

26 Altshuler, D.M., Gibbs, R.A., Peltonen, L., Dermitzakis, E., *et al.* (2010) Integrating common and rare genetic variation in diverse human populations. *Nature*, **467**, 52–58.

CHAPTER 12

Pharmacogenetic Testing in the Clinical Laboratory Environment

Mark P. Borgman, PhD and Mark W. Linder, PhD
Department of Pathology and Laboratory Medicine, University of Louisville School of Medicine, Louisville, Kentucky

Introduction

The purpose of this chapter is to provide guidance to the clinical laboratory scientist on the implementation of pharmacogenetic testing in a clinical setting. This chapter is intended to be a thoughtful guide to help answer questions such as what general information you need, what decisions need to be made, and what actions are important to take when starting pharmacogenetics testing for the purpose of clinical diagnostics (Figure 1).

Pharmacogenomics and pharmacogenetics are terms now often used interchangeably to describe the science of genetic variation and a person's response to a drug (1). More specifically, according to NCBI definitions, *pharmacogenomics* refers to the study of many different genes that determine drug behavior and *pharmacogenetics* refers to the study of inherited variations in drug metabolism and response. Interestingly, the differentiation of these two terms is linked to the technology employed. Commercially available kits for common clinical laboratory testing of specific genetic variations in drug enzymes or receptors are an example of pharmacogenetic tests. Alternatively, microarray technologies that evaluate many genes are considered pharmacogenomic tests. As the technology of molecular testing improves, the availability of testing is bolstered, cost burden is eased and certified clinical laboratories have the ability to perform more pharmacogenomic testing.

As of 2010, the FDA includes pharmacogenetic testing information in approximately 10% of drug labels and this number is expected to increase (2). The clinical laboratory will be challenged with enabling the evolving standard of care as driven by the adoption of pharmacogenetic knowledge into clinical practice (3). Clinical pharmacogenetic diagnostic services reveal fundamental biologic characteristics of the individual that may influence likeliness of a response, risk of an adverse drug reaction, or dictate modifications to standard drug therapies. Deciding on the appropriate assays involves selecting pertinent therapeutics and respective targets, determining that a genotypic result provides necessary and valuable clinical information, selecting the appropriate genetic variants to test for, and overall establishing a complete assay menu to provide services that fulfill clinical need for a patient's therapeutic drug management.

Analytical methods range from FDA approved test kits to laboratory-developed tests (LDTs) that may incorporate use of commercially available reagents. According to the College of American Pathologists, LDTs are tests developed within a Clinical Laboratory Improvement Amendments (CLIA)-certified laboratory for use in patient management, are solely performed by the clinical laboratory where the test was developed and is currently neither FDA cleared nor FDA approved. Scenarios exist where it is necessary to implement an LDT due to the lack of FDA-approved tests so long as it has gone through

Pharmacogenomics in Clinical Therapeutics, First Edition. Edited by Loralie J. Langman and Amitava Dasgupta.
© 2012 John Wiley & Sons, Ltd. Published 2012 by John Wiley & Sons, Ltd.

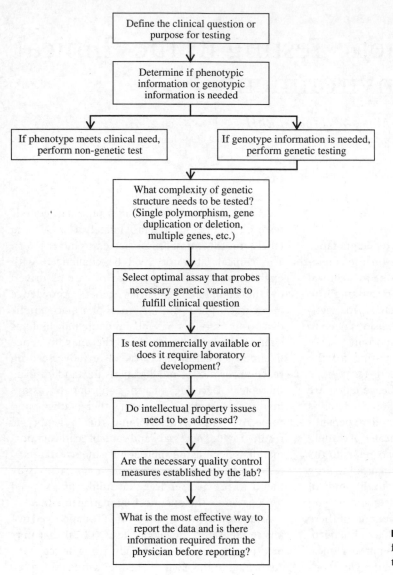

Figure 12.1 Implementation strategy for clinical diagnostic pharmacogenetic testing.

rigorous in house validation according to CLIA guidelines. The regulatory environment regarding the use laboratory designed assays for genetic testing is constantly evolving with the increasing genetic testing landscape. It is important that the clinical laboratory scientist understands this environment and conducts laboratory operations appropriately.

Finally, the delivery of accurate and often complex pharmacogenetic test results in a way that is useful and understandable to a physician, nurse or pharmacist is crucial to successful clinical application. Therefore this chapter includes a discussion on how this information can be used for reporting the information using patient-specific computerized algorithms and modelling software. Interpretive reports incorporating computer algorithms have now become available for common pharmacogenetic tests and the amount of guidance in this area is increasing.

Laboratory perspective on genotype and phenotype

It is widely recognized that *genotype* refers to the unique inherited structural makeup of a person's genetic material and *phenotype* refers to the observable physical manifestation of one's genotype through a composite of biological influences. Clearly many factors influence a phenotype, and indeed individuals with differing genotypes can be phenotypically similar. As it relates to pharmacogenetics, a person's genotype specifically means the genetic code for a given drug metabolizing enzyme or drug target protein (enzyme, cell surface receptor, etc.). Additionally, a phenotype in pharmacogenetics is an observable clinical event upon administering a drug. This phenotype is related to the genotype under routine dosing circumstances and can be altered through modifications in therapeutic regimens. Therefore, the manifestation of a biological phenotype defining a drug response is dynamic and dependent upon a variety of influences.

The goal of pharmacogenetic analysis is to link inherited genetic variants with drug metabolism and response (4). This would allow the use of pharmacogenetic information to provide a phenotypic prediction based on a person's genotype to optimize a drug regimen. It may be true that the early discoveries of a specific alteration in a genotype resulting in a well-defined phenotype has produced a simplified understanding of the genotype–phenotype relationship in pharmacogenetics (5). It should be recognized, however, that the downstream effects of a person's genotype prior to reaching the phenotype are dynamic and can be manipulated. Therefore, it is the utilization of the pharmacogenetic information prior to initiation of a new therapy that drives the desired phenotype. The clinical pharmacogenetic laboratory can have the most influence and impart the most benefit by providing information to achieve a desired phenotype and therefore successful clinical intervention. This is largely due to the lab being the last link in the information before the patient–physician interaction. Directed medical intervention following guidance from the identified genotype can be used to alter the observable phenotype. Laboratory evaluations of patient pheno-

typic responses including changes in biological processes, identification of toxicity, and drug monitoring are well established in routine clinical laboratories. This chapter will focus on laboratory techniques and considerations relative to determination of patient genotype.

Pharmacogenetic test selection

Selecting the genetic structure and the important variants to test for is a critical first step in establishing a pharmacogenetic service. The primary basis for choosing the variants to test for is determined with respect to their correlation with phenotypic responses of pharmacokinetic, pharmacodynamic, and possibly toxicological end points. This entails laboratory testing for genetic variants that alter the bioconversion or elimination of drugs as well as those variants that affect the biological response to a drug at the molecular level. Furthermore, National Academy of Clinical Biochemistry (NACB) guidelines recommend testing for genetic alterations that have a well-defined influence on the functional aspects of a gene product (6).

Calculating testing error

The NACB recommends that the overall testing error be determined for each test. Testing error in a pharmacogenetic test can be defined as the clinical sensitivity of the assay for correctly identifying phenotype, for example poor metabolizers as poor metabolizers. A mutant allele that is clinically significant but not included in the test will produce a false-negative result for patient DNA containing the mutation (identified genotype as wild type). This sensitivity therefore is based upon the selected allele for testing and the population frequency of the alleles that contribute to the observed phenotype. These calculations are based upon the Hardy-Weinberg principle of genetic equilibrium, whereby allele and genotype frequencies in a population remain constant. According to the principle using a single-locus gene with two alleles, the frequency of dominant homozygotes are represented by a^2, recessive homozygotes by b^2 and heterozygotes by *2ab* with their sum equal to 1. It is on the basis of these scientific approximations that we calculate frequencies and testing error in pharmacogenetics. Using CYP2D6 as an example, phenotypic poor metabolizers represent approximately 7% of the population. A methodology testing for *CYP2D6*3,*4,*5*, and *6 poor metabolizer alleles would identify up to 98% of poor metabolizer alleles in a Caucasian population (7). The remaining 2% of alleles not included could lead to 1 in 23 poor metabolizers misidentified as having one active allele. This calculates to approximately 1 genotyping error in 305 patients tested in a regular population.

The example described above is an ideal scenario and calculation largely attributed to the ability to assess population CYP2D6 phenotypes. Phenotypic poor metabolizers can be identified in vivo using probe compounds such as debrisoquine (reviewed in (8)) and monitoring metabolism. However, in situations where the phenotype cannot be independently verified, the true phenotype frequency is indeterminate and therefore detailed error calculations as described above cannot be performed.

Relevance of genetic structure in clinical testing

The complexity of the genetic structure tested for is ultimately determined by the target protein and the selected genetic variants as discussed above. Examples of mutations varying by the genetic structure relevant to pharmacogenetics include localized mutations such as single nucleotide polymorphisms (SNPs) or deletions. Large-scale mutations are also significant such as gene duplication or gene deletion, whereby large chromosomal regions coding the protein of interest exist in multiple copies or are lost, respectively. Pharmacogenetic testing based on the magnitude of genetic structure alteration begins with assays for small-scale mutations of one nucleotide in the genetic locus. These changes can be resulting from SNPs where a mutation of one base for another occurs, most commonly a transition between adenine and guanine $(A > G; G > A)$ or cytosine and thymine $(C > T; T > C)$. The loss or deletion of one single nucleotide can also occur. Many clinically important pharmacogenetic variations are the result of single base changes. Examples include *CYP2C9*2* allele 430C >T resulting in deficient enzyme activity and *CYP2C19*2* allele 681G>A resulting in null enzyme activity (reviewed in (9)). Additionally, *CYP2D6*3* allele 2549A>del mutation resulting in null enzyme activity is an example of a base deletion of clinical relevance. Examples of large-scale mutations include *CYP2D6*5* allele deletion resulting in a loss of enzyme activity and *CYP2D6*2xN* duplication of the *2 allele resulting in increased enzymatic activity. Pharmacogenetic testing for mutations in multiple genes responsible for biological response such as CYP2C9 and VKOR in warfarin response and metabolism is an example of multiple gene testing due to the interaction of two different gene products affecting drug response.

The NACB has recommended a limited number of variant alleles based on literature findings to evaluate for CYP2D6, CYP2C9, and CYP2C19 testing. These are included as a starting point for generating clinically applicable information in the general population (Table 12.1, adapted from Andersson (9) and NACB guidelines (6)). Further-

Table 12.1 Recommended Alleles for Clinical Testing in CYP2D6, CYP2C9, and CYP2C19 in All Population Groups

CYP2D6			CYP2C9			CYP2C19		
Alleles	Variant	Activity	Alleles	Variant	Activity	Alleles	Variant	Activity
*2xN	Duplication of *2	Ultra	*2	430C>T	Deficient	*2	681G>A	Null
*5	Deletion	Null	*3	1075A>C	Deficient	*3	636G>A	Null
*6	1707T>del	Null						
*4	1846G>A	Null						
*3	2549A>del	Null						

more, recommendations were made for testing of thiopurine methyl transferase (TPMT) and UDP-glucuronosyltransferase 1A1 (UGT1A1). Important alleles for those enyzmes would include *UGT1A1*28* (10) and *TPMT*2, *3A* and *3C* (11). In addition to these NACB recommendations, the field of clinical pharmacogenetic testing includes many additional targets important for drug action and metabolism. An extensive list of pharmacogenetic targets, assays, and associated alleles including those discussed above as well as many others is maintained by the Pharmacogenomics Knowledge Base (www.pharmgkb.org). Table 12.2 includes examples of the most relevant clinical PGx tests and the associated variants. Clinical laboratorians should be aware that patents may exist protecting a mutation and the application of the genotype information for clinical use. Licensing agreements may be necessary to offer certain diagnostic services.

Table 12.2 Pharmacogenetic Tests Available for Most-Studied Genes and Alleles Adapted from Pharmacogenomics Knowledge Base

Gene	Drug	PGx Test	Variants Assayed
ABL1	imatinib, dasatinib	BCR-ABL quantitation in CML; BCR-ABL Mutations in CML	BCR-ABL (reciprocal translocation involving chromosomes 9 and 22; t(9;22)(q34;q11))
BCR	imatinib, dasatinib	BCR-ABL quantitation in CML; BCR-ABL Mutations in CML	BCR-ABL (reciprocal translocation involving chromosomes 9 and 22; t(9;22)(q34;q11))
CYP2C9	warfarin	TrimGen Corporation eQ-PCR LC Warfarin Genotyping Kit	CYP2C9*2, CYP2C9*3
CYP2C19	clopidogrel, esomeprazole, omeprazole, phenytoin, others	Roche AmpliChip Cytochrome P450 Genotyping test and Affymetrix GeneChip Microarray Instrumentation System	CYP2C19*1, CYP2C19*2, CYP2C19*3
CYP2C19	clopidogrel, esomeprazole, omeprazole, phenytoin, others	Infiniti CYP450 2C19	CYP2C19*2, CYP2C19*3, CYP2C19*4, CYP2C19*5, CYP2C19*6, CYP2C19*7, CYP2C19*8, CYP2C19*9, CYP2C19*10
CYP2D6	codeine, fluoxetine, metropolol, risperidone, tamoxifen, others	Roche AmpliChip Cytochrome P450 Genotyping test and Affymetrix GeneChip Microarray Instrumentation System	CYP2D6*1, CYP2D6*2ABD, CYP2D6*3, CYP2D6*4ABDJK, CYP2D6*5, CYP2D6*6ABC, CYP2D6*7, CYP2D6*8, CYP2D6*9, CYP2D6*10AB, CYP2D6*11, CYP2D6*15, CYP2D6*17, CYP2D6*19, CYP2D6*20, CYP2D6*29, CYP2D6*35, CYP2D6*36, CYP2D6*40, CYP2D6*41, CYP2D6*1XN, CYP2D6*2XN, CYP2D6*4XN, CYP2D6*10XN, CYP2D6*17XN, CYP2D6*35XN, CYP2D6*41XN

(Continued)

Table 12.2 (*Continued*)

Gene	Drug	PGx Test	Variants Assayed
DPYD	capecitabine, 5-fluorouracil	TheraGuide 5-FU	Full gene sequence analysis
EGFR	erlotinib, gefitinib	DxS EGFR29 Mutation Test Kit	EGFR: 19 deletions in exon 19, T790M, L858R, L861Q, G719X (detects the presence of G719S, G719A or G719C but does not distinguish between them), S768I, 3 insertions in exon 20 (detects the presence of any of 3 insertions, but does not distinguish between them)
ERBB2	trastuzumab	PathVysion HER2-DNA Probe Kit	ERBB2 gene amplification
HLA-B	abacavir	HLA-B*5701 Test	HLA-B*5701
HLA-B	carbamazepine, phenytoin	HLA-B*1502 Carbamazepine Sensitivity	HLA-B*1502
HLA-DQB1	clozapine	Pgx Predict: Clozapine	HLA-DQB1:G6672C
KRAS	cetuximab, panitumumab	KRAS Mutation Test Kit	KRAS:Gly12Asp, KRAS:Gly12Ala, KRAS:Gly12Val, KRAS:Gly12Ser, KRAS:Gly12Arg, KRAS:Gly12Cys, KRAS:Gly13Asp
KRAS	cetuximab, panitumumab	KRAS Mutation Detection Kit	KRAS:Gly12Asp, KRAS:Gly12Ala, KRAS:Gly12Val, KRAS:Gly12Ser, KRAS:Gly12Arg, KRAS:Gly12Cys, KRAS:Gly13Asp, KRAS:Gly13Ser, KRAS:Gly13Arg, KRAS:Gly13Cys, KRAS:Gly13Ala, KRAS:Gly13Val
TPMT	azathioprine, mercaptopurine	Prometheus TPMT Genetics	Not available
TYMS	capacitabine, 5-fluorouracil	TheraGuide 5-FU	TYMS:2R, TYMS:3R, TYMS:4R
UGT1A1	irinotecan	Invader UGT1A1 Molecular Assay	UGT1A1*28
VKORC1	Warfarin	TrimGen corporation eQ-PCR LC Warfarin Genotyping Kit	VKORC1:G-1639A

*Adapted from Pharmacogenomics Knowledge Base, updated April 2009 (www.pharmgkb.org).
**Manufacturers listed for reference only and do not constitute endorsement.

Pharmacogenetic test approval and availability

As of 2010, a limited number of FDA-cleared pharmacogenetic assays are available. Examples include two Amplichip™ assays manufactured by Roche for CYP2D6 and CYP2C19 as well as five assays approved for CYP2C9/VKORC1 warfarin genotyping (12). These systems are kit based and have a proposed intended use, instructions for use, and manufacturer-established performance characteristics. When bringing an FDA approved assay in house, the laboratory is required to perform and document standard validation procedures. Alternatively, laboratories can perform and offer laboratory-developed tests (LDTs). These tests require extensive evaluation and validation of performance character-istics as regulated by the Centers for Medicare and Medicaid Services (CMS) under CLIA and as described in later sections. Clinical laboratories should be aware of current FDA policy regarding oversight of LDTs.

Analyte specific reagents

Under CLIA regulations, laboratories can purchase individual reagents from manufacturers to use on their testing platforms. These reagents are termed *analyte-specific reagents* (ASRs) and have been defined by the FDA to pertain to "antibodies, both polyclonal and monoclonal, specific receptor proteins, ligands, nucleic acid sequences, and other similar reagents which, through specific binding or chemical reac-tions with substances in a specimen, are intended for use in a diagnostic application for identification and quantification of an individual chemical substance or ligand in biological specimens" (21 CFR 864.4020[a]). ASRs are regulated by the FDA and subject to general controls including current Good Manufacturing Prac-tices (cGMPs) (13). ASRs are building blocks for assays allowing for adaptation to existing laboratory tech-nologies. Validating their use in a given pharmacoge-netic test offers laboratories an alternative route for providing a diagnostic service that can be easier to translate into routine laboratory use and offers impor-tant medical information in some cases not available through other testing means (14).

ASRs are regulated by the FDA under general controls to exempt them from stringent premarket approval procedures and must meet certain require-ments. The "ASR rule" was established in 1997 to ensure the quality of the active reagents in LDTs (13). This includes manufacturer requirements to submit medical device reports, follow labeling requirements and follow cGMPs. The rule further restricts the sale, use, distribution, labeling, advertising and promo-tion of ASRs. Lastly, manufacturers of ASRs cannot make any claims of the clinical or analytical perfor-mance of the reagents. Overall, the FDA views ASRs as having certain characteristics, including that they (a) are used to detect a single ligand or target, (b) are not labeled with instructions for use or perfor-mance claims, and (c) are not promoted for use on a specific instrument or in specific tests (13).

Also important to discuss is what does not consti-tute an ASR. These could be items such as multiple individual ASRs (e.g., probes or primer pairs) included together in a single mixture and used in an LDT (13). This is important to pharmacogenetics testing as many assays use sets of primers or probes to detect multiple genotype variants. Additionally, products that use more than one single ASR or products that are designed for use in one specific assay or on a designated instrument (e.g., bead arrays) are not considered ASRs. Research use only (RUO) and inves-tigational use only (IUO) products are in vitro diag-nostic devices (IVD) that are distinctly separate from ASRs. RUO products are in the laboratory research phase of development and are not intended for use in routine clinical diagnostic procedures. IUO products are in the clinical investigation phase of development. These products are not subject to the same cGMPs requirements as ASRs and other cleared products. The FDA established guidelines for ASRs to ensure that laboratories are able to have access to the reagents needed to for LDTs while still maintaining reagent quality through cGMP requirements.

The evolving oversight of laboratory-developed tests

Clinical laboratory services can be offered by using FDA approved assays as well as LDTs. The use of ASRs in LDTs has long been accepted provided that the test meets CLIA requirements. Hundreds of laboratories translating to nearly two thousand laboratory tests are considered LDTs. With the increased use of LDTs, particularly as it pertains to personalized medicine, the FDA has expressed interest in reevaluating their policies regarding regulatory enforcement due to the increased use and complexity of LDTs and the poten-tial public risk in the absence of appropriate over-sight (15). Increased availability is occurring through laboratories employing direct-to-consumer market-ing strategies or through the use by commercial labs distant from the point of service. According to the FDA this use expands outside the definition of an LDT and the intention that the test is to be performed within a patient's local health care setting under guidance from a treating physician.

The LDT regulation under CLIA and the increasing regulation of LDTs by the FDA represent a possible dual oversight for these tests that may pose many challenges to pharmacogenetic testing laboratories, including increased potential for regulatory costs and conflicts between dual regulatory schemes (15, 16). Although both CLIA and FDA regulatory systems share some similarity concerning the oversight of laboratory diagnostics they are in fact separate and contain differences. The impact of these pending changes to the implementation, growth, and innovation of clinical pharmacogenetic testing remains to be determined.

Regulations for pharmacogenetic testing laboratories

The field of molecular genetic testing has been rapidly expanding due to the efforts identifying genetic targets that are associated with disease states or other conditions. The expansion of the number of tests performed and the number of laboratories performing genetic testing has followed suit. Increases in the number of molecular genetic tests offered have driven the increased need for quality assessment and assurance of these laboratory tests. The Centers for Disease Control and Prevention (CDC) published a comprehensive report outlining good laboratory practices for molecular genetic testing (17). This document incorporated numerous CLIA regulations as well as Clinical Laboratory Improvement Advisory Committee (CLIAC) recommendations. Pharmacogenetics testing, a subspecialty of molecular genetic testing, is subject to these regulations.

Under CLIA, laboratories performing pharmacogenetics testing are subject to general CLIA requirements for nonwaived testing and personnel requirements for high-complexity testing. These tests require extensive clinical laboratory training and expertise due to their complex nature and high medical significance of the result. Laboratory errors are most likely to occur in the pre-analytic or postanalytic phases of testing (18), though a small percentage (0.06–0.12%) may occur during specimen handling and analytic steps performed in the laboratory (19). Furthermore, unrecognized DNA sequences or polymorphisms could affect the results

of molecular genetic testing causing false-positive or false-negative results (17). The CDC report states that problems affecting patient testing outcomes in the field of molecular genetic testing include inadequate establishment or verification of test performance specifications, inadequate personnel training or qualifications, inappropriate test selection and specimen submission, inadequate quality assurance practices, proficiency testing issues, and misinterpretation of test results. The following sections contain information relevant to pharmacogenetics testing that covers all phases of laboratory testing including pre-analytic, analytic, and postanalytic regulations as reported by the CDC and others.

Pre-analytic practices

Recommendations pertaining to the pre-analytic phase of testing include guidelines for laboratory responsibilities for providing information to users of laboratory services, informed consent, test requests, specimen submission and handling, test referrals, and pre-analytic systems assessment (17). CLIA specifies that laboratories must develop and follow written policies and procedures for specimen submission and handling, specimen referral, and test requests (42 CFR § 493.1241 and 1242). Additionally, laboratories performing nonwaived testing are required to have a qualified clinical consultant available for test-ordering assistance (42 CFR § 493.1452[b]). In general, CLIA requires laboratories to provide users of lab services on request with information on laboratory test methods, performance specifications, and method verification (42 CFR § 493.1291[e]). It is recommended, however, that laboratories performing molecular genetic testing to provide test performance information to users before test selection and ordering as opposed to waiting until after a test has been performed, as traditionally occurs. Accordingly, laboratories offering pharmacogenetic testing should provide information regarding the tests performed to users of their services, including health care professionals, patients, referring laboratories, and payers of laboratory services. Important information to include would start with that necessary for appropriate test selection. This would include information pertaining to the intended use of the test, the indications for testing, the test method in use, applicable performance characteristics for analytical and clinical validity, limitations of the test, and whether the test being performed is FDA approved or an LDT. Further information that the laboratory should provide includes appropriate specimen collection and handling, patient information necessary to perform the test and report results (relevant clinical information, age, race, gender, family history, etc.), and a statement pertaining to the availability of laboratory consultations regarding test selection, specimen submission, and interpretation of results. It is important to note that the information provided in the pre-analytic phase of pharmacogenetics testing be consistent with that which appears on interpretive test reports.

Informed consent

Informed consent is defined by the CDC for molecular genetic testing as the process by which an individual voluntarily confirms the willingness to participate in a particular test after being given all of the necessary information required to make an informed decision. CLIA does not regulate whether a laboratory must document informed consent prior to performing the requested tests, but the recommendations emphasize that all testing decisions and subsequent patient treatment be based on properly informed decision making (17). Additionally, some states require informed consent be obtained before genetic testing occurs. Summaries of state laws concerning informed consent can be accessed online (20). If informed consent is required, laboratories should assist in the process by providing relevant and necessary information as well as having methods in place for documenting informed consent on test request forms (17).

Test requests

Laboratories must follow CLIA requirements for information gathered for a test request including: the name and other identifiers of the requesting individual or laboratory, patient name or unique identifier, gender, age, and the date and time of specimen collection (42 CFR § 493.1241[c]). Additionally, as recommended by the CDC, laboratories performing molecular genetic testing should

obtain more comprehensive information on test requests (17). This includes patient name and unique identifiers, patient date of birth, indication for testing and relevant clinical or laboratory information, patient ethnic information if applicable, patient family history as applicable to the condition being evaluated, information pertaining to the conditions for which the patient is being tested, and informed consent information if applicable. Obtaining this additional information is a critical step to ensuring appropriate test selection, interpreting the test results, and finally delivering the results in an efficient manner.

Specimen requirements

CLIA requirements and further recommendations are also in place for laboratories performing molecular genetic testing pertinent to quality assurance of specimens including appropriate specimen collection, handling, transport, and submission (17). Information regarding these areas must be supplied to users of the tests including appropriate type and amount of specimen to be collected, the correct collection container or device (plasma tubes, buccal swabs, saliva, etc.), specimen preparation and handling prior to submission, stability information, appropriate conditions and timing for specimen transport, and finally reasons for specimen rejection (42 CFR § 493.1242). The NACB practice guidelines for pharmacogenetics recommend whole blood as the preferred specimen for testing, unless an alternative sample has been properly validated (6). This recommendation was based on the quantity and quality of DNA obtained from whole blood specimens. However, demand for molecular genetic technologies that can use alternative DNA sources has increased. This will ease burdens of specimen collection at the point of care when phlebotomy services are not available. Regardless, DNA from other sources may be subject to specimen variability, and it is recommended that laboratories validate assay reliability under these circumstances. Laboratories should also maintain specific written criteria for the acceptance or rejection of pharmacogenetic testing specimens. Upon specimen rejection, it is recommended that the laboratory notify the authorized person so they may take corrective action.

Possible criteria may include improper handling or transport, insufficient quantities, inappropriate collection device, possible cross contamination of specimens, mislabeled specimens, and lack of information on test requests. Additionally, it should be seen that information on requests for molecular genetic tests be retained accurately across the entire testing process.

Finally, encompassing all of these pre-analytic requirements and recommendations is the requirement that laboratories maintain written policies and procedures for the quality assessment of the pre-analytic systems (17). For molecular testing, it is recommended that laboratories seek to correct missing or unclear information from test requests, take corrective actions for test requests submitted with inappropriate specimens or test requests made inconsistent with the appropriate use of the test results.

Analytic practices

CLIA requirements exist that govern the analytic phase of testing and pertain to the establishment or verification of the analytic performance of non-waived tests prior to patient testing (42 CFR § 493.1253). This includes demonstrating that accuracy, precision, reportable range of results, and reference ranges are reproducible according to manufacturer-established specifications. Additionally, more stringent requirements occur for laboratories using modified laboratory test systems and LDTs. The CDC published in their report recommended practices for establishing laboratory developed molecular genetic tests so these assays produce valid and reliable results. Five general principles for establishing performance specifications of a new molecular genetic (including pharmacogenetic) test include conducting a literature review of available scientific studies, defining the patient population for the test, selecting the appropriate test methodology, establishing analytic performance specifications, determining quality control procedures, and ensuring that test results can be interpreted and test limitations are defined (21). Sample selection for establishing performance specifications is highly important and appropriate selection will ensure that limitations of testing and test results are known. It is recommended that factors such as the prevalence of mutations or variants, inclusion of all specimen formats, inclusion of all possible genotypes to be reported, and the types of control materials used in test procedures are considered when selecting samples to use for establishing performance specifications.

Laboratory-developed tests

Laboratory-developed molecular genetic tests and other tests not cleared or approved by the FDA require that performance specifications including accuracy, precision, analytic sensitivity, analytic specificity, reportable range of test results, and normal values be determined prior to patient testing (17). Qualitative molecular genetic tests must be accurate. According to typical definitions that is a high degree of closeness between measured values and the true result. For pharmacogenetic testing, this refers to agreement between the new method and an established method, typically sequencing assays. This is best assessed through testing of reference material for a given assay. A laboratory should demand 100% accuracy in detecting genetic variants or mutations compared to the true genotype for a new method due to the medical risks and implications of a misidentified genotype.

Precision is considered the closeness of agreement between independent results obtained under fixed conditions (22). Certain molecular assays (e.g., PCR-ASPE) generate allele ratios as the result output. The precision of the allele ratio must be determined by analyzing multiple replicates for each SNP present in wild type and well as heterozygous and homozygous variant samples. With this numerical output, calculations of the mean allele ratio, standard deviation, and percent coefficient of variation are used to establish allele ratio ranges in which the genotype determination (or "call") is made for each SNP. FDA guidance on establishing pharmacogenetic testing highlights the requirements for performing precision studies (23). For LDTs this would include repeatability of the assay (same day, operator, and lot) and reproducibility (between runs, days, operators, and lots). Furthermore, precision studies should be designed to evaluate the effect of the lowest and highest nucleic acid concentrations allowed for the assay or reagents. Repeatability and reproducibility can be assessed using known samples such as quality control materials or previously confirmed waste genomic DNA specimens (24). Predetermined allele ratio ranges for each SNP should be established which result in 100% precision in genotype call. It is preferable to perform these precision experiments with multiple technologists utilizing multiple reagent lots and with a variety of SNPs.

Analytic sensitivity in pharmacogenetic testing is considered the ability of the assay to detect a given SNP based on the amount of genetic material present. In other words, analytic sensitivity is the limit of detection (LOD). An LOD in pharmacogenetic testing is the amount of DNA required to produce a positive result (agreement with established genotype of sample) in greater than or equal to 95% of the studies. Determination of the LOD should occur for each of the specimen types used for an assay. Dilutions of sample DNA should be made to concentrations below the recommended DNA concentration. Higher DNA concentrations than recommended can also be included to evaluate the upper end of the DNA range. Analytic specificity is defined by practice guidelines as the ability of a genetic test to distinguish target sequences, alleles, or mutations from other sequences in the sample being analyzed (25). Other factors affecting analytic specificity are interfering substances in the patient sample influencing DNA extraction or amplification. All LDTs require establishing appropriate reference ranges (24). However, for molecular genetic tests normal values may refer to normal alleles or variants of the gene in question or a reference DNA sequence for sequencing assays (6). Reportable range of an assay for pharmacogenetic testing is a qualitative measure and includes all possible genotypes that can be detected by the assay.

The CDC recommends that laboratories document information on the clinical validity of the pharmacogenetic tests that they run to demonstrate that they are clinically usable and can be interpreted in terms of specific patient scenarios (17). Clinical validity documentation can include such things as clinical sensitivity or predictive value of the genetic

tests obtained from literature resources. High-complexity testing as is the case for pharmacogenetics testing requires that laboratory directors or technical supervisors are responsible for the appropriateness of the clinical test for providing quality results that can be clinically interpretable, and that these individuals are available for consultation regarding these issues (26). Furthermore, recommendations indicate that laboratory directors must use professional judgment as further scientific information is gained regarding clinical validity or more gene targets are discovered that can be utilized for clinical tests (17).

Quality control

Quality control procedures are of high importance when performing molecular genetic testing. These steps are pivotal in the analytic phase of pharmacogenetic testing. Laboratories performing molecular genetic testing are required to meet CLIA quality control requirements for nonwaived testing (42 CFR § 493.1256) (26). This pertains to the following laboratory requirements as summarized by the CDC (17). Control procedures must be in place to monitor the accuracy and precision of the entire analytic process for each test. This includes specimen processing (DNA extraction and amplification), analyte detection, and reporting. Control procedures including the frequency and type of control material must be established using performance specifications established by the laboratory. Furthermore, control procedures must be able to immediately identify testing errors. This allows for monitoring test performance between reagent lots and from assay to assay, propagates rapid identification of testing errors, and avoids patient result delays.

The requirements for implementation of quality control testing on a daily basis are quite extensive. Focusing specifically on qualitative pharmacogenetic testing discussed in this chapter, the requirements would include each day that patient samples are tested running a negative control sample and a positive control. Additionally, two control materials must be used including one that can detect errors in the extraction process for each test that requires an extraction phase. This will help to monitor the quality of the extraction and determine if the extraction yield is appropriate for the given test. Finally, two control materials must be used that can detect errors in DNA amplification procedures, especially if inhibition of amplification leads to false negative results (17). NACB recommendations indicate that according to these regulations controls that detect potential inhibitors in genetic assays such as allele-specific amplification, restriction enzyme digestion or cleavase-based assays be tested on each run. This includes performing validation studies on each type of specimen (whole blood, buccal swabs, etc.) to determine the performance characteristics.

The CDC recommends additional quality control measures necessary to maintain quality of molecular genetic testing. This includes using quality control materials that are similar to patient specimens during all of the analytic steps and to perform experiments to validate and also monitor that no carryover occurs while using sampling instruments or automated instrumentation. Carryover can be evaluated during the method validation phase by alternating positive and negative samples on 96-well plate format assays to determine if the instrument probe contaminates a negative sample well. The direction of travel for the probe along the plate determines if the probe contaminates in a horizontal (between columns) or vertical manner (between rows) manner. Contamination in the opposite direction to probe movement can occur from splashing and should also be evaluated.

It is also recommended that laboratories ensure that the control material used is as comprehensive as possible and representative of all the genotypes expected for the patient population. For a single mutation, a heterozygous allele sample or a normal sample along with a homozygous variant may be sufficient (17). However, typical pharmacogenetic testing involves many different mutations being tested for a variety of alleles. Under these circumstances, alternative control procedures can be accepted such as using positive control samples for each variant and mutation and rotating all of them within a reasonable timeframe while still being able to monitor test performance over time and to be able to detect immediate errors (17). This method is supported by NACB practice guidelines. Practice guidelines also state that assay validation should

include whole genomic samples that are homozygous normal, heterozygous, and homozygous variant if possible. These validation materials need to be in quantities sufficient to reduce the potential for interference by rare polymorphisms in probe or primer binding sites (6).

NACB recommendations suggest that validation of pharmacogenetics tests should use samples in which the genotype has been independently verified. Additionally, these materials should be from renewable and sustainable sources. These types of sources would include lymphoblastoid cell lines that have been immortalized through Epstein-Barr virus transformation, thus allowing for sustainable production of reference DNA. Resources for high-quality reference materials for pharmacogenetic testing quality control are available. The CDC maintains a program called the Genetic Testing Reference Materials Coordination Program (GeT-RM). Their purpose is to provide assistance to the genetic testing community for obtaining appropriate and characterized reference materials (27). Specifically, they maintain cell line DNA information for numerous alleles for common pharmacogenetic tests including but not limited to CYP2D6, CYP2C19, CYP2C9, VKORC1, and UGT1A1. The cell lines and cell DNA material cataloged by GeT-RM are maintained by the Coriell Institute for Molecular Research Human Genetic Cell Repository sponsored by the National Institute of General Medical Sciences. Each specimen is characterized using multiple-assay technologies for each target gene.

Practice guidelines for pharmacogenetics recommend that analytic sensitivity and specificity are determined for each assay, allowing for identification of result discrepancies (6). Systemic errors can be identified based on genotyping frequency trends and comparison with anticipated frequencies. For additional measures of quality assurance the NACB recommends that all results that are inconsistent with clinical information or patient population genotype frequencies be investigated. This requires maintaining statistics of patient test population frequencies to monitor these changes.

The CDC also included in their recommendations for analytic testing phase practices measures to ensure quality in molecular amplification processes (17). It is a CLIA requirement that laboratories have procedures in place to monitor and minimize biological contamination during the analytical process (42 CFR § 493.1101) (26). The laboratory must ensure that amplification procedures not contained in closed systems are performed in a unidirectional workflow. A closed system is one in which all aspects of the testing system (purification, amplification, detection, etc.) are automated and self-contained. Unidirectional workflow requirements include having separate areas for specimen preparation, amplification, detection, and reagent preparation. More specific guidelines are provided for use during amplification procedures not in closed systems such as including at least one no-template control (NTC) sample each time patient specimens are tested (17). An NTC sample should also be included in extraction steps if possible. Laboratories should also ensure that procedures are established to monitor the unidirectional workflow and to prevent cross-contamination of tests using successive amplification procedures. Using agents such as DNAZap™ to destroy amplicons from previous PCR runs is also recommended.

Proficiency testing

Proficiency testing is a vital practice laboratories conduct to ensure quality of testing and competence. CLIA regulations require proficiency testing to be performed on all tests that a laboratory performs (42 CFR § 493.1236[c]). For most common laboratory assays, many private agencies are available to provide proficiency testing services. Proficiency testing for molecular genetic assays is less common. Furthermore, CLIA does not have specific regulations on proficiency testing for specific molecular genetic tests. However, the general requirement for laboratories to be conducting proficiency testing on all laboratory tests supersedes. Therefore, pharmacogenetic laboratories must participate in proficiency testing for every test they offer at least twice per year. In their set of recommendations, the CDC provided more specific and stringent measures than CLIA outlining proficiency testing practices (17). Their recommendations include first participating in any available proficiency testing at least twice per year for each molecular genetic test performed, consistent with CLIA requirements. They encourage laboratories to regularly review proficiency testing

program information to monitor for the development of additional programs. Second, they support CLIA requirements for performing proficiency testing challenges within the laboratory's regular patient testing workload and by the personnel who routinely run the assays. Proficiency testing results should always be evaluated as reported by the proficiency testing program and steps taken to investigate and correct incorrect results. Furthermore, the CDC recommends when possible proficiency testing samples to resemble patient specimens. They realize that when laboratories are provided purified DNA samples for proficiency testing they do not perform all analytic steps typically required to generate a patient result. Therefore, establishing proficiency testing programs that evaluate the entire testing process are recommended. The NACB recommends, for pharmacogenetic proficiency testing, to use whole genomic specimens that have been tested by other laboratories for each assay. For pharmacogenetic genotyping assays, they attest that there is no difference between proficiency testing for these tests compared to other molecular diagnostic tests. Currently, the College of American Pathologists (CAP) offers pharmacogenetics proficiency testing. Their standard testing includes extracted DNA for CYP2C19, CYP2C9, CYP2D6, UGT1A1, and VKORC1 testing (28). Challenges for these common pharmacogenetic allele detection tests occur twice per year. Additionally, CAP sends two interpretive challenges per year.

NACB guidelines suggest that if no proficiency testing programs or samples are available for a given pharmacogenetic test that laboratories perform internal proficiency testing by using previously tested samples that have been de-identified. Following the challenge, a key to the samples can be released to compare with previous results. In these samples, they recommend having the genotype initially validated using a reference method. Alternative proficiency testing assessments must be conducted twice per year as required by CLIA. Alternative assessment could also include interlaboratory exchange of patient specimens. CAP maintains an internet-based resource called the Sample Exchange Registry for Alternative Assessment. This service connects three or more laboratories that perform esoteric genetic testing to assist in sample exchanges. Additionally, CAP recently added a service whereby participating laboratories can submit purified DNA to them; subsequently, CAP is responsible for distributing the material to participating laboratories testing for the same genotype. In this service, CAP also produces anonymous summary reports for all participants. According to the CDC, laboratories should make certain that alternative assessments are conducted comparing the same testing methodologies and that the total number of samples for each assessment is large enough to confirm accuracy and reliability of the testing (17).

Postanalytic practices

Personnel qualifications

Practice guidelines base the classification of pharmacogenetics testing on the CLIA scoring system. Those tests that score greater than 12 are classified as *high complexity* (26). The NACB guidelines estimate a complexity score of 18 to 21. Scoring criteria include the following based on their complexity required to perform the test: scientific knowledge; training and experience; reagent preparation; characteristics of operational steps; calibration, QC, and proficiency testing materials; test system troubleshooting and maintenance; and interpretation and judgment. According to this classification and recommendations from NACB for pharmacogenetics testing, laboratory personnel must be qualified to perform high-complexity testing as defined by CLIA or as required by individual states.

The CDC lists numerous personnel qualifications in their report (17). They include recommendations for qualifications and responsibilities for positions such as laboratory director, technical supervisor, clinical consultant, general supervisor, and finally testing personnel. It is recommended to consult these guidelines based on specific laboratory needs. CLIA requires laboratories that perform high-complexity testing to have directors who (a) are a doctor or medicine or osteopathy and board certified in anatomic or clinical pathology or both; (b) are a doctor of medicine, osteopathy, or podiatry who has at least 1 year of laboratory training during

residency or a minimum of 2 years experience directing or supervising high-complexity testing; or (c) have earned a doctoral degree in chemical, physical, biological, or clinical laboratory science from an accredited institution and board certified as approved by the Department of Health and Human Services (42 CFR § 493.1443). Directors of pharmacogenetics laboratories should consider additional training and experience to fulfill their knowledge base and responsibilities based on the types of tests they offer. CLIA dictates specific requirements of laboratory directors that perform high-complexity testing including ensuring the quality of all aspects of test performance and results reporting for all laboratory tests, ensuring safe laboratory environment conditions, ensuring proficiency testing enrollment, employing the appropriate laboratory personnel required for patient testing, specifying duties for each laboratory employee and maintaining personnel competence, and ensuring compliance with requirements and regulations governing laboratory operations.

For laboratory personnel performing pharmacogenetics testing CLIA requires that they meet one of these sets of qualifications: (a) are a doctor of medicine, osteopathy, or podiatry; (b) have earned a doctoral, master's, or bachelor's degree in chemical, physical biological, or clinical laboratory science from an accredited institution; (c) have earned an associate's degree in laboratory science or medical laboratory technology from an accredited institution; or (d) meet CLIA requirements for employment before 1992 (42 CFR § 493.1489) (17). CLIA then requires these individuals to follow laboratory protocols for test performance, quality control, results reporting, and troubleshooting (42 CFR § 493.1495). Additionally, laboratory management should ensure that testing personnel receive adequate on-the-job training and demonstrate competency in pharmacogenetic testing before running patient samples. Assessing personnel competency is a CLIA requirement, and laboratory directors must be responsible to ensure that this is an established practice. Laboratories should follow the Centers for Medicare and Medicaid Services (CMS) guidelines for ensuring the competency of all laboratory personnel including technical supervisors, clinical consultants and testing personnel. It is recommended to assess performance of laboratory personnel at least semiannually during the first year of employment and subsequently at least annually. Personnel performance should be reevaluated in the event that the laboratory adds or changes test methodology or instrumentation. It is noted that these types of performance evaluations will help to identify the training needs of the laboratory and ensures that laboratory personnel receive the correct type of continued education appropriate for their job responsibilities (17).

Report and specimen retention

Retaining reports and tested specimens is important practice for pharmacogenetics laboratories. While CLIA requires laboratories to retain the original test report for a period of at least 2 years after date of reporting (42 CFR § 493.1105), the CDC recommends a longer timeframe. For molecular genetics tests they recommend that test reports be retained for at least 25 years following the report date (17). They suggest that this extended timeframe for molecular genetic test reports is important because of the long-term and possibly lifetime implications that the results can have for patients or their families. Also, with the advances in technology and pharmacogenetics, it is possible that the initial interpretation of a genotype may change, possibly making it necessary to amend a past report or suggest retesting. Laboratories must ensure that procedures and policies are in place for test report retention and that in addition to CLIA requirements and CDC recommendations they follow state laws or other requirements. This may mean that it is necessary to retain reports for longer than 25 years. Following these recommendations implies that test reports are archived and retrievable. Electronic records are seemingly the most efficient and cost-effective means of fulfilling this requirement and laboratories should make certain they have the policies and infrastructure in place to achieve this. Furthermore, retaining records of laboratory testing must also follow CLIA requirements such that test requests, procedures, records of analytic systems and test system performance specifications, and proficiency testing records are retained for a minimum of 2 years.

For tested specimen retention, the CDC recommends maintaining the specimen for as long as possible after completing the testing and reporting results. The minimum recommendation is to retain the sample until the next proficiency testing cycle is complete in case action must be taken on samples that may have been subject to testing error identified in proficiency testing. These decisions will depend on the specimen stability, space, and cost.

Confidentiality

Finally, ensuring confidentiality of all patient information throughout the testing process is a CLIA requirement. However, the Health Insurance Portability and Accountability Act of 1996 (HIPAA) provides more stringent requirements for patient confidentiality that laboratories should follow for patient information pertaining to pharmacogenetic testing. Pharmacogenetic laboratories must maintain policies to govern employee responsibility to protect patient information and ensure that appropriate access, documentation, storage, release, and transfer of confidential information as well as protection against unauthorized access is maintained. These practices are additionally supported by NACB recommendations for protecting patient confidentiality.

Genetic test reports

The CDC recommends an extensive list of information to include in molecular genetic testing reports that is applicable to pharmacogenetics. Specific practice guidelines and recommendations as well as examples for pharmacogenetics testing interpretive reports are discussed in a separate section. First, an overview of CLIA requirements and general CDC recommendations is included. CLIA requires test reports for nonwaived testing to include the following information: patient name and unique identifier, name and address of testing laboratory, test performed and report date, specimen source, test results with interpretation if applicable, and relevant information if the specimen did not meet acceptability criteria (42 CFR § 493.1291). Importantly, CLIA also requires the following statement concerning the test to appear on the report if the test used was laboratory-developed using analyte-specific reagents: "This test was developed and its performance characteristics determined by (laboratory name). It has not been cleared or approved by the U.S. Food and Drug Administration" (21 CFR § 809.30[e]). Additional information is recommended for genetic tests relevant to pharmacogenetics testing including: patient date of birth, indication for testing, date and time of specimen collection and arrival, name of referring physician or authorized person who ordered the test, test method, test performance specifications and limitations, test results with interpretation, references to literature if applicable, implications of test results for family members, and finally a statement addressing that the test results and interpretation are based on current knowledge and technology (17). Information pertaining to the test method should include the nucleic acid targets for the test (which mutations are detected), and laboratories should provide the performance specifications and limitations of the test on the report at all times as opposed to "by request." The NACB recommends that the report contains sufficient information about the assay to establish the structural features of the tested gene and the results of that testing (6). All of the structural features of the genetic locus tested for in a given genetic assay should be identified in the report. Likely, most of this information can be referenced to the test kit used in the assay. Additionally, it is not recommend to report a phenotype interpretation or allele designation if the corresponding structural finding is not identified. The CDC also recommends that test results and interpretation be written using current recommended standard nomenclature and should include clarification if necessary. The language used including terminology should be understandable by all health professionals and users of the tests and not just trained pharmacogeneticists. For pharmacogenetic tests that have more than one common name, it is advised to report all versions. This is especially true for cytochrome P450 genes (e.g., P450 2D6, CYP2D6, etc.).

According to CLIA, laboratories must provide updates on testing information to users when changes occur altering the test results or interpretation. This includes providing a revised test report if the interpretation changes based on the measured variant later is shown to have a different effect or if a better interpretation is available according to scientific advancement for the detected variant. Finally, a qualified person must review all reports before being released and a written or electronic signature should document this review.

Interpretive reports for pharmacogenetics testing

Interpretive reporting of pharmacogenetic results is pivotal to successful laboratory utilization and patient care. These reports in the context of a medical problem can be used by the clinical team to guide appropriate therapy. Making the interpretation as specific to the patient's clinical scenario as possible maximizes the effectiveness of the report and the pharmacogenetic information contain therein. Specific guidelines for what information should be included in the interpretive report were provided by the NACB (6). First, they recommend that pharmacogenetic genotype results be accompanied with information on the metabolic pathways involved. Additionally, this information could be made available as part of a consultation service to allow for correct evaluation of drug metabolic pathways for selection of the appropriate genetic test. They also recommend that the laboratory should supply information on drug substrates in the interpretive report. The phenotypic identification depends on the genotype measured as well as the drug. Therefore, without specific data for a given drug and its genotype interaction it is unadvised to assign a metabolic classification (poor metabolizer, extensive metabolizer, etc.) or phenotype. For example, variant alleles of CYP2C9 (*CYP2C9*2* or *CYP2C9*3*) were shown to have varying metabolic capacities for different drugs (29). An opposite scenario would be for CYP2D6. The CYP2D6 enzyme system is complex and has a large number of variants. In such a complex system, it may be useful as a first step to report metabolic status (*CYP2D6*1/*1* = fast, *CYP2D6*/1*4* = intermediate, *CYP2D6*5/*5* = slow, *CYP2D6*1xN* = ultra) (14). This is accomplished if the patient's genotype is easily classified; however, difficulty arises if the genotype is heterozygous for alleles that have the opposite effect (e.g., *1xN/*4). Further complicating the interpretations currently and into the future will be the continued discovery of new variant alleles (14). One method to overcome the complications inherent in categorizing a patient's metabolic status based on genotype for inclusion in the interpretive report is to follow methods presented by Gaedigk et al. (30). These investigators devised a scoring system to classify the activity of CYP2D6 based on the tested genotype and the metabolism of a CYP2D6 probe substrate dextromethorphan. Each CYP2D6 allele is assigned a value (0, 0.5, 1, or 2), and the combined value is the *activity score*, with a value of 1 representing the fully functional *CYP2D6*1* allele. This activity score allows for a more accurate way to predict phenotypic classification and can be implemented for interpretive reports.

Interpretive reports should also contain analytical information as described in a previous section. The NACB recommends documenting the analytical methodology used in the test and addressing limitations of the test that may influence the robustness, interpretation, sensitivity, and specificity. Gene duplication allele detection and assessing the actual number of duplication can affect the robustness of the assay, particularly for CYP2D6. For example, in one commercial assay, a duplicated allele can be detected but in heterozygous patients it is not able to distinguish which allele has been duplicated (31). However, another assay can determine which allele has been duplicated in a heterozygous patient, but neither system can identify the exact copy number (32). This has an impact on the metabolic status of the patient made in the interpretation.

Interpretive reports should include an analysis of the patient's current and possibly past drug regimens to identify any potential cytochrome p450 interactions. This step could mitigate some risk involved with drug–drug interactions that may occur for the genotype tested. Alternatively, the report could include examples of drug interactions at cytochrome p450 enzymes potentially transforming a genotyped extensive metabolizer to a poor metabolizer by way of enzyme competition. This would alert a clinician

to possible adverse drug reactions. The NACB advises against including a specific drug dosage in an interpretive report for a given patient due to the many variables that can influence dosing requirements for each patient. This can include age, weight, comedications, medical history and other comorbidities, administration route, and so forth.

In some specific cases a suggested drug dosage could be indicated for a specific patient if all necessary clinical information is gathered and the dosage information is strongly supported by literature studies. For example, dosing algorithms have been developed for warfarin therapy that include relevant nongenetic factors including age and height as well as genetic factors including CYP2C9 and VKORC1 genotypes (33). Together, the algorithm could account for up to 55% of variability in warfarin dosing. Similar algorithms can account for up to 61% of warfarin dosing variability (34). This type of algorithm could be used to predict an estimated maintenance dose for a patient and be included on the interpretive report provided that the laboratory has done due diligence gathering all of the required nongenetic information required for the calculations. In 2009, the International Warfarin Pharmacogenetics Consortium published the most comprehensive dosing algorithm for a pharmacogenetics test (35). The algorithm calculates warfarin dosing and is based on the largest study population ever present for pharmacogenetic testing. Calculations using this model are available online at www.warfarindosing.org.

Interactive models are also available that expand pharmacogenetic test interpretations beyond a single report. These models incorporate nongenetic and genetic factors similar to the dosing algorithms but also provide a visual representation of warfarin pharmacokinetics (36). Models such as PerMIT:Warfarin (www.permitwarfarin.com) can be used to estimate loading and maintenance doses based on the targeted biological response (target INR). Additionally, the interactive model allows for representation of plasma S-warfarin concentrations after repeated dosing and maps the temporal changes in concentration as the drug approaches steady state (Figure 12.2). Not only can the model then be used to guide standard dosing, but can also be used to rapidly achieve alternative steady-state drug concentrations or INR targets required to maintain the patient on stable therapy.

The future of pharmacogenetics in the clinic is partially dependent upon the development of additional drug-specific dosing models for use in routine clinical practice (14). These models substantiate the pharmacogenetic testing performed and can benefit patients who are prescribed drugs with narrow therapeutic indices.

Cost-effectiveness and reimbursement

Determining the cost-effectiveness of a pharmacogenetic test is challenging. The main difficulty is assigning cost value to patient care improvement or reduction in risk following drug interventions. According to the NACB, pharmacogenetic testing should be undertaken at the time of therapeutic interventions and not as a general population screening tool (6). They propose that the use of pharmacogenetic testing services be based on convincing rationale for offering the test and not solely based on cost-effectiveness. Improved outcomes in pharmacogenetic testing could include predicting blood concentrations of a drug, reducing drug-related adverse events, improving therapeutic response, reducing the cost of overall treatment, and having an impact on the global heath care economy (37). They recommend that laboratories establish criteria to demonstrate the utility of the tests. However, this is a challenge because of a lack of agreement between regulatory and professional groups as to what constitutes convincing rationale. Some believe that convincing rationale could be identifying phenotypic characteristics (estimated drug clearance, recommended dosage, etc.) of a patient for a given drug therapy while others believe that convincing rationale needs to be viewed on a large scale such as improved clinical outcomes that demonstrate cost-effectiveness (6). Additional criteria for providing a pharmacogenetic test has been offered by the FDA in that they have recommended certain tests due to the mitigation of risk that the results can provide for certain medications. Included

in that the FDA recognizes importance of testing for CYP2C9 and VKORC1 for warfarin therapy, TPMT for azathioprine therapy and UGT1A1 for irinotecan therapy (38). Their recommendation was based on the increased risk of adverse drug events inherent to genetic variants of the genes listed and not based directly on cost-effectiveness. The FDA offers further information regarding valid pharmacogenetic biomarkers and testing on their website (2). Drug label statements are provided and in some instances give specific recommendations for pharmacogenetic testing (e.g., *HLA-B*1502* and *HLA-B*5701*). However, the majority of genes listed are included for their recognized impact and do not constitute a specific testing recommendation from the FDA.

Despite NACB guidelines and select FDA recommendations, some believe the future of increased implementation of pharmacogenetic testing in clinical practice includes the requirement for demonstrating cost-effectiveness. Finite health care budgets are driving the need to evaluate which health care interventions to use, and therefore there is a need to demonstrate pharmacogenetic interventions add value to health care management compared to current practice (39). Cost-effectiveness analysis is useful in this situation with the primary aim to provide robust information to decision makers whose responsibility is to allocate resources to health care interventions (40). Pharmacogenetic testing is apt to be cost-effective under conditions where (a) the polymorphism being tested for is prevalent in the population and has a high degree of penetrance (good association between genotype and phenotype), (b) pharmacogenetic testing is highly sensitive and specific and cheaper testing strategies are not available, (c) the disease has poor morbidity or mortality if left untreated, and (d) treatment outcomes directed by genotype-guided interventions results show a significant benefit (38).

Medical interventions are considered cost-effective when new technology produces health benefits at costs comparable to the other common accepted treatments. Cost assessment should include all medical and nonmedical expenses incurred in the care process including the cost of performing the genetic test, treatment expenses with and without the use of

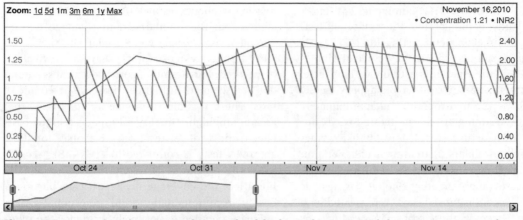

Figure 12.2 Screen shot of PerMIT:Warfarin graphical display tracking estimated plasma concentrations of *S*-warfarin (left axis) and measured INR response (right axis). Computerized tool incorporates pharmacogenetic information to estimate drug dose and allows for visual monitoring of patient's warfarin therapy.

the genetic test, the cost of adverse drug reactions, and costs of other treatment effects (38). The *quality-adjusted life year* (QALY) is a measure of disease burden used in assessing cost-effectiveness based on the quality and quantity of life lived added through a medical intervention. Interventions that produce one additional QALY of benefit for less than $50,000 have been traditionally considered cost effective and those that are estimated between $50,000 and $100,000 per QALY are of equivocal cost-effectiveness (38). However, it is recognized that these ranges are too low and the threshold for cost-effectiveness should be increased closer to the $200,000 range (41).

Unfortunately, data supporting the use of pharmacogenetic testing based on cost-effectiveness remains fragmented. In one summary, a literature review of the cost-effectiveness of pharmacogenetic studies revealed that 22 out of 30 studies (73%) reported favorable economic evidence supporting the implementation of pharmacogenetic testing (42). However, due to varying methods of economic data analysis and cost calculations, final conclusions on cost-effectiveness cannot be reached. Examples of studies on cost-effectiveness have also shown mixed results. In the first, researchers describe the cost-benefit of *HLA-B*5701* pharmacogenetic testing to select for patients that are likely to have a hypersensitivity reaction to abacavir (43).

Their study found that *HLA-B*5701* testing was cost-effective only if abacavir treatment had equal efficacy and cost less compared to other antiretroviral therapies. Alternatively, a study demonstrated that CYP2C9 and VKORC1 genotyping prior to warfarin initiation in patients with nonvalvular atrial fibrillation was not cost effective (44). The theoretical simulation predicted a less than 10% chance testing would be cost-effective at less than $50,000 per QALY. However, under certain conditions warfarin genotyping could be cost-effective. These conditions include restricting testing to patients at high risk for hemorrhage, be able to prevent greater than 32% of major bleeding events, be available within 24 hours, and cost less than $200 (44). A limitation in their analysis was low evidence of the effect of genotype-guided dosing on bleeding events. Therefore, in the scope of nonvalvular atrial fibrillation the testing may not be cost-effective, while in other conditions the testing can be warranted on the basis of cost-effectiveness or other convincing rationale. Other estimations on warfarin genotyping have shown that testing could prevent 17,000 strokes, 85,000 serious bleeding events, and 43,000 emergency room visits each year (45). Calculations of cost savings indicate that at a cost of $125 to $500 per test and with 2 million people starting warfarin therapy each year cost savings could be upward of $1.1 billion dollars annually.

Finally, a recent UGT1A1 genotyping cost-effectiveness study demonstrated the utility of testing (46). Pharmacogenetic testing for *UGT1A1*28* homozygous patients reduces the dosage of irinotecan by 25% in these patients with the variant allele. This treatment strategy could avoid approximately 85 cases of severe neutropenia and approximately five deaths resulting from irinotecan toxicity for every 10,000 patients tested. This results in a savings of $2.7 million dollars in treatment costs, and an estimated savings of nearly $8 million dollars per year if all cases (approximately 29,000) of metastatic colorectal cancer diagnosed each were treated with irinotecan. However, these cost savings estimations are only valid if the dose reduction in homozygotes is as effective as full dose therapy, which remains to be fully evaluated.

Cost-effectiveness analysis to date has primarily been focused on testing for single genes. In the future, more complex methods of cost-effectiveness will be needed to evaluate multiplex technologies that offer information on multiple genes and treatment pathways resulting from a single test (39).

Pharmacogenetic testing reimbursement

Payers of health care services are interested in the utilization of pharmacogenetic testing to ensure that drug therapies are safe and effective in light of rising health care costs. However, reimbursement of pharmacogenetic services is an area of controversy largely due to the lack of justification for the testing. To clarify the terms used in health care economics, the term *coverage* refers to "the scope of services a payer will pay for and under what circumstances" while the term *reimbursement* refers to "the level of payment" (47). Favorable coverage policies are a requirement for reimbursement. These coverage policies have been traditionally based on medical necessity considerations. However, while medical necessity for some pharmacogenetic testing is controversial, payers have been applying more evidence-based methods for coverage decision making (47).

A recent study published by Meckley and Neumann evaluated factors that affect the reimbursement of personalized medicine tests including pharmacogenetics testing (48). In general, they concluded that the reimbursement coverage policies among several payers were similar and that a test with stronger evidence for its use was more likely to be covered. Furthermore, cost-effectiveness studies did not seem to influence the reimbursement of tests. There was also no evidence to suggest that greater and higher quality information on the cost-effectiveness of a test was available for FDA approved tests as compared to LDTs (48). Accordingly, the regulatory pathway for a given test did not affect the coverage by health care payers. A positive recommendation from professional society guidelines tended to positively influence the reimbursement for individual tests. Interestingly, with limited health care payers covering pharmacogenetic testing, direct to consumer marking of testing is on the rise. For example, warfarin and irinotecan pharmacogenetic testing are available online offered by independent laboratories but still require physician ordering (48). These trends indicate the willingness of the health-conscious population to take control of their medical management and determine if the drug regimen they need to take will cause side effects, at their own expense.

Reimbursement for pharmacogenetic tests is currently governed by the CMS Clinical Laboratory Fee Schedule using processes of matching reimbursement for new tests to reimbursement for existing tests based on arbitrarily related testing features and technologies (47). Actual reimbursement for testing occurs through the use of Current Procedural Terminology (CPT) codes and rates have been determined by the costs to provide a test and not based on the clinical value the information has to offer. CPT codes for many pharmacogenetic tests have not been established (14). Therefore, the only method for laboratory billing of pharmacogenetic tests is by each step of the testing process required to produce a result. This could include DNA extraction, amplification, DNA analysis by probes, mutation scanning and test interpretation (14). An example of pharmacogenetic testing reimbursement for CYP2C9/ VKORC1 genotypes by CPT code was published by Wu *et al.* (14). Laboratories can bill for each mutation probed for in a given test (CPT code 83914); however, they must be able to justify their billing practices in lieu of an audit by the CMS. In their calculation, a total of six CPT codes (with two of the codes used multiple times for multiplex PCR reactions and multiple mutation identifications) were used to bill for reimbursement of a warfarin sensitivity CYP2C9/VKORC1 genotyping assay using allele-specific primer extension. Total reimbursement was calculated to be approximately US$240. In 2010, the CMS proposed for consideration a standard reimbursement rate of US$174 for warfarin genotyping.

Overall, a lack of standard reimbursement systems and standard reimbursement rates can limit the implementation of pharmacogenetic testing. Additionally, not having specific reimbursement codes for the testing gives the appearance of less importance for pharmacogenetics tests and can result in less coverage by payers (14). A revision of the reimbursement system for molecular diagnostics with pharmacogenetics included is needed. It is suggested that administrative pricing be eliminated and reimbursement rates for each pharmacogenetic test be negotiated based on its relevance to clinical decision making (48). This type of system is termed *pay for performance* or *value-based purchasing*. Value-based purchasing methods may be effective for implementing pharmacogenetic testing coverage. This strategy uses reimbursement of testing to support effective health care procedures and avoids payment for ineffective care (47). Using this strategy is dependent on the amount of quality evidence available to support payment coverage decision making. As such, cost-effectiveness analysis of pharmacogenetic testing is required to base reimbursement coverage in value-based purchasing schemes. Due to the lack of clinical data supporting pharmacogenetic testing and clinical outcomes, as well as a lack of unity in cost-effective analysis in pharmacogenetic testing, informed payer decision making in the value-based purchasing model has been limited (47). Therefore, an improved future of pharmacogenetics testing reimbursement under value-based purchasing schemes will depend upon quality data supporting the use of the tests by establishing value in relationships between genetic variation and clinically relevant outcomes. This need encourages rapid demonstration of relevance and additionally pushes the reimbursement system to respond to a growing demand for testing.

Conclusion

The clinical laboratory implementation of pharmacogenetics testing has faced many challenges. A steady increase in the clinical utilization of genetic information in relation to drug therapy has been promising. However, the field will continue to be challenged as clinical implementation of diagnostic services, laboratory technology, and genetic discovery constantly evolve. In recent years, guidelines from government agencies as well as current practice guidelines have solidified the foundation for clinical molecular genetic and pharmacogenetic testing. Despite concerns of pharmacogenetic testing justification and cost-effectiveness, it is anticipated that the utilization of pharmacogenetic information in patient care and management will continue to see growth. As such, quality laboratory results delivered in a highly impactful and beneficial manner will be necessary. Thoughtful recognition of these challenges paired with diligent execution of diagnostic clinical services will impart great benefit to this growing field.

Acknowledgments

The authors would like to thank Dr. Kristen Reynolds of PGXL Laboratories for her thoughtful discussions and manuscript review.

References

1 NCBI (2010) *One size does not fit all: the promise of pharmacogenomics* [WWW document]. URL http://www. ncbi.nlm.nih.gov/About/primer/pharm.html [accessed on 12 June 2011]

2 U.S., Food and Drug Administration (2011) *Table of valid genomic biomarkers in the context of approved drug labels* [WWW document]. URL http://www.fda.gov/Drugs/ ScienceResearch/ResearchAreas/Pharmacogenetics/ ucm083378.htm [accessed on 12 June 2011]

3 Linder M.W., Prough R.A., Valdes R., Jr., (1997) Pharmacogenetics: a laboratory tool for optimizing therapeutic efficiency. *Clinical Chemistry*, **43**(2), 254–266.

4 Reynolds, K., Valdes, R., Jr., Hartung, B., Linder, M. (2007) Individualizing warfarin therapy. *Personalized Medicine*, **4**(**1**), 11–31.

5 Meyer, U.A. (1994) Pharmacogenetics: the slow, the rapid, and the ultrarapid. *Proceedings of the National Academy of Sciences of the United States of America*, **91**(**6**),1983–1984.

6 Valdes, R., Jr., Payne, D.P., Linder, M.W., *et al.* (2010) *Laboratory Medicine Practice Guidelines: Laboratory Analysis and Application of Pharmacogenetics to Clinical Practice, 2010*. National Academy of Clinical Biochemstry, Washington, DC.

7 Sachse, C., Brockmoller, J., Bauer, S., Roots, I. (1997) Cytochrome P450 2D6 variants in a Caucasian population: allele frequencies and phenotypic consequences. *American Journal of Human Genetics*, **60**(**2**), 284–295.

8 Frank, D., Jaehde, U., Fuhr, U. (2007) Evaluation of probe drugs and pharmacokinetic metrics for CYP2D6 phenotyping. *European Journal of Clinical Pharmacology*, **63**(**4**), 321–333.

9 Andersson, T., Flockhart, D.A., Goldstein, D.B., Huang, S.M., Kroetz, D.L., Milos, P.M., *et al.* (2005) Drug-metabolizing enzymes: evidence for clinical utility of pharmacogenomic tests. *Clinical Pharmacology & Therapeutics*, **78**(**6**), 559–581.

10 Marcuello, E., Altes, A., Menoyo, A., Del Rio, E., Gomez-Pardo, M., Baiget, M. (2004) UGT1A1 gene variations and irinotecan treatment in patients with metastatic colorectal cancer. *British Journal of Cancer*, **91**(**4**),678–682.

11 Krynetski, E.Y., Evans, W.E. (2000) Genetic polymorphism of thiopurine S-methyltransferase: molecular mechanisms and clinical importance. *Pharmacology*, **61**(**3**), 136–146.

12 Pharmacogenomics Knowledge, Base. (2011) *Pharmacogenonmic tests* [WWW document]. URL http://www.pharmgkb.org/resources/forScientificUsers/pharmacogenomic_tests.jsp [accessed on 12 June 2011]

13 U.S., Food and Drug Administration (2007) *Guidance for industry and FDA staff: commercially disributed analyte specific reagents (ASRs) frequently asked questions* [WWW document]. Document no. 1590. URL http://www.fda.gov/cdrh/oivd/guidance/1590.pdf [accessed on 12 June 2011]

14 Wu, A., Babic, N., Yeo, K. (2009) Implementation of pharmacogenomics into the clinical practice of therapeutics: issues for the clinician and the laboratorian. *Personalized Medicine*, **6**(**3**), 315–327.

15 Gibbs, J. (2010) *Regulating laboratory-developed tests* [WWW document]. *Genetic Engineering and Biotechnology News*. URL http://www.genengnews.com/gen-articles/regulating-laboratory-developed-tests/3414/ [accessed on 12 June 2011]

16 Gibbs, J. (2010) *The cost of regulating LDTs* [WWW document]. *Genomics Law Report*. URL http://www.genomicslawreport.com/index.php/2010/08/25/the-cost-of-regulating-ldts/ [accessed on 12 June 2011]

17 Centers for Disease Control and Prevention (2009) Good laboratory practices for molecular genetic testing for heritable diseases and conditions. *Morbidity and Mortality Weekly Report*, **58**(**No. RR–6**), 1–37.

18 Bonini, P., Plebani, M., Ceriotti, F., Rubboli, F. (2002) Errors in laboratory medicine. *Clinical Chemistry*, **48**(**5**), 691–698.

19 Hofgartner, W.T., Tait, J.F. (1999) Frequency of problems during clinical molecular-genetic testing. *American Journal of Clinical Pathology*, **112**(**1**), 14–21.

20 NCSL (2011) *Genetic privacy laws* [WWW document]. URL http://www.ncsl.org/default.aspx?tabid=14287 [accessed on 12 June 2011]

21 U.S., Food and Drug Administration (2011) *Guidance on pharmacogenetic tests and genetic tests for heritable markers* [WWW document]. URL http://www.fda.gov/MedicalDevices/DeviceRegulationandGuidance/GuidanceDocuments/ucm077862.htm [accessed on 12 June 2011]

22 Burtis, C.A., Ashwood, E.R., Border, B., Tietz, N.W. (2001) *Tietz Fundamentals of Clinical Chemistry*, 5th ed. W.B. Saunders, Philadelphia, PA.

23 U.S. Food and Drug Administration (2007) *Guidance for industry and FDA staff: pharmacogenetic tests and genetic tests for heritable markers* [WWW document]. Document no. 1549. URL http://www.fda.gov/MedicalDevices/DeviceRegulationandGuidance/GuidanceDocuments/ucm077862.htm [accessed on 12 June 2011]

24 Centers for Medicare & Medicaid, Services. (2011) *Appendix C: survey procedures and interpretive guidelines for laboratories and laboratory services* [WWW document]. URL https://www.cms.gov/CLIA/03_Interpretive_Guidelines_for_Laboratories.asp [accessed on 12 June 2011].

25 American College of Medical Genetics (2011) *ACMG standards and guidelines for clinical genetic laboratories* [WWW document]. URL http://www.acmg.net/am/template.cfm?section=laboratory_standards_and_guidelines&template=/cm/htmldisplay.cfm&contentid=2511 [accessed on 12 June 2011]

26 Centers for Disease Control and Prevention (2004) *Current CLIA regulations, 42 C.F.R. Part 493* [WWW document]. URL http://wwwn.cdc.gov/clia/regs/toc.aspx [accessed on 12 June 2011]

27 Centers for Disease Control and Prevention (2011) *Reference materials availability* [WWW document]. URL http://wwwn.cdc.gov/dls/genetics/rmmaterials/MaterialsAvailability.aspx [accessed on 12 June 2011]

28 College of American Pathologists (2011) *2011 Surveys and Anatomic Pathology Education Programs catalog* [WWW document]. URL http://www.cap.org [accessed on 12 June 2011]

29 Kirchheiner, J., Brockmoller, J. (2005) Clinical consequences of cytochrome P450 2C9 polymorphisms. *Clinical Pharmacology & Therapeutics*, **77**(**1**), 1–16.

30 Gaedigk, A., Simon, S.D., Pearce, R.E., Bradford, L.D., Kennedy, M.J., Leeder, J.S. (2008) The CYP2D6 activity score: translating genotype information into a qualitative measure of phenotype. *Clinical Pharmacology & Therapeutics*, **83**(**2**), 234–242.

31 Schaeffeler, E., Schwab, M., Eichelbaum, M., Zanger, U.M. (2003) CYP2D6 genotyping strategy based on gene copy number determination by TaqMan real-time PCR. *Human Mutation*, **22**(**6**), 476–485.

32 Gaedigk, A., Bradford, L.D., Alander, S.W., Leeder, J.S. (2006) CYP2D6*36 gene arrangements within the cyp2d6 locus: association of CYP2D6*36 with poor metabolizer status. *Drug Metabolism and Disposal*, **34**(**4**),563–569.

33 Sconce, E.A., Khan, T.I., Wynne, H.A., Avery, P., Monkhouse, L., King, B.P., *et al.* (2005) The impact of CYP2C9 and VKORC1 genetic polymorphism and patient characteristics upon warfarin dose requirements: proposal for a new dosing regimen. *Blood*, **106**(**7**),2329–2333.

34 Zhu, Y., Shennan, M., Reynolds, K.K., Johnson, N.A., Herrnberger, M.R., Valdes, R., Jr., *et al.* (2007) Estimation of warfarin maintenance dose based on VKORC1 (−1639 G>A) and CYP2C9 genotypes. *Clinical Chemistry*, **53**(**7**), 1199–1205.

35 Klein, T.E., Altman, R.B., Eriksson, N., Gage, B.F., Kimmel, S.E., Lee, M.T., *et al.* (2009) Estimation of the warfarin dose with clinical and pharmacogenetic data. *New England Journal of Medicine*, **360**(**8**), 753–764.

36 Linder, M.W., Bon Homme, M., Reynolds, K.K., Gage, B.F., Eby, C., Silvestrov, N., *et al.* (2009) Interactive modeling for ongoing utility of pharmacogenetic diagnostic testing: application for warfarin therapy. *Clinical Chemistry*, **55**(**10**), 1861–1868.

37 Bertilsson, L., Dahl, M.L., Dalen, P., Al-Shurbaji, A. (2002) Molecular genetics of CYP2D6: clinical relevance with focus on psychotropic drugs. *British Journal of Clinical Pharmacology*, **53**(**2**), 111–122.

38 Flowers, C.R., Veenstra, D. (2004) The role of cost-effectiveness analysis in the era of pharmacogenomics. *Pharmacoeconomics*, **22**(**8**), 481–493.

39 Payne, K., Shabaruddin, F.H. (2010) Cost-effectiveness analysis in pharmacogenomics. *Pharmacogenomics*, **11**(**5**),643–646.

40 Claxton, K. (2008) Exploring uncertainty in cost-effectiveness analysis. *Pharmacoeconomics*, **26**(**9**), 781–798.

41 Ubel, P.A., Hirth, R.A., Chernew, M.E., Fendrick, A.M. (2003) What is the price of life and why doesn't it increase at the rate of inflation? *Archives of Internal Medicine*, **163**(**14**), 1637–1641.

42 Paci, D., Ibarreta, D. (2009) Economic and cost-effectiveness considerations for pharmacogenetics tests: an integral part of translational research and innovation uptake in personalized medicine. *Currents in Pharmacogenomics and Personal Medicine*, **7**(**4**), 284–296.

43 Schackman, B.R., Scott, C.A., Walensky, R.P., Losina, E., Freedberg, K.A., Sax, P.E. (2008) The cost-effectiveness of HLA-B*5701 genetic screening to guide initial antiretroviral therapy for HIV. *AIDS*, **22**(**15**), 2025–2033.

44 Eckman, M.H., Rosand, J., Greenberg, S.M., Gage, B.F. (2009) Cost-effectiveness of using pharmacogenetic information in warfarin dosing for patients with non-valvular atrial fibrillation. *Annals of Internal Medicine*, **150**(**2**), 73–83.

45 McWilliam, A., Nardinelli, C., Lutter, R. (2006) *Health care savings from personalizing medicine using genetic testing: the case of warfarin* [WWW document]. URL http://ideas.repec.org/p/reg/wpaper/538.html [accessed on 12 June 2011]

46 Gold, H.T., Hall, M.J., Blinder, V., Schackman, B.R. (2009) Cost effectiveness of pharmacogenetic testing for uridine diphosphate glucuronosyltransferase 1A1 before irinotecan administration for metastatic colorectal cancer. *Cancer*, **115**(**17**), 3858–3867.

47 Deverka, P.A. (2009) Pharmacogenomics, evidence, and the role of payers. *Public Health Genomics*, **12**(**3**), 149–157.

48 Meckley, L.M., Neumann, P.J. (2010) Personalized medicine: factors influencing reimbursement. *Health Policy*, **94**(**2**), 91–100.

Index

Pharmacogenomics in Clinical Therapeutics, First Edition. Edited by Loralie J. Langman and Amitava Dasgupta.
© 2012 John Wiley & Sons, Ltd. Published 2012 by John Wiley & Sons, Ltd.